Treating Psychological Trauma and PTSD

TREATING PSYCHOLOGICAL TRAUMA AND PTSD

Edited by

John P. Wilson
Matthew J. Friedman
Jacob D. Lindy

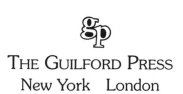

THE GUILFORD PRESS
New York   London

Library of Congress Cataloging-in-Publication Data

Treating psychological trauma and PTSD / edited by John P. Wilson, Matthew J.
Friedman, Jacob D. Lindy.
    p. ; cm.
   Includes bibliographical references and index.
   ISBN 1-57230-687-4
   1. Post-traumatic stress disorder—Treatment.   2. Psychic trauma—Treatment.   3.
Psychotherapy.   I. Wilson, John P. (John Preston).   II. Friedman, Matthew J.   III. Lindy,
Jacob D., 1937–.
   [DNLM: 1. Stress Disorders, Post-Traumatic—therapy. WM 170 T78465 2001]
RC552.P67 T764 2001
616.85′21—dc21   2001040601

About the Editors

John P. Wilson, PhD, is Professor of Psychology at Cleveland State University. An internationally recognized expert on PTSD, he is a past president of the International Society for Traumatic Stress Studies. Dr. Wilson is the coeditor of *Assessing Psychological Trauma and PTSD* (with Terence M. Keane) and *Countertransference in the Treatment of PTSD* (with Jacob D. Lindy).

Matthew J. Friedman, MD, PhD, is Executive Director of the National Center for PTSD, based at the VA Medical Center in White River Junction, Vermont. He is also Professor of Psychiatry and Pharmacology at Dartmouth Medical School. His eight books and more than 100 scientific and clinical publications address the psychobiology of stress, clinical psychopharmacology, ethnocultural aspects of PTSD, disaster mental health interventions, and treatment of PTSD. Dr. Friedman is the coeditor of *Effective Treatments for PTSD: Practice Guidelines from the International Society for Traumatic Stress Studies* (with Edna B. Foa and Terence M. Keane).

Jacob D. Lindy, MD, is a training and supervising analyst at the Cincinnati Psychoanalytic Institute. For 27 years, he has adapted psychoanalytic clinical theory to the special circumstances of the trauma survivor. As a trauma clinician and researcher, he has studied and treated survivors of natural and man-made disasters (Buffalo Creek, Beverly Hills fire), war (Vietnam), and political repression (Eastern Europe). He is a past president of the International Society for Traumatic Stress Studies and has just completed 5 years as Director of the Cincinnati Psychoanalytic Institute. Dr. Lindy's publications include the coedited *Countertransference in the Treatment of PTSD* (with John P. Wilson).

Contributors

Matthew Dobson, PhD, University of New South Wales, Sydney, New South Wales, Australia

Lee A. Fitzgibbons, PhD, Center for the Treatment and Study of Anxiety, Allegheny University of the Health Sciences, Philadelphia, PA

Edna B. Foa, PhD, Center for the Treatment and Study of Anxiety, Allegheny University of the Health Sciences, Philadelphia, PA

David W. Foy, PhD, Graduate School of Education and Psychology, Pepperdine University, Culver City, CA; Headington Program in International Trauma, Fuller Graduate School of Psychology, Pasadena, CA

Matthew J. Friedman, MD, PhD, National Center for PTSD, Veterans Affairs Medical Center, White River Junction, VT; Department of Psychiatry and Pharmacology, Dartmouth Medical School, Hanover, NH

Shirley M. Glynn, PhD, Research Service, Greater Los Angeles Veterans Affairs Healthcare System at West Los Angeles, Los Angeles, CA

Fred D. Gusman, MSW, National Center for PTSD, Veterans Affairs Medical Center, Palo Alto, CA

Laurie Harkness, PhD, West Haven VA Medical Center, New Haven, CT

J. David Kinzie, MD, Department of Psychiatry, University of Oregon Health Sciences Center, Portland, OR

Jacob D. Lindy, MD, Cincinnati Psychoanalytic Institute, Cincinnati, OH

Charles R. Marmar, MD, Department of Psychiatry, University of California at San Francisco, San Francisco, CA; Veterans Affairs Medical Center, San Francisco, CA

Alexander C. McFarlane, MD, Department of Psychiatry, Adelaide University, The Queen Elizabeth Hospital, Woodville, South Australia

Kim T. Mueser, PhD, New Hampshire–Dartmouth Psychiatric Research Center, Concord, NH

Kathleen Nader, PhD, private practice, Cedar Park, TX

Laurie Anne Pearlman, PhD, Traumatic Stress Institute, Center for Adult and Adolescent Psychotherapy, South Windsor, CT

Beverley Raphael, MD, Department of Health, New South Wales Center for Mental Health, North Sydney, New South Wales, Australia

Stanley D. Rosenberg, PhD, Department of Psychiatry, Dartmouth–Hitchcock Medical Center, Lebanon, NH

Paula P. Schnurr, PhD, National Center for PTSD, Veterans Affairs Medical Center, White River Junction, VT; Department of Psychiatry, Dartmouth Medical School, Hanover, NH

Melissa S. Wattenberg, PhD, Psychology Service, Department of Veterans Affairs Healthcare System, Outpatient Clinic, Boston, MA; Department of Psychiatry, Tufts University, Boston, MA

Daniel S. Weiss, PhD, Department of Psychiatry, University of California at San Francisco, San Francisco, CA; Veterans Affairs Medical Center, San Francisco, CA

John P. Wilson, PhD, Department of Psychology, Cleveland State University, Cleveland, OH

Noka Zador, MSW, West Haven VA Medical Center, New Haven, CT

Lori A. Zoellner, PhD, Department of Psychology, University of Washington, Seattle, WA

Preface and Acknowledgments

This book was born of a collaborative vision to create a reference volume on the treatment approaches for posttraumatic stress disorder (PTSD) within a contemporary psychobiological perspective of prolonged stress responses to traumatic events. The collaborative effort between the editors and contributors has been a richly rewarding endeavor. Together, the editors attempted to build a new theoretical scaffold in Part I by which to understand PTSD as an allostatic psychobiological process from which sound principles of clinical treatment could be established. The result of our effort was a holistic, dynamic, organismic approach to the therapeutic techniques for treating PTSD in its simple and complex forms. As a result of the collaboration, we have expanded the diagnostic criteria of PTSD to 65 symptoms within five clusters that define the syndrome dynamics. We have also identified 80 specific treatment objectives for the domain of PTSD symptoms that can be treated by 11 different psychotherapeutic approaches. We believe that the theoretical models, level of specificity of the five domains of PTSD symptoms, and the clearly delineated treatment goals provide practitioners with useful knowledge and tools to assist them in their work with trauma clients. Chapter 3 presents 30 principles for the treatment of PTSD, reflecting the entire spectrum of issues that confront practitioners in the process of posttraumatic therapy. In Chapter 15, we present a meta-analysis of 25 case histories that were provided by the authors in their respective chapters. This meta-analysis provides "lessons learned" about each of the treatment approaches and their relative effectiveness in treating PTSD. In Chapter 16, we review and summarize each of the treatment modalities and organize them into a set of practical guidelines for the practitioner. As such, this chapter is a straightforward condensation of the treatment methods, goals, and clinical applications to trauma populations. It is our hope that this book will stimulate thoughtful examination of processes of posttraumatic therapies and be of use to clinical practitioners, researchers, academics, and PTSD clients in search of healing and recovery from trauma.

Our appreciation and thanks extend to many persons and institutions who have supported our collaborative efforts in writing this book. No single person has labored with more dedication than Kathy Letizio of the Forensic Center for Traumatic Stress and Post-Traumatic Stress Disorders in Cleveland, Ohio (*www.fc-ptsd.com*). Kathy typed and retyped the manuscripts to perfection. She oversaw the revisions and organization of the book and went beyond the call of duty so many times we cannot count them all. Without her dedication, this book would not have been completed.

At Cleveland State University, thanks extend to the College of Arts and Sciences and the Department of Psychology for granting the senior editor a sabbatical leave of absence to work on this project. Support was received from Vice Provost William Shorrock, Dean Karen Steckel, and Chairperson Mark Ashcraft. Jill McNiven, the department secretary, oversaw correspondence and early drafts of the chapters.

We extend our appreciation to the staff of the National Center for PTSD of the VA Medical Center and Regional Office in White River Junction, Vermont. Special kudos are extended to Fred Lerner, information specialist (*www.ncptsd.org*), who aided in providing needed reference materials. Time and time again invaluable assistance was provided by Jan Clark, Sandy Mariotti, and other staff of the National Center for PTSD to ensure the progress and quality of the work being done.

In Cincinnati, we acknowledge the ongoing support of the staff of the Center for Psychoanalysis, who saw to it that the numerous revisions were properly done and available to the contributors as needed.

Finally, a special thank-you to our wives, Diane, Gayle, and JoAnn, for enduring the expectable travails and late-night telephone calls as the work was in progress. On more than one occasion, Matt and Gayle Smith made their home in Woodstock, Vermont, a sanctuary for thought, reflection, and writing.

Contents

I

THEORY, MODELS, AND CLINICAL PARADIGMS OF TREATMENT

1

Treatment Goals for PTSD

JOHN P. WILSON, MATTHEW J. FRIEDMAN, and JACOB D. LINDY

It has been more than 20 years since the term "posttraumatic stress disorder" (PTSD) was included in the third edition of the *Diagnostic and Statistical Manual of Mental Disorders* (DSM-III) of the American Psychiatric Association (1980). The inclusion of PTSD under the rubric of the anxiety disorders was not without political controversy, academic and theoretical debate, or outright skepticism as to its scientific validity as an illness (see Krystal, 1968, and Wilson, 1994, for reviews). Despite the catastrophic stress-related events which served to define nodal world crisis points in the 20th century (e.g., World War I; World War II; the Holocaust; Hiroshima and Nagasaki; state terrorism and political tyranny; the Korean War; the Vietnam War; the Cambodian genocide and more recent ethnic massacres in Bosnia, Rwanda, Kosovo, and East Timur; technological disasters such as that in Bhopal, India; and the threat of nuclear accidents such as the meltdown and explosion at Chernobyl), the *absence* of a separate diagnostic category for trauma-related psychiatric syndromes was simply a fact from DSM-I (American Psychiatric Association, 1952) to DSM-III (American Psychiatric Association, 1980). Beyond a doubt these historical and tragic catastrophic events had life-altering sequelae to persons, cultures, governments, and nations. It is only reasonable, therefore, that the absence of a specific diagnostic category for PTSD had medical and psychiatric consequences for the quality of health care and treatment of trauma victims. While it is possible to speculate on the reasons for this void in scientific and medical classification, the advent of PTSD as a separate diagnostic category (American Psychiatric Association, 1980) was a distinct and critical turning point in the advancement of knowledge. Today the legacy of these traumatic experiences are still present in

3

memory, spirit, and being for many individuals who persist in their search for meaning in an effort to understand their victimization within the fabric of modern civilization.

In many respects it remains a puzzle that a "cloistered" group of mental health professionals charged with the responsibility of revising the psychiatric criteria of DSM-I (American Psychiatric Association, 1952) (i.e., DSM-II 1968 APA publication committee) would have difficulty in recognizing and accepting the necessity of scientifically classifying PTSD as a distinct psychiatric disorder, especially given the profound worldwide and historic traumatic events which punctuated the 20th century. Moreover, prior to DSM-II, there was voluminous scientific literature on traumatic stress (see Laughlin, 1967, for a review). We have to wonder, collectively and individually, why it took so long to acknowledge "officially" that psychic trauma can lead to a distinct psychiatric illness of a chronic nature or cause alterations in personality functioning which may be pathological or transformative in ego functioning and identity (Wilson, 1988). Indeed the field of stress medicine and psychoanalytic investigations established parameters of prolonged stress effects to the organism well before PTSD was classified in DSM-III (e.g., Selye, 1976; Laughlin, 1967; Freud, 1895, 1917; Janet, 1900; Cannon, 1929; Fenichel, 1945).

To place these issues in a broader historical context, it is instructive to note that Sigmund Freud grappled extensively with the concept of PTSD (i.e., traumatic neurosis) from 1895 to 1920. In his book *Beyond the Pleasure Principle* (1920), he labored to distinguish between the core dynamics of traumatic neuroses and their relation to ego defense, anxiety, the concept of the stimulus barrier, and threat anticipation. In this work Freud elaborated on the idea that trauma could breach the stimulus barrier and overwhelm ego defenses, producing psychic trauma that could influence behavior, including manifestations of compulsions to repeat elements of the traumatic experience. Despite theoretical difficulties in resolving the differences between the traumatic neuroses, the war neuroses, and the anxiety-based neuroses, Freud understood that "mechanical violence of the trauma would liberate a *quantity* of 'sexual excitation' (i.e., stress response or pre-existing intrapsychic conflict) which, owing to the lack of preparation for anxiety, would have a traumatic effect" (Freud, 1920, p. 38; emphasis added). If a traumatic event had a *magnitude* of impact which overwhelmed coping resources, "the mechanism of the ego, including efforts to master the trauma in dream work, might not succeed" (Freud, 1920, p. 38). The potential for long-term stress effects on the dynamics of the psyche became obvious to Freud prior to World War II, long before the insertion of PTSD in the DSM-III (1980) diagnostic classification system. Moreover, as early as 1917 (i.e., during World War I), during his lectures in Vienna to the medical society, Freud identified and discussed *all* of the PTSD criteria that are listed in the current DSM-IV (1994); see his *Introductory Lectures on Psychoanalysis* (Freud, 1917), Chapter XVIII, "Fixation to Traumas—The Unconscious," for a detailed discussion of traumatic neuroses.

It is not our purpose in this introductory chapter to review the history and debate surrounding PTSD as a diagnostic entity, phenomenon, or process. Rather, it is to establish a framework in which to present the treatment goals for PTSD—a formidable and an extraordinarily interesting task, as will become evident in the chapters that follow. Clinicians, academics, and researchers face a multitude of considerations when attempting to understand and treat PTSD, as do patients trying to come to grips with and heal from its impact on their lives. As the book unfolds we hope that these factors will become evident and provide a sense of direction and understanding for practitioners, as well as for patients and their families affected by personal trauma.

Thoughtful examination will show that the complexity of the phenomena of PTSD will raise more questions than science can provide answers to at the present time, despite 16,925 articles in the international scientific database known by the acronym of PILOTS (Published International Literature on Traumatic Stress).[1] By the time this book reaches print, we expect that the worldwide database will contain between 18,000 and 20,000 annotated and indexed articles on the subject of traumatic stress and PTSD. So perhaps the most utilitarian, pragmatic, and scientific consequence of placing PTSD in the DSM-III of the American Psychiatric Association (1980) was that it opened the door to research scientists and other inquiring minds as to the nature, meaning, and structure of psychological trauma. What has happened since then speaks for itself in terms of scientific research, epidemiological studies, educational curricula and certification, the development of professional societies concerned with PTSD, and the urgency of understanding traumatic stress and PTSD in modern life.

We believe that it is important to clarify that posttraumatic phenomena are not limited to psychiatric diagnoses or decision making algorithms as defined in professional reference manuals (e.g., DSM-IV; American Psychiatric Association, 1994). PTSD symptoms listed in DSM-IV are primarily for use by clinicians who attempt to help their patients suffering from traumatic life experiences. We believe that it is necessary to expand these basic groupings of symptoms which define the *triad* of PTSD symptoms in order to maximize treatment effectiveness. Posttraumatic phenomena and their permutations are rich in their tapestry and are woven of thousands of threads whose fibers are spun from unique and sometimes exotic, secretive, horrific, and forbidden sources of discovery. Working clinically or in research settings with PTSD is a journey of puzzlement, curiosity, fascination, and uncertainty. At one end of the continuum, the work often exacts an enormous toll on therapists, draining their inner empathic resources (Dalenberg, 2000; Wilson & Lindy, 1994). At the other end of the continuum is the realization of the human capacity for resilience and self-actualization, and the power of the human spirit to heal itself. Practitioners working with PTSD clients often oscillate between the emotional extremes of this continuum. There is nothing easy in their task; they often confront the worst horrors of human cruelty and malevolence. Listening to trauma stories is emotionally draining and hard work. As recent research has confirmed, clinical moments of dedication, inspiration, and hoped-for wisdom through education and training alternate with private reflections of self-doubt, insecurity, despair, and fantasies of escape from the heavy professional responsibility entailed in this task (Wilson & Thomas, 1999). Confronting human suffering through trauma work is often a painful process. It may result in professional burnout (Figley, 1995). The challenge and responsibility of the therapist who chooses to work with PTSD clients is to overcome burnout, empathic strain, maladaptive countertransference, and ineffective modalities of treatment. To do so demands endurance, commitment, and perseverance.

A second aim of this book is to identify areas of research, treatment, and clinical outcome which are not being addressed by the field of traumatic stress studies (Raphael & Wilson, 2000). This statement should not be construed as a criticism of the many excellent programs in the United States, Australia, Canada, Europe, Israel, and elsewhere where dedicated scholars labor to answer cutting-edge issues ranging from the epidemiological prevalence of PTSD (e.g., Kessler, 1995; Breslau, 1998) to the neuroscience of stress disorders (Bremner, 1999) to cross-cultural dynamics at work in processing psychological trauma (Kinzie, 1993).

In order to advance the field of studies in traumatic stress and PTSD, it is important to ask a series of critical questions. What are the voids in our knowledge base at this time? What fundamental sets of studies are necessary to define commonly agreed-upon advances in methodology, techniques of assessment, and neuroscience approaches? What are the consequences of traumatic experiences to epigenesis and life-stage development? What new educational endeavors need to be implemented in academic and professional training? What organizations (e.g., International Society for Traumatic Stress Studies [ISTSS]; National Center for Post-Traumatic Stress Disorders [NC-PTSD]; National Institute of Mental Health [NIMH]; United Nations International Children's Fund [UNICEF]; World Health Organization [WHO]; United Nations High Commission on Refugees [UNHCR]; International Critical Incident Stress Foundation [ICISF]; American Psychiatric Association; American Psychological Association; and American Academy of Experts in Trauma Studies [AAETS]) are going to undertake the responsibility of building bridges and foundations for cooperation, systematic planning, and program development in *all* of the areas which embrace and encompass the domains of trauma, stress disorders, and the myriad of related social-psychological and clinical phenomena?

As we enter the new millennium, how will such proactive programs be developed and facilitated in light of higher moral concerns for the future well-being of humankind and the quality of life worldwide? Dealing with human-induced traumas is a health-care priority as serious as any major medical illness (U.S. Surgeon General, 1999). We believe that a broad and imaginative vision is critically needed if we are to advance to the further reaches of knowledge of the pathways to healing and recovery from PTSD and other related psychiatric phenomena (Maslow, 1971; Mack, 1999). With the acceleration of societal change brought on by the information age, we have seen that the new technologies are inducing rapid shifts in the patterns of day-to-day living and the rate at which ordinary people can access information on which to make decisions affecting their lives. In the field of traumatic stress studies, we must coordinate interorganizational/interagency cooperation to implement visionary agendas for the future and move in proactive ways beyond outdated models that limit innovative thinking and research.

When we consider the pressing issues which confront the field, it is evident that there is so much new ground to be unearthed and properly tilled that the task can sometimes seem daunting and even overwhelming. However, among the legacies of the 20th century is a "collective energy" to address these profoundly serious human concerns though many might wish to ignore them. Imagination, courage, risk taking, and the willingness to follow intuition are often accompanied by subjective feelings of danger and foreboding. As Abraham Maslow (1968) noted with brilliant lucidity, human growth motivation toward greater degrees of self-actualization enhances our attraction to the unknown, the uncertain, and less well-understood concepts in many areas of knowledge acquisition, especially as regards pressing contemporary issues. In contrast, fear, anxiety, insecurity, uncertainty, and the need for safety maximize our desire for the comfort of the known, the secure, and simple methods of plodding along, doing that which is conventional, unimaginative, and noncontroversial.

In the field of traumatic stress studies the current zeitgeist and momentum of the field impel us onward, realizing the humanitarian urgency of the task. Such a move toward greater scientific coordination and planning is a challenge and a mission. In this book we have chosen to take a small step in that direction and are hopeful that the issues presented by the contributors will stimulate new ways of thinking about treatment of trauma and PTSD, leading to healing. Our approach is conceptually holistic, dynamic, and rooted in the foundations of modern science, an approach driven by the marriage of theory, data, and clinical experience.

THE SPECTRUM OF PTSD AND STRESS DISORDERS

The treatment approaches for PTSD recognize that it is a complex, dynamic entity rather than a unidimensional set of symptoms in a psychiatric reference manual. It is a premise of this book that PTSD represents a dramatic and complex shift in the steady state of the organism. The concept of a spectrum of PTSD means that it can appear in different structural configurations. For example, the disorder may be expressed in a relatively "pure" sense of symptom presentation as defined in DSM-IV (1994). It may appear with other Axis I or Axis II disorders or be manifested as *complex PTSD*, with impacts on the inner core of the self-structure (Wilson & Zigelbaum, 1986; Marmar, Foy, Kazan, & Pynoos, 1993; Herman, 1992; Wilson, 1995). PTSD affects psychophysiological functioning in subtle and "masked" presentations, as illustrated by dissociative identity disorder (DID). The spectrum of PTSD is thus more than a diagnostic classification. There are relatively predictable forms of the disorder such as "pure" PTSD as a distinct, discrete anxiety phenomenon. There are also nonstatic, fluctuating PTSD states with extreme hyperarousal phenomena and complex defenses against underlying psychobiological processes (see Friedman, Chapter 4, this volume, and Wang, Wilson, & Mason, 1996). PTSD phenomena are manifested at multiple levels of synergistic processes: (1) stress-based emotional responses; (2) effects on cognitive-appraisal and information processing mechanisms; (3) psychobiological changes (i.e., neurohormonal), with feedback "loops" to organismic and system functioning (McEwen, 1998); (4) altered adaptation and coping behaviors; (5) effects on motives and goal-directed behaviors; and (6) shifts in spiritual and existential perspectives of day-to-day living and in the individual's sense of meaning and purpose (Wilson & Moran, 1997). The spectrum of PTSD therapy includes attempts to understand levels of consciousness and awareness (LCA) as part of the phenomenon itself. Most therapists who have experience in treating PTSD know that *unconscious* reenactment behaviors are not atypical (Blank, 1985; Wilson, 1989; Bremner & Marmar, 1998; Marmar, Weiss, & Metzler, 1997; Putnam, 1989). In terms of traumatic memories, van der Kolk (1999) and Goodwin (1993) described this phenomenon rudimentarily by the statement "emotional memories are forever." This research shows that traumatic residues exist within the memory bank of life experiences. As is well known, trauma can transform individual identity, the trajectory of the life cycle itself, and even subsequent generations (Wilson, 1980, 1988; Laufer, 1988; Danieli, 1994, 1998; Horowitz, 1999). Those who study trauma *ontologically* examine the vicissitudes of traumatic events and their transformation throughout life.

In Chapter 2, we present a holistic–dynamic model of PTSD and related psychological processes. We also present new models of PTSD as an allostatic organismic process (discussed further in the next section). These models are not only new forms of conceptualizing PTSD as a process but build on more than 20 years of accumulated scientific data. The "new paradigms" of emerging science and information utilization in the 21st century demand holistic, nonlinear models of complex stress-related phenomena. Among other historical legacies of the past century, PTSD has arisen rapidly to the attention of scientists and humanitarian workers because of its significance for human evolution. Wars around the world and massive traumas such as the Holocaust and other genocidal outbreaks have increasingly threatened our existence as a species. Humankind may well not survive another century of annihilative conflicts employing ever-enhanced weapon systems of mass destruction. Paradoxically, the study of PTSD is ultimately about the need to find proactive mechanisms to eradicate those conditions which cause human sources of trauma in the first place (Wilson, 1995).

TOWARD A NEW THEORETICAL PARADIGM OF PTSD

In the past few years, a series of research programs carried out by Bruce S. McEwen and his associates at Rockefeller University has explored the concept of allostasis and allostatic load in terms of the psychobiology of stress. Allostasis and allostatic load are related concepts and important to the understanding of PTSD and its treatment by one of the core treatment approaches. *Allostasis, unlike homeostasis, refers to the body's effort to maintain stability through change when loads or stressors of various types place demands on the normal levels of adaptive biological functioning.* According to McEwen (1998), allostasis is a response to the "wear and tear" that is produced by environmental demands (i.e., stressors of all types) which subsequently create allostatic loads challenges to the system to maintain itself in a healthy and potentially optimal mode of functioning. The failure to "switch off" allostatic mechanisms once the threat or requirement to respond has terminated, however, begins a complex process of "wear and tear" on the nervous and hormonal systems.

As McEwen states (1998):

> The core of the body's response to challenge—whether it is a dangerous situation, an infection, living in a crowded and unpleasant neighborhood, or a public speaking test—*is twofold, turning on an allostasis response that initiates a complex adaptive pathway, and then shutting off this response[, which] involves the sympathetic nervous system and HPA [hypothalamic–pituitary–adrenal] axis.* For these symptoms, activation releases catecholamines from nerves and adrenal medulla and leads to secretion of corticotropism from the pituitary. . . . Inactivation returns the systems to baseline levels of cortisol and catecholamine secretion, which normally happens when the danger is past. . . . *However, if the inactivation is inefficient, there is over-exposure to stress hormones, over weeks, months or years, exposure to increased secretion of stress hormones can result in allostatic load and its pathophysiologic consequences.* (pp. 171–172, emphasis added)

The relevance of allostasis and allostatic load to PTSD phenomena is fundamental to the understanding of stress-related psychobiological behaviors. For many victims of trauma, the failure to resolve (i.e., integrate) the traumatic experience within a new healthy baseline of normal psychobiolog-ical functioning renders them vulnerable in repeated ways to experience en-vironmental cues (i.e., triggers) that can lead to a stable but abnormal adjust-ment characterized by intensification of the existing pathological stress responses which never fully terminated after the threatening (i.e., traumatic) situation ended. One of the major challenges of the core therapies for PTSD is to facilitate a reduction or "switching off" of *persistent hyperarousal mechanisms* associated with allostatic load that are readily reactivated and amplified by traumatic memories (conscious or unconscious) stored in the brain. Stated somewhat differently, persons suffering from PTSD are vulnerable to abrupt changes in their sense of well-being. They find themselves rapidly switching between states of relative calmness to states of hypervigilance, anxiety, anger, and extreme arousal. Sometimes the rapid switch is not readily understand-able in terms of triggers or cues. As shown by van der Kolk (1999), Eitinger (1971), Freud (1917), and others, "the body keeps score." But unlike a base-ball scoreboard where there are only two scores posted for each inning of play for the opposing teams, the body's "scoreboard" for allostasis in subtypes of PTSD is more like a powerful search engine of the most complex comput-er software in the organism's "internet" repertoire. Allostasis can affect virtu-ally any domain of stored information and challenge the integrity of the sys-tem to execute its preprogrammed functions. When this occurs, a potential cascade of psychobiological processes can become "target" specific, as docu-mented by Seeman and McEwen (1996) in their empirical study of health outcomes for subjects with higher versus lower degrees of allostatic load as operationally defined by psychobiological parameters (see Friedman, Chap-ter 4, this volume, for more detail).

Building on the seminal work of McEwen and his associates, we can apply the concept of allostasis and allostatic load directly to PTSD with spe-cific implications for the core treatment approaches to PTSD. Initially, there is the normal, healthy response pattern to allostatic load: stress leads to cop-ing and adaptation, followed by recovery and *homeostatic restability*. The healthy steady state is restored and continues in an optimal mode until called upon to respond again, with efficacy and mastery (White, 1959; McEwen, 1998; Antonovsky, 1979).

McEwen (1998) classifies four subtypes of allostatic load which produce "wear and tear" on the capacity to deal with stress, especially in PTSD be-cause of the extreme nature of the traumatic stressor events. Briefly, these four patterns include the following: (1) *repeated hits* from multiple stressors in which the normal response pattern is frequently and repetitively activated, placing recurring demands on the system, which in turn tax effective coping; (2) the *lack of adaptation response* is similar to the above "repeated hits" subtype except that the effectiveness of normal adaptation starts to break down as the system's capacity to meet the load generated by the stressor is worn out, so that the system begins to fail at its genetically driven task; (3) the *prolonged stress response,* in which the duration, frequency, or intensity of the traumatic event persists, as seen, for example, in war veterans, Holocaust survivors, political internees, and repeatedly abused children (Wang et al., 1996; Simpson, 1993; Pynoos & Nader, 1993; van der Kolk & Sapporta, 1993) (in these cases, the physiological response of allostatic adaptation continues, chronically activating the HPA axis [i.e., the biological stress response system] without relief and causing the stress hormones to persist in efforts to meet the ever-present demands of the stressors; in such cases, there may be no timely, proper, or adequate development and recovery period, thereby setting in motion *a synergistic pattern of pathological events in the brain and body*[2] that may have long-term deleterious consequences, some of which may become irreversible, permanent changes in both the structure and function of cortical, subcortical, and neurohormonal mechanisms [DeBellis et al., 1999]); (4) *inadequate response,* by which McEwen (1998) is referring to system failure, for example, the "inadequate secretion of glucocorticoids, resulting in increased concentrations of cytokines that are normally counter-regulated by glucocorticoids" (p. 174). McEwen argues convincingly that the various forms of allostatic load affect the brain and cardiovascular, metabolic, and immune systems.

When applied to the analysis of PTSD, we believe that it is possible to add a fifth subtype of allostatic load—the *combined-fusion model,* in which features of the other four subtypes coexist in relative degrees in different psychobiological systems: (1) repeated hits (multiple stressors); (2) lack of capacity for adaptation; (3) prolonged stress response; and (4) inadequate response, or system failure. Furthermore, they not only may exist in different degrees but may *alternate* with "rest" periods, even brief ones, of normal stress response periods, only to be followed by one or more of the allostatic load patterns. Wilson (1981, 1988) has clinically described this phenomenon in Vietnam combat veterans with heavy war zone exposure (i.e., prolonged stress response) and identified nine typologies of PTSD. For example, after repatriation, many Vietnam veterans had repeated problems of postwar adjustment, such as divorce, unemployment, substance abuse, social alienation, and loss of self-worth in society (i.e., repeated hits; multiple stressors), coupled with lack of adaptation due to inadequate stress response (i.e., system dysregulation, breakdown, and failure) (Lindy, 1986; Kulka et al., 1990). In such cases, the combined-fusion pattern of allostatic load led not only to "complex PTSD" but also to comorbidity (Lindy, 1986; Yehuda, 1998).

PSYCHOLOGICAL THERAPIES FOR PTSD AND THE CRITERIA FOR RECOVERY, HEALING, AND REINTEGRATION OF THE SELF

What are the criteria by which to measure the healing and recovery from trauma? This question is germane to each of the treatment approaches outlined in this book. How is a specified treatment used to ameliorate allostatic load in PTSD? How is maximum stabilization achieved and the return toward optimum functioning restored to the individual? When does integration of the traumatic experience become a part of the general life perspective of the person rather than a fragmented, ego-alien, and unresolved bitter chapter in the life story (Horowitz, 1999)? How do therapists deal with persons who are so fragmented in their ego functioning that they have powerful unconscious self-destructive motives that subtly undermine the therapeutic process by attempting to re-create object-relational patterns which "justify" self-destructiveness, suicidality, and the malignant disruption of useful boundaries that have been established in therapy, friendships, family relationships, and the workplace (see Lindy & Wilson, Chapter 17, this volume, for a discussion)?

There can be no doubt that PTSD clients can create exceptionally difficult therapeutic relationships which engender powerful transference and countertransference relationships (Dalenberg, 2000; Wilson & Lindy, 1994). We believe that successful posttraumatic therapy (PTT) must know how to use the dynamics of the transference–countertransference matrix that exists in treatment settings in order to enter one of the five portals to the innercore phenomena of PTSD which are the targets of treatment (see Wilson, Friedman, & Lindy, Chapter 2, this volume, regarding portals of entry for all domains of symptom treatment). It is our view that from a dynamic and holistic perspective the diversity and spectrum of PTSD typologies has three critical elements pertaining to the ego state of clients: (1) their perception of the trauma and its impact on their identity and personhood; (2) the allostatic disruption of their lives in terms of affect regulation and capacity to recognize and modify noneffective allostatic processes that perpetuate the syndrome rather than truncating nonadaptive stress response mechanisms; and (3) restoration of a meaningful sense of self-sameness and self-continuity (Erikson, 1968; Lifton, 1976, 1993; Wilson, 1989), which encompasses their view of themselves as persons having worth, dignity, wholeness, purpose, and an essential feeling of vitality. The healed self that was once traumatized can project itself into the future with joy, serenity, and a measure of wisdom. Persons who have transformed trauma can do so because of an awareness that the boundary separating the fear of threat from quiescence is more often than not illusory and only creates allostatic load when induced by cognitive appraisals of threat to the psychological basis of existence. The specter of loss of one's self through injury, or the death of a loved one can lead to a radical shift in the existential plane of beliefs and consciousness, as noted brilliantly by R. J. Lifton (1979), M. J. Horowitz (1999), and others in their pioneering contributions to the field. A shift in consciousness may lead to many different forms of behavior change, including a sense of spirituality. Writers of literature, many of whom endured war trauma, have given us poetry and fiction with new insights and sensitivity as to the frailty and resiliency of the human spirit. Psychotherapists and counselors use words such as "grounded," "centered," "integrated," "recovered," "healed," "transformed," "rejuvenated," "together," "transcended," "self-actualized," "psychosocially accelerated," and "spiritually connected" to characterize the extraordinary changes that occur when those afflicted by trauma emerge with a human radiance, energy, and dignity that is the total antitheses of illness, despair, suffering, and fragmentation of personality. Healthy and resilient survivors of trauma are persons who have found pathways to reverse or attenuate the destructiveness of psychic burdens which affect their health. They have freedom of consciousness to create active minds and bodies. They are also potential guides, healers, and teachers, and may be subjects of scientific inquiry concerning resiliency, salutogenesis, and self-efficacy. The study of healthy PTSD survivors (Krystal, 1968; Wilson, 1989; Antonovsky, 1968, 1979) ultimately may be more important than the study of those whose deterioration can only be stabilized or moderately reversed in the advanced stages of decompensation (Friedman, 2000; Wang, Wilson, & Mason, 1996).

The effort to find answers to questions of how recovery from PTSD occurs challenges those who are ready to move beyond the 20th-century models of trauma and coping dominated by psychopathology and illness (Wilson, Harel, & Kahana, 1988). Of course, understanding stress disorders remains of critical importance, but expanding our knowledge of regenerative health and vitality is now an imperative in an era of innovations in humankind's capacity to shape itself in ways never before imagined.

Transforming the psychobiological expressions of stress-related illness and enlarging our capacity to restore the well-being of clients are tangible possibilities. Traumatic and untreated stress, in the broadest medicopsychological sense, can cause (1) physical illness, (2) the loss of self-realization or growth, (3) and a disruption of the life-course trajectory. The core therapeutic approaches to PTSD seek inroads to facilitate innovative and effective modalities of healing traumatic injury. We suggest that a transformation of consciousness can be a key part of PTSD therapy (Wilson, 1980; Wilson & Moran, 1997).

THE SCIENTIST–PRACTITIONER: CRITERIA AND STANDARDS FOR DEFINING THE SUCCESSFUL TREATMENT OF PTSD

It has been traditional in the history of psychotherapy, especially in debates surrounding the most effective approach to helping clients with PTSD, to argue as to what "works best" in alleviating symptoms (Nathan & Gorman, 1998). On the one hand, there are the pragmatists who take the view that if a clinical technique "works" to produce the relief of symptoms, then its use and practice is justified, especially if clients report that they "feel better" (Williams & Sommer, 1994). On the other hand, there are the "hardheaded" researchers who demand technical–scientific proof of therapeutic efficacy through controlled and repeated clinical trials which are subject to the most rigorous and conservative standards of modern research methodology (Foa & Meadows, 1997). These opposing views are readily appreciated and understood because they reflect different professional roles and responsibilities, despite the fact that both positions are committed to the ethical principles of "doing no harm" to the patient and upholding the highest standards of practice. However, when it comes to the treatment for PTSD, we must move toward a synthesis of the two divergent and well-justified approaches.

Foa and Meadows (1997), in the *Annual Review of Psychology*, Volume 48, argue that there are "Gold Standards" by which to determine treatment outcome studies of PTSD. They suggest seven general methodological procedures: (1) *clearly defined target symptoms* (e.g., distressing intrusive recollections—traumatic memories; (2) the use of *reliable and valid measures*; (3) use of *blind evaluations* (i.e., independent raters with no biases) in measuring symptom improvement; (4) *assessor training*, which includes such things as interrelator reliability and familiarity with the clinical syndrome; (5) *manualized, replicable treatment programs* (i.e., structural, standardized protocols); (6) *unbiased assignment to treatment* (i.e., the use of randomization); and (7) *treatment adherence* (i.e., monitoring compliance with the treatment program being used).

To begin, it is useful to specify some of the areas in which the objectives of successful treatment of PTSD are in concurrence in the clinical and scientific literature. Our approach builds on the model of allostasis and allostatic load in the subtypes of PTSD (discussed earlier), woven within a theoretical fabric of a holistic–dynamic approach to the treatment of PTSD.

Objectives of the Treatment Approaches for PTSD

In the simplest formulation, the central objectives in the treatment of PTSD are as follows: (1) normalization of the stress response, that is, attenuate allostatic load and allostatic processes that perpetuate maladaptive and prolonged psychobiological stress responses within the organism to alleviate anxiety, tension, and levels of distress; (2) facilitate a reduction or elimination of maladaptive psychobiological processes which include cognitive distortion, hyperarousal processes, hypervigilance, startle responses, sleep disturbance, and affective instability ranging on a continuum from anger to depression to diverse forms of anxiety. In terms of anxiety management, Keane (1998) and Foa and Meadows (1997) (see also Zoellner, Fitzgibbons, & Foa, Chapter 7, this volume) have reviewed the various techniques for clinically managing the anxiety spectrum of PTSD, including cognitive-behavioral treatments (CBT), exposure procedures (EP), *in vivo* exposure procedures (VP), anxiety management treatment (AMT) programs, and stress inoculation training

(SIT). In their 1997 summary based on a review of the literature, Foa and Meadows concluded:

> Overall, cognitive-behavioral treatments enjoy the greatest number of controlled outcome studies, and have been the most rigorously tested. Those studies converge to demonstrate that both prolonged exposure procedures and stress inoculation training are effective in reducing symptoms of PTSD. CPT (cognitive processing treatment) has shown promising initial findings, but it awaits the results of more rigorously controlled studies before its efficacy can be determined. (p. 474)

Keane (1998) reaches virtually the same conclusion in his review, suggesting that there is a concurrence of information pointing toward the conclusion proposed above that reductions in allostatic load has generalizable effects in the psychobiologically based dimensions of the anxiety–depression hyperarousal spectrum.

The various techniques (CBT, AMT, PE, etc.) that have shown effectiveness in treating the salient symptoms of PTSD, measured by different techniques (see Foa & Meadows, 1997), are consistent with Friedman's view (see Chapter 4, this volume) of PTSD as a psychobiological state. The use of the term "psychobiological" is important since there is no dualism being proposed between mind and body. Stated simply, *allostatic processes are inextricably linked to the spectrum of PTSD phenomena.* The therapeutic technologies reviewed by Foa and Meadows (1997) may be effective for the anxiety-based dimensions of PTSD, but are they sufficient for other aspects of the disorder, such as the client's impaired sense of integrity, wholeness, self-esteem, and personal identity, as well as his or her proneness to dissociation and high-risk-taking behaviors?

Viewed from a different perspective, what treatments work best for which kind of PTSD client and under what circumstances? Table 1.1 illustrates this relationship and is particularly important when therapists are considering the use of any of the core treatment approaches for PTSD.

PTSD as a Psychobiological Stress Response Syndrome: Implications for Treatment

Serving as a brief summary, Table 1.1 encapsulates how the subtypes of allostatic load are associated with PTSD processes. In Chapter 4 of this volume, Friedman expands upon these psychobiological mechanisms and related issues in greater detail, considering their many implications for treatment.

1. *Altered thresholds of response.* Allostasis implies that there are degrees of altered thresholds of response. Behaviorally, these include the degrees of readiness to respond, levels of hyperarousal, and altered appraisal processes,

TABLE 1.1. PTSD as Psychobiological Allostasis: Treatment Implications

Allostatic process	Associated PTSD symptoms	DSM-IV PTSD criteria
1. Altered *threshold* of response	Readiness to respond; hypervigilance; altered appraisal processes; increased threat appraisal; proneness to reenactment or reexperience; lower stress tolerance	B1, B3, B4, B5, C1, C2, D1, D2, D3, D4, D5
2. *Hyperreactivity*: allostatic dysregulation	Irritability; proneness to aggression; physiological and psychobiological hyperreactivity; startle response; insomnia; avoidance tendencies; inability to modulate arousal and affect	B1, B3, B5, D1, D2, D3, D4, D5
3. Altered *initial* response patterns	Decreased safety appraisal; decreased stress tolerance; overreaction to external or internal cues; proneness to fight-or-flight response	B3, B4, B5, C1, C2, D2, D4
4. Altered *capacity* of internal monitoring	Decreased capacity for accurate self-monitoring; increased vulnerability of cognitive and emotional response	B3, B4, B5, C6, D4
5. Altered *feedback* based on distorted information	Decreased capacity for accurate monitoring of interpersonal events and effects on others; altered cognitive schemas; erroneous cognitions of self and world	B3, C1, C2, C3, C5, C6, D2, D4
6. Altered *continuous* response	Increased proneness to avoidance and dissociation, amnesia, hyperarousal, cognitive dysregulations and somatic expressions of distress; insomnia; startle response	B1, B2, B3, B4, B5, C1, C2, C3, D1, D4, D5
7. *Failure to habituate*: failure of system to "shut down" and restore homeostasis (i.e., allostatic load)	Increased proneness to reenactment, traumatic memory, fluctuating levels of arousal; proneness to act out and reenact posttraumatic events; sleep disturbance; avoidance patterns; startle response	B1, B3, B4, B5 C1, C2, D1, D2 D4, D5
8. Establishment of new level of allostatic steady-state adaptations	Encompasses all of the above. (1–7)	All B, C, D

especially threat appraisals. The perception and appraisal of threat is *trauma specific in nature* (Wilson & Lindy, 1994; Dalenberg, 2000). Thus, depending on the particular event witnessed, endured, or survived, a PTSD client will have different sensitivity thresholds and memories as to cues associated with the appraisal process and its implication for thresholds of behavioral responsiveness in allostatic mechanisms.

2. *Hyperreactivity: Allostatic dysregulation.* Hyperreactivity is one component of the psychobiology of PTSD. Hyperreactivity refers to allostatic dysregulation and is associated with an inability to modulate arousal and affect. This lack of capacity for regulating arousal and affect is associated with irritability, proneness to aggression, exaggerated startle response, insomnia, hypervigilance, and excessive autonomic nervous system arousal. Persons prone to modes of hyperreactivity in PTSD may alternate between displays of threat, aggression, and intimidation, on the one hand, and isolation, detachment, and withdrawal from others, on the other. In either mode, there is a behavioral attempt to impose structure and control which is missing in situations due to dysregulation. Prolonged states of hyperreactivity may lead to fatigue, exhaustion, and depressive symptoms (i.e., hypersomnia, loss of initiative and striving, weight loss or gain, feelings of being "blue" and "down in the dumps," and the like). Clinically, persons suffering from high levels of hyperreactivity behaviors may be misdiagnosed as having bipolar disorder because states of high arousal and energy may appear manic-like and, when fatigue occurs leading to detachment, withdrawal, and isolation, may manifest a depressed-like state in demeanor and affect.

3. *Altered initial response thresholds.* Allostatic loads influence the predisposition to initial response patterns in PTSD. This includes such examples as decreased capacity for accurate self-monitoring of emotional states (e.g., anger, psychic numbing, affective constriction or effects of alcohol consumption). More essential is that altered response threshold as disposition is experienced as subjective vulnerability, which in turn affects cognitive appraisals, ego defensiveness, and readiness to respond to cognitive appraisals. As will be discussed further by Lindy and Wilson (see Chapter 17, this volume), ego vulnerability is at the core of the most severe and radical of PTSD disturbance. But what constitutes "vulnerability" is a complex question compounded by genetics, personality, and trauma-based experiences. *However, once situated within the personality, the individual's subjective perception of personal vulnerability has enormous implications for cognitive schemas, especially threat appraisal and risk-taking behaviors* (Wilson, 1989; Aronoff & Wilson, 1985; Krystal, 1968; Lifton, 1993; Dalenberg, 2000).

4. *Altered capacity of internal monitoring.* Another allostatic process common to PTSD is an altered capacity to monitor internal states. This refers to a decreased capacity to accurately "read" (i.e., self-monitor) levels of hyperarousal as well as affective states. The inability to monitor and experience af-

fective states includes degrees of psychic numbing, emotional blunting, or anesthesia in which feelings are absent or inaccessible to individual perception and recognition. Moreover, the altered capacity for self-monitoring has implications for cognitive processing, interpersonal relations, and subjectively experienced states of vulnerability. The failure to accurately monitor and process internal states creates the possibility for misperceiving others' intentions and emotional states by cognitive distortion or simply as failure to feel empathically their emotional state of being. In PTSD ego states increased vulnerability occurs because a loss of capacity for internal monitoring results in faulty information processing and "signal" detection from cues in others and the environment. When the capacity to adequately monitor internal states leads to faulty, distorted, or inadequate person perception or situational cue analysis, a heightened sense of vulnerability may result. As discussed by Lindy and Wilson in Chapter 5 of this volume, increased vulnerability leads to defensive adaptations to ward off anxiety, fear and uncertainty.

5. *Altered feedback based on distorted information.* Allostatic load is associated with the phenomena described in the last section, but also includes cognitive alterations in schemas. Elsewhere, Wilson (1989) identified five common subtypes of cognitive alterations in response to traumatic stressors: (a) *denial/avoidance* of the stressor or stressors as events or specific stimulus cues; (b) *cognitive and/or perceptual distortions* (e.g., augmentation or reduction of a perceptual modality—visual, auditory, olfactory, or kinesthetic); (c) *accurate appraisal of the traumatic events*; (d) *dissociation* (e.g., derealization, depersonalization, or amnesia); and (e) the *peritraumatic onset of memories* associated with the event itself—in other words immediate, intrusive recollections of what just took place in the traumatic situation (Bremner & Marmar, 1998; Singer, 1990; Cohen, Lewis, Berzoff, & Elin, 1997).

6. *Altered Continuous Responding.* Allostatic load has also been associated with the consequence of increasing proneness to dissociation (due to system overload in information processing) in any of its well researched forms (see Steinberg, 1997, for a review). Further, altered continuous responding is related to the threshold of responsiveness of behavioral adaptation. Hence, hypervigilance and alterations or transformations in cognitive processes (i.e., memory, problem solving, executive functioning, data interpretation, and categorization of newly acquired information, etc.) are but a few examples of how cognitive-perceptual and motivational dimensions of PTSD can combine in complex psycho-algorithmic formulas to affect allostatic processes.

7. *Altered continuous response.* Altered continuous response is another form of allostatic processes. In this process, the continuous flow of behavior, coping, and adaptation is disrupted. Disrupted response tendencies are manifest in psychobiological ways which include emotional lability and distress, somatic expressions (e.g., fatigue, headaches, bodily complaints or sleep disturbance), exaggerated startle response, and hyperaroused states. Furthermore, other forms of altered continuous response patterns may be seen in dissocia-

tion (i.e., altering conscious mental activity), amnesias, increased proneness to avoidance (e.g., geographic isolation, emotional detachment, and/or social noninvolvement with others) Finally, altered cognitive processes, such as information processing, attention, memory, and higher-order executive functions, may be expressed allostatically as well.

8. *Nonhabituation: The failure of the allostatic system to "shut down" and restore homeostasis.* The presence of allostatic load drives the entire autonomic nervous system and related endocrine functions to varying degrees. By this we mean that allostatic load can have a profound impact on the IIPA axis, as noted by McEwen (1998) and Friedman (1990), but eventually have systemic effects as well, often to organ systems. The failure of the system to shut down thus increases the full spectrum of PTSD behaviors from reenactment phenomena to fluctuating levels of hyperarousal, which may alternate in affective manifestations in varying combinations (e.g., hyperarousal → depression → anxiety → anger → withdrawal or acting out inner tensions). Thus, the failure to habituate encompasses all other forms of allostatic processes but must be categorized separately because it reflects what McEwen termed inadequate response to return to homeostasis. The failure to habituate implies much more than the original stress formulation proposed in the brilliant early work of Hans Selye (1976), namely, alarm reaction (A), resistance (R), and exhaustion (E). The general adaptation syndrome (GAS = A, R, E) described by Selye is both organ specific and cognitive in nature. Indeed, the GAS is one of the earliest formulations of the process of allostasis and its effects within the organism. However, Selye considered the GAS as nonspecific responses to stressors, whereas allostasis specifies the pathways of disturbed functions caused by system overload.

ALLOSTATIC TRANSFORMATIONS IN PTSD

As Freud noted in *Beyond the Pleasure Principle* (1920), the breach of the stimulus barrier may lead to "hypercathexis" and other consequences delineated in psychoanalytic terminology (Lindy, 1993; Wilson & Lindy, 1994). The failure to return to equilibrium or homeostatic states due to allostatic load has two basic principles which are the psychobiological "brick and mortar" of the stress syndrome: (1) *lowered stress tolerance,* which may trigger a cascade of PTSD phenomena; and (2) *the psychobiological memory of trauma,* which produces behavioral states of overreadiness to respond to situations due to hyperarousal, hypervigilance, decreased accurate self and other-monitoring and cognitive dysregulations in memory, thinking, information processing, judgment, perception, and appraisal processes, especially those of perceived threat. Lowered stress tolerance renders the trauma client even more vulnerable; a wider range of stimuli may act as triggers or cues evoking one or more of the syndrome dynamics outlined in Table 1.1. From a psychodynamic perspective, this makes the human psyche even more complicated because each of the forms of PTSD as allostatic transformations has the potential to interact and intensify, augment (amplify), or attenuate one aspect of the system. As discussed later in this chapter, relational patterns, ranging from total isolation to active group membership, may play a significant role in recovery and restoration of the self. *Healthy recovery involves the capacity to find a role in a significant group or society that allows a sense of personal integrity without the loss of selfhood and self-fragmentation, as well as the ability to sustain commitments and responsibilities that define the survivor's continuity of daily life.*

PSYCHOLOGICAL TREATMENTS FOR PTSD

It is one of the primary objectives of this book to present the treatment approaches for PTSD and to do so within a holistic–dynamic theoretical perspective. To provide adequate care for someone suffering from PTSD requires an understanding of the dynamics and complexity of the phenomenon (Matsakis, 1994). In this final section, we present a framework of the internal and external manifestations of the stress disorder.

As noted by Friedman (2000) the exponential growth of research on PTSD has enabled educators, consumers, scientific researchers, and others to select from a fairly vast array of information in the following areas most relevant to the treatment approaches for PTSD: (1) diagnostic criteria; (2) psychological assessment and clinical interview procedures; (3) differential diagnoses (i.e., taking into account how PTSD is similar to or different from other psychological disorders); (4) the various treatment options available; (5) specialized treatments for children; and (6) medical and pharmacological options that are available, ranging from medications to inpatient treatment programs.

TREATMENT GOALS FOR TRAUMATIC
STRESS SYNDROMES

What are the common treatment goals for PTSD? Marmar et al. (1993), in the *Review of Psychiatry* (Volume 12), presented one of the first attempts to present "an integrated approach for treating post-traumatic stress" (pp. 239–272). Among the important contributions of their review was the identification of 13 common treatment goals by psychodynamic, cognitive-behavioral, and pharmacological approaches. These treatment goals were more or less universal in nature; that is, they apply to simple and complex forms of PTSD which correspond remarkably closely to McEwen's subtypes of allostatic processes. Marmar et al. (1993) classified traumatic stress categories into five groupings: (1) normal stress response; (2) acute catastrophic stress reaction; (3) PTSD without comorbidity; (4) PTSD with Axis I comorbidity; and (5) PTSD with Axis II comorbidity. In their review, the authors discuss the application of the three types of psychotherapies (i.e., psychodynamic, cognitive-behavioral, and pharmacological) to these five categories of traumatic stress. Thus, despite the type of traumatic event or psychotherapeutic approach, the 13 common treatment goals share common objectives in terms of reducing allostatic load. Included in the list of the 13 treatment objectives are such factors as reduced levels of hyperarousal, accurate threat appraisal, return to the normal pathway of psychosocial development, reduction in traumatic memories; reduction of comorbid problems, restoration of integrity and self-esteem, and education about the stress process associated with PTSD as a disorder.

Table 1.2 presents a summary of the five core areas of PTSD and the general treatment goals for them. Later, in Chapters 2 and 3, we discuss these areas in much greater detail from a psychodynamic and psychobiological perspective. Moreover, each of the individual chapters on the core treatment approaches presents even more detail and discussion than space permits here. A general summary is useful as an introduction to the later chapters.

Each domain of PTSD has a set of target objectives which Wilson discusses in Chapter 3 of this volume in greater detail. Here, however, we can identify treatment goals by the symptom clusters. First, in terms of psychobiological alterations, the two primary goals are (1) to reestablish the normal (healthy) stress response to the extent possible and (2) to identify allostatic changes such as sleep disturbances, hypervigilance, irritability, proneness to anger, problems of concentration, and vulnerability to medical illness.

In terms of traumatic memory, the treatment goals from an allostatic perspective include identifying triggers for intrusive, distressing recollections of the trauma; uncoupling traumatic memory from debilitating affects and gaining authority and mastery over anxiety-provoking processes through cognitive reappraisal mechanisms and desensitization procedures.

The treatment goals for the avoidance, numbing, and denial cluster are primarily centered around the development of insight into maladaptive avoidance activities as part of PTSD and learning positive coping skills of various sorts that increase a sense of self-control, autonomy, and capacity for healthy self-esteem in the day-to-day transactions of living.

When traumatic events produce damage to ego processes (i.e., the self-structure, personal identity, and adequacy of the self-concept) the treatment goals are to reduce narcissistic injury to the self and to promote the integration of the traumatic experience within the self-schema of the individual so that it is not experienced as ego alien but as part of the life-history of the person. The primary treatment goals for this cluster of symptoms includes correcting faulty cognitions about self and world and gaining insight into states of experienced vulnerability and the use of ego-defense mechanisms to protect areas of injury to the coherency to the self-structure.

TABLE 1.2. Common Goals in Treatment for PTSD and Their Relation to Allostasis

PTSD dimension	PTSD treatment goal
1. *Psychobiological alterations:* hypervigilance, irritability, proneness to anger, depression, emotional lability, exaggerated startle response, sleep disturbance, problems of concentration, dissociation, somatic expressions of PTSD, vulnerability to medical illness	Reestablish normal stress response; normalize PTSD as psychobiological process; medicate as necessary; restore sleep and relaxation mechanisms (e.g., biofeedback, exercise); understand dissociation as hyperarousal; gain insight into medical/somatic expressions of PTSD
2. *Traumatic memory:* intrusive recollections, nightmares, emotional (somatic) memories, acting-out/reliving trauma, reenactment play, perceptual illusions, dissociation, memory retrieval	Identify "triggers" for memories; active cognitive reappraisal; understand dissociative episodes; integrate memories of trauma; uncouple memory from debilitating affect; gain mastery over fear and distress; learn accurate appraisal of anxiety and threat stimuli
3. *Avoidance, numbing, and denial:* avoidance, emotional constriction/numbing, amnesia, loss of active social interpersonal engagement, substance abuse, social/geographic isolation, desexualization, estrangement and detachment, obsessive–compulsive, attention diversion as defense	Gain insight into development and use of avoidance/numbing/denial mechanisms; facilitate recall of fragmented, amnestic, repressed, or blocked memories; treat substance abuse concurrent with PTSD; restore self-esteem and identity as survivor rather than victim; find ways to reconnect to self, others, and meaningful activities; reduce maladaptive coping behavior; uncouple memory from fear response
4. *Self-concept, ego states, personal identity, and self-structure:* demoralization, ego fragmentation, identity diffusion, proneness to dissociation, hopelessness and helplessness, vulnerability, loss of spirit and vitality, dysphoria, shame, guilt, misanthropic beliefs, faulty cognitions about self and world	Reduce narcissistic injury to self; restore self-esteem; restore personal integrity and vitality; decrease sense of vulnerability; integrate trauma experience in self-concept; identify risks of suicidality; place trauma within developmental perspective; facilitate normal psycho-social development and understand changes in life-course developmental trajectory; correct faulty cognitions about self and world
5. *Attachment, intimacy, and interpersonal relations:* Alienation; mistrust, detachment; self-destructive relationships; somatic tension; "boundary" problems with others; issues of loss, abandonment, impulsiveness, and object relations deficits	Restore good personal relations; learn to establish healthy boundaries; confront emotional feelings associated with vulnerability, detachments, and problem areas associated with bodily tension, invoke self-trust and capacity for meaningful personal relationships

PTSD includes, in many cases, impacts on attachment behaviors, capacity for intimate relations, and the quality of interpersonal encounters. Treatment objectives for this domain of symptoms includes learning to establish or maintain boundaries; reducing alienation, isolation, detachment, mistrust, and self-defeating behaviors. In order to restore or maintain good personal relations, it is necessary for the client to understand the connection between vulnerability states (e.g., fears, feelings, perceived threats) and dispositional tendencies in social encounters. Clearly, the link between *intra*personal dynamics in ego states and *inter*personal dynamics is an important one, and treatment goals should attempt to identify the manner in which they influence each other in reciprocal ways.

As a general summary, Table 1.2 presents the common goals for the treatment of PTSD symptoms classified according to the five domains which constitute the disorder viewed as an allostatic process.

NOTES

1. Personal correspondence with Dr. Fred Lener, November 30, 1999, National Center for PTSD, White River Junction, VT. The PILOTS database is available on-line at:

www.ncptsd.org

2. This might be construed as fatigue or somatic weariness, which has been referred to often in the PTSD literature (Wilson & Raphael, 1993).

REFERENCES

American Psychiatric Association. (1952). *Diagnostic and statistical manual of mental disorders* (1st ed.). Washington, DC: Author.

American Psychiatric Association. (1968). *Diagnostic and statistical manual of mental disorders* (2nd ed.). Washington, DC: Author.

American Psychiatric Association. (1980). *Diagnostic and statistical manual of mental disorders* (3rd ed.). Washington, DC: Author.

American Psychiatric Association. (1987). *Diagnostic and statistical manual of mental disorders* (3rd ed., rev.). Washington, DC: Author.

American Psychiatric Association. (1994). *Diagnostic and statistical manual of mental disorders* (4th ed.). Washington, DC: Author.

Antonovsky, A. (1968). Social class and the major cardiovascular diseases. *Journal of Chronic Diseases, 21,* 65–106.

Antonovsky, A. (1979). *Health, stress and coping.* San Francisco: Jossey-Bass.

Aronoff, J., & Wilson, J. P. (1985). *Personality in the social process.* Hillsdale, NJ: Erlbaum.

Blank, A. S., Jr. (1985). Irrational reactions to posttraumatic stress disorder and Vietnam veterans. In S. M. Sonnenberg, A. S. Blank, Jr., & J. A. Talbott (Eds.), *The trauma of war: Stress and recovery in Vietnam veterans* (pp. 21–34). Washington, DC: American Psychiatric Press.

Bremner, J. D. (1999). Alternations in brain structure and function associated with posttraumatic stress disorder. *Seminars in Clinical Neuropsychiatry, 4,* 249–255.

Bremner, J. D., & Marmar, C. R. (1998). *Dissociation.* Washington, DC: American Psychiatric Press.

Breslau, N. (1998). Epidemiology of trauma and posttraumatic stress disorder. In R. Yehuda (Ed.), *Psychological trauma* (pp. 1–27). Washington, DC: American Psychiatric Press.

Breslau, N., & Davis, G. C. (1992). Posttraumatic stress disorder in urban populations of young: Risk factors in for chronicity. *American Journal of Psychiatry, 149,* 671–675.

Cannon, W. B. (1929). *Bodily changes in fear, hunger, pain and rage.* New York: Appleton-Century.

Cohen, S., Lewis, M., Berzoff, J. N., & Elin, M. R. (1997). *Dissociative identity disorder: Theoretical and treatment controversies.* Northvale, NJ: Aronson.

Dalenberg, C. L. (2000). *Countertransference in the treatment of trauma.* Washington, DC: American Psychological Association Press.

Danieli, Y. (1994). Countertransference, trauma, and training. In J. P. Wilson & T. J. Keane (Eds.), *Assessing psychological trauma and PTSD* (pp. 368–389). Westport, CT: Greenwood Press/Praeger.

Danieli, Y. (Ed.) (1998). *International handbook of multigenerational legacies of trauma.* New York: Plenum Press.

DeBellis, J. M., Baum, A. S., Birnaber, B., Kesharan, M. S., Eccard, C. H., Boring, A., Jenkins, F. J., & Ryan, N. (1999). Developmental traumatology, Part I: Biological stress systems. *Biological Psychiatry, 45,* 1259–1270.

Eitinger, L. (1980). The concentration camp syndrome and its late sequela. In J. E. Dimsdale (Ed.), *Survivors, victims, and perpetrators: Essays on the Holocaust.* New York: Hemisphere Press.

Erikson, E. (1968). *Identity, youth and crisis.* New York: Norton.

Fenichel, O. (1945). *Psychoanalytic theory of neurosis.* New York.: W.W. Norton.

Figley, C. (1995). *Compassion fatigue.* New York: Brunner/Mazel.

Foa, E. B., & Meadows, E. A. (1997). Psychosocial treatments for posttraumatic stress disorder: A critical review. In J. T. Spence, J. M. Dorley, & D. J. Foss (Eds.), *Annual review of psychology* (Vol. 48, pp. 449–480). Palo Alto, CA: Annual Reviews.

Freud, S., & Brewer, J. (1895). *Studies on hysteria.* New York: Avon Press.

Freud, S. (1917). *Introductory lectures on psychoanalysis* (J. Strachey, Trans.). New York: Norton.

Freud, S. (1920). *Beyond the pleasure principle* (J. Strachey, Trans.). New York: W.W. Norton.

Friedman, M. J. (1990). Interrelationships between biological mechanisms and pharmacotherapy of post-traumatic stress disorder. In M. E. Wolfe & A. D. Mosnian (Eds.), *Post-traumatic stress disorder: Etiology, phenomenology and treatment* (pp. 204–205). Washington, DC: American Psychiatric Press.

Friedman, M. J. (2000). *Post-traumatic and acute stress disorders.* Kansas City, MO: Compact Clinicals.

Goodwin, J. M. (1993). *Rediscovering childhood trauma.* Washington, DC: American Psychiatric Press.

Herman, J. (1992). *Trauma and recovery.* New York: Basic Books.

Horowitz, M. J. (1986). *Stress response syndromes.* New York: Aronson.

Horowitz, M. J. (1999). *Essential papers on post-traumatic stress disorder.* New York: New York University Press.

Janet, P. (1900). *L'automatismre psychologique.* Paris: Ballière.

Keane, T. M. (1998). Psychological and behavioral treatments for post-traumatic stress disorder. In P. E. Nathan & J. M. Gorman (Eds.), *Treatments that work* (pp. 398–408). New York: Oxford University Press.

Kessler, N. C., Sonnega, A., & Bromet, E. (1995). Post-traumatic stress disorder in the national co-morbidity survey. *Archives—General Psychiatry, 52,* 1048–1060.

Kinzie, J. D. (1993). Posttraumatic effects and their treatment among Southeast Asian refugees. In J. P. Wilson & B. Raphael (Eds.), *International handbook of traumatic stress syndromes* (pp. 311–321). New York: Plenum Press.

Krystal, H. (1968). *Massive psychic trauma.* New York: International Universities Press.

Kulka, R., Schlenger, W., Fairbank, J., Hough, R., Jordan, B. D., Marmar, C. R., & Weiss, D. (1990). *Trauma and the Vietnam war generation.* New York: Brunner/Mazel.

Laufer, R. S. (1988). The serial self: War trauma, identity and adult development. In J. P. Wilson, Z. Harel, & B. Kahane (Eds.), *Human adaptation to extreme stress: From the Holocaust to Vietnam* (pp. 33–53). New York: Plenum Press.

Laughlin, H. (1967). *The neuroses.* Washington, DC: Butterworth.

Lifton, R. J. (1976). *The life of the self.* New York: Simon & Schuster.

Lifton, R. J. (1979). *The broken connection: On death and the continuity of life.* New York: Basic Books.

Lifton, R. J. (1993). From Hiroshima to the Nazi doctors: The evaluation of psychoformative approaches to understanding traumatic stress syndromes. In J. P. Wilson & B. Raphael (Eds.), *International handbook of traumatic stress syndromes* (pp. 11–25). New York: Plenum Press.

Lindy, J. D. (1986). *Vietnam: A carebook.* New York: Brunner/Mazel.

Lindy, J. (1993). Focal psychoanalytical psychotherapy of post-traumatic stress disorder. In J. P. Wilson & B. Raphael (Eds.), *International handbook of traumatic stress syndrome* (pp. 803–811). New York: Plenum Press.

Mack, J. D. (1999). *Passport to the cosmos.* New York: Crown Books.

Marmar, C. R., Foy, D., Kazan, B., & Pynoos, R. S. (1993). *An integrated approach for treating posttraumatic stress.* In T. M. Oldham, M. B. Riba, & A. Tasman (Eds.), *Review of psychiatry* (Vol. 12, pp. 239–273). Washington, DC: American Psychiatric Press.

Marmar, C. R., Weiss, D. S., & Metzler, T. M. (1997). The Peritraumatic Dissociative Experiences Questionnaire. In J. P. Wilson & T. M. Keane (Eds.), *Assessing psychological trauma and PTSD* (pp. 412–429). New York: Guilford Press.

Maslow, A. H. (1968). *Towards a psychology of being.* New York: Van Nostrand.

Maslow, A. H. (1971). *The farther reaches of human nature.* New York: Viking Press.

Matsakis, A. (1994). *Post-traumatic stress disorder.* Oakland, CA: New Harbinger.

McEwen, B. S. (1998). Protective and damaging effects of stress mediators. *Seminars in Medicine of the Beth Israel Deaconess Medical Center, 338*(3), 171–179.

Nathan, P. E., & Gorman, J. M. (1998). *Treatments that work.* New York: Oxford University Press.

Putnam, F. W. (1989). *Diagnosis and treatment of multiple personality disorder.* New York: Guilford Press.

Pynoos, R., & Nader, K. (1993). Issues in the treatment of posttraumatic stress in children. In J. P. Wilson & B. Raphael (Eds.), *International handbook of traumatic stress syndromes* (pp. 527–535). New York: Plenum Press.

Raphael, B., & Wilson, J. P. (2000). *Psychological debriefing: Theory, practice, evidence*. Cambridge, UK: Cambridge University Press.

Seeman, T. E., & McEwen, B. S. (1996). The impact of social environment characteristics on neuroendocrine regulations. *Psychosomatic Medicine, 58,* 459–471.

Selye, H. (1976). *The stress of life*. New York: McGraw-Hill.

Simpson, M. (1993). Traumatic stress and the bruising of the soul: The effects of torture and coercive interrogation. In J. P. Wilson & B. Raphael (Eds.), *International handbook of traumatic stress syndromes* (pp. 659–667). New York: Plenum Press.

Singer, J. L. (Ed.). (1990). *Repression and dissociation: Implications for personality theory, psychopathology and health*. Chicago: University of Chicago Press.

Steinberg, M. (1997). Assessing posttraumatic dissociation with structural clinical interviews for DSM-IV dissociative disorders. In J. P. Wilson & T. M. Keane (Eds.), *Assessing psychological trauma and PTSD* (pp. 429–448). New York: Guilford Press.

U.S. Surgeon General. (1999, December). *Mental health: A report of the Surgeon General*. Washington, DC: U.S. Public Health Service, Department of Health & Human Services.

van der Kolk, B. (1999). The body keeps score: Memory and the evolving psychobiology of posttraumatic stress. In M. Horowitz (Ed.), *Essential papers on posttraumatic stress disorder* (pp. 301–327). New York: New York University Press.

van der Kolk, B., & Sapporta, J. (1993). Biological response to psychic trauma. In J. P. Wilson & B. Raphael (Eds.), *International handbook of traumatic stress syndromes* (pp. 25–35). New York: Plenum Press.

Wang, S., Wilson, J. P., & Mason, J. (1996). Stages of decompensation in combat related PTSD: A new conceptual model. *Integrative Physiological and Behavioral Science, 31*(3), 237–253.

White, R. W. (1959). *The ego and reality in psychoanalytic theory*. New York: International Universities Press.

Williams, M. B., & Sommer, J. F., Jr. (Eds.). (1994). *Handbook of posttraumatic therapy*. Westport, CT: Greenwood Press/Praeger.

Wilson, J. P. (1980). Conflict, stress and growth. In C. R. Figley & S. Leventman (Eds.), *Strangers at home* (pp. 123–165). New York: Praeger.

Wilson, J. P. (1981). *Cognitive control mechanism in stress response syndromes and their relation to different forms of the disorder*. Paper presented at the Hospital and Community Psychiatry Conference, San Diego, CA.

Wilson, J. P. (1988). Understanding the Vietnam veteran. In F. Ochberg (Ed.), *Posttraumatic therapy and victims of violence* (pp. 227–254). New York: Brunner/Mazel.

Wilson, J. P. (1989). *Trauma, transformation and healing: An integrative approach to theory, research and post-traumatic therapy*. New York: Brunner/Mazel.

Wilson, J. P. (1994, October). Historical evolution of the diagnostic criteria for posttraumatic stress disorder—From Freud to DSM-IV. *Journal of Traumatic Stress, 7*(4), 681–698.

Wilson, J. P. (1995). Traumatic events and PTSD prevention. In B. Raphael & G. Barrows (Eds.), *The handbook of preventative psychiatry* (pp. 281–296). Amsterdam: Elsevier.

Wilson, J. P., Harel, Z., & Kahana, B. (Eds.). (1988). *Human adaptation to extreme stress: From the Holocaust to Vietnam.* New York: Plenum Press.

Wilson, J. P., & Lindy, J. D. (Eds.). (1994). *Countertransference in the treatment of PTSD.* New York: Guilford Press.

Wilson, J. P., & Moran, T. (1997). Psychological trauma: PTSD and spirituality. *Journal of Psychology and Theology, 26*(2), 168–178.

Wilson, J. P., & Raphael, B. (Eds.). (1993). *International handbook of traumatic stress syndromes.* New York: Plenum Press.

Wilson, J. P., & Thomas, R. (1999). *Empathic strain and countertransference in the treatment of PTSD.* Paper presented at the 14th annual meeting of the International Society for Traumatic Stress Studies, Miami, FL.

Wilson, J. P., & Zigelbaum, S. D. (1986). PTSD and the disposition to criminal behavior. In C. R. Figley (Ed.), *Trauma and its wake* (Vol. II, pp. 305–321). New York: Brunner/Mazel.

Yehuda, R. (Ed.). (1998). *Psychological trauma.* Washington, DC: American Psychiatric Press.

2

A Holistic, Organismic Approach to Healing Trauma and PTSD

JOHN P. WILSON, MATTHEW J. FRIEDMAN, and JACOB D. LINDY

> Healing from trauma requires a reverence for life. Reverence requires a state of meditative reflection on life's goodness. Meditative reverence is a consciousness of ultimate being and daily presence. Transformation of trauma is spiritual reverence. Spiritual reverence is the embodiment of soul and the sanctity of life.
> —JOHN. P. WILSON (2000)

The considerations concerning the psychological treatments for posttraumatic stress syndromes (PTSS) are complex and multidimensional in nature. The treatment of posttraumatic stress disorder (PTSD) involves contact with forces that inflict psychological injury and attack the human spirit and efforts to remain psychically whole. In the day-to-day reality of the clinical practitioner, the basic needs, anxieties, pain, anger, depression, and life conflicts of the trauma client are paramount. With few exceptions, their levels of psychological distress are undeniably evident and reflect internal struggles to come to grips with what happened to them in trauma. In the most basic sense, clinical intervention centers around the question of how to be most helpful to ameliorate distressing symptoms in posttraumatic psychological states.

What forms of support, counseling, psychotherapy, or human relatedness will be effective in assisting traumatized individuals in processing and integrating what has happened to them in the aftermath of a traumatic life event? How do they come to an emotional and spiritual understanding of what being a survivor means? How do they overcome the profound and often long-lasting effects of traumatization? What are the pathways to healing? What treatments exist for PTSD? How will clients become integrated in their spirits? What treatments will empower their capacity to once again function optimally with a joy and reverence for life? How will patients discover their own pathways to healing?

It is clear and beyond doubt that there are many crucial issues which confront those who choose to engage in posttraumatic therapies (Friedman, 2000; Ochberg, 1993; Herman, 1992; Wilson & Lindy, 1994; Foa, Keane, & Friedman, 2000). There is nothing easy in the work, although through it therapists may deepen their insight into themselves as persons and their wisdom as healers. It must be recognized that therapeutic recovery from PTSD is a complex interactive process between the therapist and the client during which both struggle together to find pathways to healing. Traumatic events may fracture a person's sense of wholeness and his or her willingness to persevere and go on with life. In that regard, there are no well-defined "road maps" that reveal the direction the therapist and client must pursue together in order to find the place of peace, restoration of vitality, psychological integration, and mental health. The therapist and the client walk a jointly created path to find ways that will enable the transformation of trauma.

Now, at the dawn of the 21st century, as we discussed in Chapter 1, we can see more clearly the legacy of trauma in the past century: massive global conflicts, both "hot" and "cold," including catastrophic wars, threats of nuclear annihilation, genocidal massacres (now called "ethnic cleansings"), major technological disasters, escalating terrorist assaults and reprisals, and other horrors have challenged the human spirit worldwide in ways that defy comprehension. Nevertheless, a retrospective look is important so that we never forget the magnitude of devastation that has been wrought by humankind. Yet, as malevolent as humanity has sometimes been through acts of utter cruelty and extreme violence, we also can see that a *counterforce* exists among us to promote healing, self-actualization, states of well-being, and psychic integration.

The process of understanding the way that the core treatment approaches work to ameliorate PTSD is a scientific effort which is establishing workable parameters to assist victims of trauma. As an empirical process, it is moving us closer, step by step, to the integration of theory, the creation of practice standards, and the coordination of scientific studies (e.g., clinical outcome trials), which ultimately will enhance the data-base on forms of organismic modes of recovery and healing (Friedman, 2000). Our goal in this chapter is to present a holistic, organismic approach to healing trauma and PTSD.

TOWARD NEW CONCEPTUAL PARADIGMS OF PTSD: INTRAPSYCHIC DYNAMICS

The scientific understanding of PTSD has evolved steadily during the 20th century, with a notably rapid acceleration of progress in research in the

1980s and especially in the 1990s (Friedman, 2000; Foa et al., 2000; Wilson & Keane, 1997; Raphael & Wilson, 2000; Wilson & Raphael, 1993). Such progress was inevitable once mental health scientists and clinicians began to focus on ways to assess the impact of catastrophic wars, natural disasters, acts of domestic violence, and other types of trauma that resulted in needs for crisis interventions, health care programs, counseling innovations, psychotherapy, social policy programs, and research studies. *Traumatic events tax human coping abilities and produce acute, chronic, delayed, and complex forms of PTSD.* Traumatic stress syndromes encompass but are not limited to psychiatric definitions of PTSD and its most common sequelae, such as major depression and alcohol abuse and generalized anxiety (Breslau, 1999). Posttraumatic change in psychosocial functioning also occurs and includes altered ego states and a shift in life-course developmental trajectories.

PTSD is a multidimensional construct of stress response syndromes. In a dynamic psychobiological sense, PTSD consists of many subsystems that interact in complex ways which are manifest in affective reactions, altered ego states, and fluctuating psychological phenomena (Green, Wilson, & Lindy, 1985; van der Kolk & Sapporta, 1993). The symptoms reflect the level of pain. Trauma impacts the psychic core—the very soul—of the survivor and generates a search for meaning as to why the event had to happen. A state of "dispiritedness" may cause a profound questioning of existence and force belief systems to change (Wilson & Moran, 1997). The alteration of psychoformative processes may lead to a decentering of the self, a loss of groundedness and of a sense of sameness and continuity (Lifton, 1976, 1979, 1993; Erikson, 1968; Putnam, 1997). In extreme cases, a radical discontinuity may occur in ego identity, leaving scars to the inner agency of the psyche (Watkins & Watkins, 1997; Krystal, 1968, Spiegel, 1994; Steinberg, 1997). Fragmentation of ego identity has consequences for psychological stability, well-being, and psychic integration, resulting in a proneness to dissociation (van der Kolk, McFarlane, & Weisaeth, 1996). In many cases of PTSD, the fragmentation of ego identity is a fracturing of the soul and spirit of the person (Lifton, 1979; Wilson & Lindy, 1994). As noted by Krystal (1968) and Lifton (1979), such a "broken connection" in an individul's existential sense of meaning may be a precursor to major depression, psychological surrender, and, in extreme cases, suicidality and death.

We clinicians undertaking therapeutic approaches to PTSD need to recognize that it is not a static psychopathological entity or quantity (Green, Wilson, & Lindy, 1985; Wang, Wilson, & Mason, 1996). Rather, like the changing colors of a kaleidoscope, its form, structure, and "flow" vary according to the principles associated with stress response interactions within the brain. For this reason, the clinical presentations of traumatized clients may vary significantly. Levels of severity of the condition can range from mild to disabling. There may be marked differences in degrees of traumatic impact on adaptive functioning in areas of psychosocial behavior. Diverse life-span and developmental effects may be produced by traumatic stressors (e.g., depending on the age, level of ego strength). The patterning of post-traumatic effects may range from relatively slight to profound consequences for psychological well-being and the degree of efficacy in coping at different epigenetic stages in the life cycle (Erikson, 1968; Wilson, 1980; Wilson, Harel, & Kahana, 1988; Harel, Kahana, & Wilson, 1993). Complex forms of PTSD have also been recognized in the literature, dating from Freud's various discussions of traumatic neuroses (e.g., 1895, 1917, 1920) to Lifton's (1967) description of radical traumatization in Hiroshima survivors and to more recent accounts of interpersonal violence and abuse (Herman, 1992).

Clearly, then, treatment approaches for traumatic stress syndromes must recognize the diversity, complexity, and transformability of posttraumatic conditions. While most practitioners would agree on some general treatment principles, such as the need to reduce physiological hyperarousal, depressive states, and debilitating traumatic memories, the techniques and methods which demonstrate scientific standards of effectiveness for the treatment of PTSD in its complexity are less well established or agreed upon at the present time (Foa & Meadows, 1997; Foa et al., 2000). For example, what set of techniques is most useful for treating a person who is experiencing emotionally overwhelming visual flashbacks to a trauma scene? What if the client can only report fragments of the distressing, intrusive recollections, which have a depth of allusions to many other elements of the stressors that created the memories in the first place? At the other end of the continuum, what of cases in which patients have so sealed over traumatic memories that they are psychically numb, angry, or depressed and may have classic forms of denial, repression, resistance, and counterphobic behaviors? These three examples illustrate that the configuration of posttraumatic states may vary among many subdimensions depending on such factors as the following: (1) the context of the traumatic event and the person's role in it; (2) cognitive coping and appraisal styles (e.g., Lazarus & Folkman, 1984; Wilson, 1989); and (3) cultural and prior history "risk" or "resiliency" factors (Antonovsky, 1979; Flannery, 1992). *Nevertheless, it is the structural configuration of dynamic ego states in PTSD and similar conditions that commands the attention and therapeutic efforts of the clinician* (Watkins & Watkins, 1997).

TRAUMATIC STRESS AND ORGANISMIC FUNCTIONING

Figure 2.1 illustrates traumatic impacts on organismic functioning. The figure depicts complex forms of PTSD processes within the organism. As shown, the triad ($\triangle$) of core PTSD symptoms (i.e., DSM-IV B, C, and D criteria) interact synergistically, impacting the dynamics of ego states, self-structure, and identity configuration. The structural configurations of trauma-

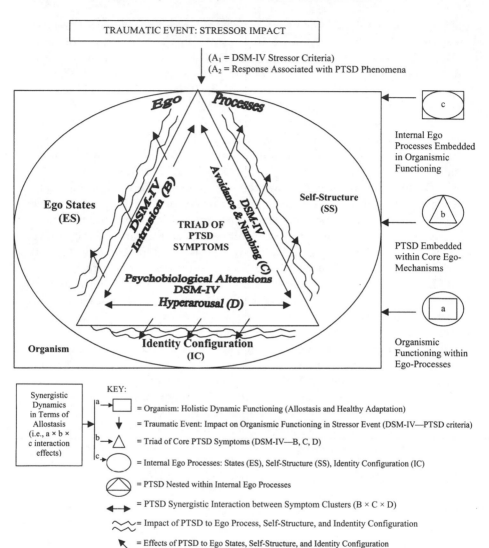

FIGURE 2.1. Traumatic impacts to organismic adaptations: PTSD, ego states, self-structure, and identity configuration.

tized ego states are epiphenomenal manifestations of the psychobiology of PTSD (i.e., allostasis). At the organismic level, posttraumatic adaptations include individual subjective responses and reaction patterns in terms of five interrelated psychological processes: (1) emotional regulation (i.e., affect modulation); (2) cognitive processes and information processing at different levels of conscious awareness (LCA); (3) motivational predispositions (i.e., need-based, goal-directed behaviors); (4) psychobiological processes; and (5) ego defenses, coping patterns, and the systems of belief, meaning, and spirituality.

We now consider the organismic model and conceptual nature of PTSD symptoms which constitute the structure of the disorder. Later in this volume, in Tables 3.2 to 3.6 of Chapter 3, Wilson identifies 80 specific objectives for the treatment of PTSD. In this chapter, we identify 65 separate PTSD symptoms within five clusters. Clearly, PTSD is a multidimensional phenomenon and the clinical symptoms which a client exhibits are products of psychobiological processes. While allostatic manifestations of PTSD take various forms and the configurations blend more than one type of behavioral adaptation, there *is* a core process in PTSD. Figure 2.1 represents the triadic relationship (△) of the core PTSD criteria and their relationship to ego states (ES), self-structure (SS), and identity configuration (IC). As illustrated in Figure 2.1 there is a dynamic interrelationship between the core PTSD processes and their impact on organismic functioning, especially on those internal processes which are intrapsychic in nature (i.e., ego states, memory, cognition, self-structure, and identity configuration). Figure 2.1 illustrates how a traumatic event impacts organismic functioning. The examination of the possible interrelations within the organism allow us to redefine and expand the core triad of symptoms presented in DSM-IV (American Psychiatric Association, 1994) to a more comprehensive set of symptoms (see Tables 2.1–2.5 and Figure 2.1).

TRAUMATIC IMPACTS ON ORGANISMIC ADAPTATIONS: PTSD AND EGO PROCESSES

Examination of Figure 2.1 reveals a model of how the core triad of PTSD symptoms impacts organismic functioning and ego processes. Inspection of the figure reveals three basic dimensions of psychological functioning: (1) the entire organism (□); (2) the triad of core PTSD symptoms per the DSM-IV criteria (△); (3) internal ego processes, including ego states (ES), self-structure (SS), and identity configuration (IC). The three dimensions depicted in the model interact synergistically in terms of allostatic processes. For convenience, each part has been identified with a lower case letter: *a*, organism; *b*, PTSD triad; and *c*, ego processes. Thus, synergistic dynamics involve all possible interaction effects among the dimensions (e.g., $a \times b \times c$, as depicted in Figure 2.1).

The model in Figure 2.1 also illustrates that the core triad of PTSD symptoms (△) impact ego processes in terms of ego states, self-structural dynamics, and the structure of identity configuration. In other words, PTSD symptom clusters can and do impact basic ego processes, cognition, information processing, memory, and ego-defensive operations within the organism. Moreover, Figure 2.1 illustrates that in terms of intrapsychic dynamics and clinical presentation the following are possibilities: First, internal ego process-es (*c*) embedded in organismic functions directly impact somatic and integrat-ed biological–organismic system functioning (*a*). Second, the triad of PTSD symptoms is embedded within core ego processes (*b*). Therefore, the existence of PTSD symptoms deterministically influences ego processes, cognition, self-reference, ego identity, and the operation of ego-defensive mechanisms. Third, the organismic functioning (*a*) is intrinsically embedded in ego processes. Thus, the psychobiological processes of the organism are repre-sented in ego states, ego processes, and elements of the self-structure, individ-ual persona (i.e., mask of self-presentation), and the entire range of dynamics in personality processes (Aronoff & Wilson, 1985).

The model presented in Figure 2.1 is a rather oversimplified but useful way of thinking about "mind–body" phenomena, or (as we prefer to say) complex psychobiological interrelationships, in PTSD.

A HOLISTIC, ORGANISMIC MODEL OF PTSD PHENOMENOLOGY

Figure 2.2 presents a graphic illustration of the psychodynamic phenomenol-ogy of PTSD from a holistic perspective (Maslow, 1968, 1970; Wilson, 1989; Friedman, 2000). The model of PTSD is designed as a tetrahedral represen-tation of the organism with five symmetries, the well-known mathematical representation of living systems (Hoagland, 1992; Mack, 1999). The tetrahe-dral model depicts organismic functioning in posttraumatic states. The model represents multiple levels of posttraumatic ego and psychobiological states and encompasses all aspects of organismic adaptations. An integrated theoretical approach to the facets of PTSD, social behavior, and personality processes, the model provides a theoretical basis for understanding natural, organismically based healing of traumatic injury.

First, as explained in Figure 2.2., the tetrahedral shape of the organis-mic model represents the human organism. Second, inscribed in the center of the model is an inverted tetrahedron formed by the five-pointed star creat-ed by the arc angles of the tetrahedral structure. The central inverted tetra-hedron contains the core PTSD phenomenology, reflecting complex allostat-ic adaptations. Third, the core PTSD phenomenology is formed by the three triangles (marked B, C, and D) which represent the triad of PTSD symptoms (i.e., DSM-IV PTSD criteria B, C, D). Fourth, the bold arrows (emanating from the PTSD symptom clusters point (→) to the interior core tetrahedron, indicating *variability* in their contributions to specific configurations of post-traumatic processes in the core phenomenology of the syndrome. For exam-ple, person *A* experiences frequent traumatic memories, whereas person *B* has extreme denial and repression of the traumatic experience and person *C* manifests anxiety and hyperarousal. Thus, persons *A*, *B*, and *C* may have *dif-*

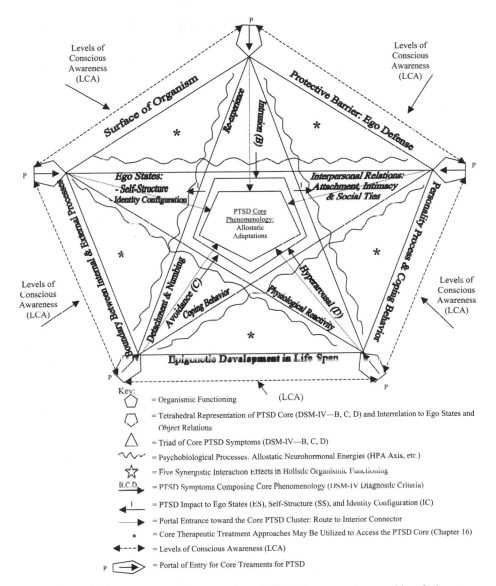

FIGURE 2.2. Organismic representation of PTSD phenomenology and its relations to ego states and interpersonal relations.

ferent degrees of PTSD symptoms manifest in coping adaptations; hence, different syndrome dynamics in PTSD and subtypes of the disorder would be discernible. Fifth, the arrows marked by an "I" that extend laterally from the interior core tetrahedron to the exterior triangles represent the impact (I) of PTSD on ego states (including self-structure and identity configuration) and interpersonal relations (including attachment, intimacy, and social ties); or the triad ($\triangle$) of core PTSD phenomenology thus respectively impacts *intra*personal or *inter*personal processes. Sixth, the five-pointed star (depicting the symmetrical systematic organismic interactions) is bordered by a single "wavy" or "vibrating" line, representing psychobiological processes (i.e., allostasis, neurohormonal HPA [hypothalamic–pituatary–adrenal axis energies] that operate within the entire organism afflicted with PTSD. These neurohormonal energies (wavy lines) reflect fluctuating allostatic states and influence PTSD symptom expression, ego states, and object-relational capacities (Friedman, 1994, 1998, 2000; Yehuda, 1998). Seventh, the exterior of the tetrahedron contains five portals (P) of entry into the core PTSD phenomenology. *The portals indicate areas of access to the treatment, understanding and analysis of PTSD phenomena.* These portals of entry include the core triad ($\triangle$) of PTSD symptom clusters as well as ego states and interpersonal relations. If one considers them in terms of a three-dimensional organismic model (i.e., a pyramidal tetrahedron), the portals of entry are passageways to interior connectors in ego states which reflect the totality of organismic functioning at any given moment. Moreover, each of the five triangles surrounding the five-pointed star are areas in which a core treatment technique can be used as a guide in the treatment process (see Wilson, Chapter 3, this volume). Thus, the model provides a method by which it is possible to determine how treatment should be approached for each of the five PTSD symptom clusters. Stated simply, the model illustrates synergistic interconnection in posttraumatic states.

The exterior of the tetrahedron contains five domains of organismic functioning which are related to each other by structure and function. The domain levels of organismic functioning include the following: (1) the surface (i.e., the totality) of the organism, representing holistic–dynamic adaptation; (2) the protective barrier of the organism (i.e., ego defenses and coping strategies to deal with traumatization); (3) personality processes and coping behavior; (4) the boundary between internal and external organismic and ego-level processes; and (5) epigenetic development and the potential impact of trauma to the trajectory of life-course development. Finally, enclosing the exterior are long double-headed dashed arrows representing levels of conscious awareness (LCA) among and within the domains of organismic functioning.

To summarize, the organismic model of PTSD phenomenology encapsulates the complexity and interrelatedness of posttraumatic adaptation. The model illustrates the multidimensional ways in which trauma impacts human adaptation and functioning in terms of internal psychological states (e.g., ego states), and external behavioral manifestations, (e.g., hyperarousal, startle response, response readiness, and sleep disturbance). The utility of the tetrahedral organismic model is that it illustrates the psychobiological connection at cellular, hormonal, psychological, behavioral, and cultural levels (Friedman, 2000; Bremner, 1999). In regard to the cultural level, it must be recognized that it influences many aspects of healing and recovery (Wilson, 1989; Kinzie, 1988). *In terms of the treatment approaches for PTSD (*), the portals of entry into the interior core phenomenology allow the therapist different pathways by which to assist the client in transforming traumatization through organismic healing.* In terms of treatment, the portals of entry have both trauma-specific and culture-specific implications for healing and recovery as well as transformation of the self. The ultimate meaning of the transformation of the self has no meaning without a cultural content. The utility of the organismic model presented in Figure 2.2 is that it allows the therapist/clinician to envision and access at least five separate portals of entry to the complex phenomenology of PTSD in its integrated or fragmented states as seen in either ego functions, symptom manifestations, or somatic (i.e., physical) states.

PTSD AND DISSOCIATION: AN EXPANDED ORGANISMIC TETRAHEDRAL REPRESENTATION

Figure 2.3 is an expansion of Figure 2.2 to include the relationship between PTSD and dissociation. The perimeter of the tetrahedral model contains the five common forms of dissociation: amnesia, depersonalization, identity confusion, derealization and identity alteration (i.e., dissociative identity disorder or DID) (Putnam, 1997; Steinberg, 1997; Spiegel, 1994). The central inverted pentagon represents the core PTSD triad and dissociative ego states. The arrows emanating from the core to the five perimeter triangles reflect alternative pathways of dissociation in PTSD. The exterior surface of the tetrahedron (i.e., the organismic whole) contains five sets of basic psychological processes associated with the forms of dissociation and include the following:

1. Memory and information processing
2. Self-detachment, altered awareness, and sensory changes
3. Discontinuity in ego processes
4. Sensory, perceptual, kinesthetic, and levels of awareness phenomena
5. Ego-fragmentation processes within the organization of the self

Furthermore, the dotted-line arrows emanating outward from the core PTSD triad and dissociated ego states to the five triangles inside the tetrahedron create a second inverted pentagon which overlaps and intersects the PTSD triad, the five forms of dissociation, and ego states and interpersonal relations. The third, larger tetrahedron represents the multiple possibilities of the relations between PTSD and dissociated ego states and their relation to the underlying psychobiological processes defined by the data on the exterior surface of the tetrahedron. There are five portals of entry (P) indicating pathways to the core PTSD processes and/or dissociated ego states.

The addition of the representation of dissociated ego states in PTSD

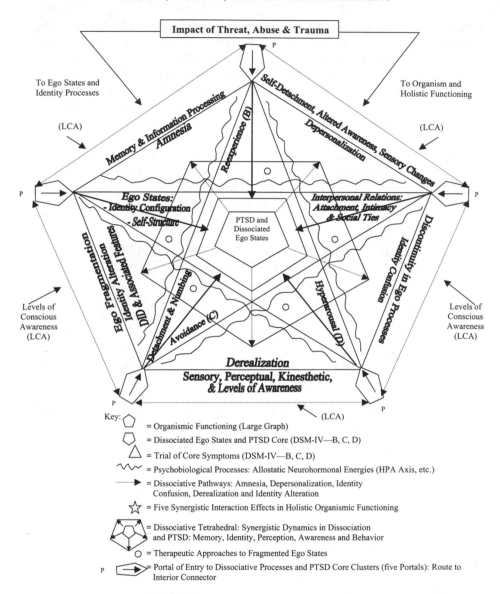

FIGURE 2.3. PTSD and dissociation.

permits a more complex analysis of psychic traumatization. As Figure 2.3 illustrates, it is the impact of threat, abuse, and trauma to organismic functioning, especially to ego states and identity processes, that creates combinations of PTSD symptoms and dissociative processes. For example, there are cases of amnesia for childhood sexual abuse with unconscious reenactment behavior activities in adulthood which are derivatives of the earlier abuse and are split-off ego states (e.g., repetitive self-destructive relationships; Watkins & Watkins, 1997). In this example, the underlying psychological processes include memory and information processing which have, through learning and conditioning, impacts on social relations, especially in terms of attachment, intimacy attempts, and the patterning of interpersonal relationships. Alternatively, there are other cases, at the other end of the spectrum, in which individuals have clear, vivid, intrusive traumatic memories which are associated with extreme levels of hyperarousal and proneness to dissociation (e.g., depersonalization) upon exposure to trigger events containing trauma-specific stimuli. These two examples are just a few of the forms of allostatic adaptation in organismic adaptation. Through systematic analysis, it is possible to discern the subtypes of the PTSD-dissociative spectrums and their configuration in ego states in victims of trauma.

TRAUMA-SPECIFIC CONFIGURATIONS OF EGO STATES AND DISSOCIATION IN PTSD

Wilson and Lindy (1994) have noted that one clue to understanding the configuration of ego states associated with PTSD are trauma-specific transference (TST) manifestations. Stated differently, persons afflicted with traumatic stress syndromes will manifest specific sets of cues in their behavior which reveal the meaning of the trauma-related behavior and its origin in dysregulated subsystems of functioning (see Putnam, 1997; Bedosky, Wilson, & Iskra, 1996; Wilson & Lindy, 1994; and Friedman, 1998, for a review). In TST, the patient engages in transference behaviors with the therapist. *The nature of the transference reveals content representations of unmetabolized elements of the traumatic event* (Haley, 1974; Danieli, 1988; Lindy, 1987). Dalenberg (2000), Ochberg (1988), Wilson (1989), and Wilson and Lindy (1994) suggest that an important therapeutic consideration is the proper timing of interpreting the underlying meaning of PTSD-related behaviors which are components of TST.

The parsimony of Figure 2.3 allows the therapist to further understand and interpret PTSD/dissociative phenomena. The core triad of PTSD symptoms impacts ego states and organismic functioning. Also, dissociative symptoms and phenomena are related to five basic psychological processes: (1) memory and information processing; (2) altered awareness, detachment, and memory/changes; (3) sensory and other changes in kinesthetic awareness; (4) ego fragmentation; and (5) discontinuity in ego processes. Moreover, the domain of the five PTSD symptom clusters (criteria B, C, D, plus ego states and interpersonal dispositions) interact with dissociative mechanisms to create an extraordinarily rich combination of posttraumatic adaptations. These adaptational configurations span the range of clinically and anthropologically observed phenomena in dissociation, dissociative disorders, personality alteration, PTSD in all its combinations with other Axis I or Axis II disorders, paranoid phenomena, and anomalous forms of adaptation (Laibow & Laue, 1993). In this sense, what looks like an impossibly difficult task of unraveling the organization of mental processes associated with posttraumatic states of adaptation can be placed within a meaningful conceptual framework as depicted in Figure 2.3. Although at first glance several geometric structures nested within each other might seem rather confusing, with closer examination they reveal pathways into the ego space of the PTSD client. If we saw Figure 2.3 as a three-dimensional object, that is, a pyramid, the directional arrows would indicate passageways and entry portals to different "floors" of the structure containing different processes and types of information regarding the unique ways in which the client's response to traumatic injury is organized. Visualized in that way, the model should seem much less complex.

DEFINITION OF CORE TREATMENT APPROACHES FOR POSTTRAUMATIC THERAPIES

As noted earlier, PTSD is a dynamic and complex form of stress-response syndrome (Horowitz, 1999). The core treatment approaches target symptom reduction and enable conditions of safety and equilibrium which permit trauma healing. Such a treatment approach aims at mastering specific reexperiencing phenomena, reducing physiological hyperarousal, and/or restoring capacity for attachment and integrity of self-structure. *A core treatment approach removes obstacles so that the organism can heal on its own.* Such a treatment proceeds from a body of clinical evidence demonstrating effectiveness, is consistent with a disciplined body of applicable theory, subjects its results to scientific criticism, and approaches PTSD through a valid entry portal (see Figure 2.2). A core treatment approach reduces allostatic load and produces positive changes in homeostatic regulation (McEwen, 1998). (See our Chapter 1, this volume, for a discussion of allostasis.)

THE TARGET SYMPTOMS OF POSTTRAUMATIC THERAPIES

Target I. The core triad of PTSD symptoms
1. Traumatic memory and stress-reexperiencing phenomena (Table 2.1).
2. Avoidance, numbing, depression, and coping adaptations (Table 2.2).
3. Psychobiological alterations in behavior (Table 2.3).

Target II. Ego states, identity, and interpersonal relations
4. Impact on attachment, intimacy and interpersonal relations (Table 2.4).
5. Impact on the self, identity, and life-course development (Table 2.5).

In this section we undertake a task that is twofold in nature. First, to revisit and review the triadic clusters of the B, C, and D criteria for PTSD in DSM-IV of the American Psychiatric Association (1994) and associated features. Second, to reconceptualize those primary triadic clusters in terms of recent advances in the scientific database (Friedman, 2000; Raphael & Wilson, 2000) and attempt to further define and integrate core symptom clusters which comprise the structural foundations of the "three legs" of the triad that define PTSD as presented in the DSM-IV. Furthermore, we attempt to move beyond the DSM-IV criteria to add other core psychological processes that are intrinsic to posttraumatic adaptations (see Tables 2.4 and 2.5). Some researchers (e.g., Horowitz, 1999; Yehuda, 1998; Herman, 1992; Wilson, 1995) refer to these dimensions as complex PTSD since by definition the symptom clusters and styles of behavioral adaptation transcend the diagnostic criteria set forth in the DSM-IV.

As with any diagnostic syndrome, new empirical information calls for an evaluation of the adequacy, complexity, and inclusivity of the diagnostic criteria. In that regard, we have expanded in Tables 2.1–2.5 the core criteria of PTSD symptoms into five distinct and separate categories. We consider PTSD not so much as a traditional psychiatric illness but as an adaptational pattern to traumatic stress. A holistic, dynamic perspective implicitly recognizes the synergistic nature of the phenomena. A synergistic perspective is consistent with approaches to understanding allostatic changes within the organism that have specific pathways of adaptation to trauma-related stress (McEwen, 1998). Consequently, the core treatment approaches must be tailored to the client's clinical presentation. Treatment protocols need to be designed around the adaptations of allostatic patterns of trauma syndromes (see Chapters 1, 3, 4, 5, and 16, this volume). *To be effective, treatment protocols should therefore recognize the need to individualize therapy to the patterned specificity of the patient's PTSD profile.*

BEYOND DSM-IV: REVISION, EXPANSION, AND RECONCEPTUALIZATION OF PTSD SYMPTOMS

To begin our reformulation, the set of criteria presented in Tables 2.1–2.5 each contain 13 symptoms for five interrelated dimensions of PTSD, or 65 separate but interrelated components of posttraumatic stress phenomena. The permutation of the five factors defines allostatic patterns of PTSD syndrome dynamics suggested by McEwen (1998). Like the amino acid peptide strands that define the DNA code in biological science, PTSD has its own "stress response psychobiological code" which defines the combinations of elements that can cohere in adaptational configurations. The understanding of these psychobiological processes eventually will lead to scientific advances in the understanding of PTSD in all of its complex behavioral and psychosocial manifestations (Yehuda, 1998). Allostatic adaptations refer to the subtypes of PTSD which are different forms of psychic integration after trauma. Clinicians who treat PTSD confront dynamic clinical phenomena for which there are no universally standardized protocols for treatment. In that sense, they face professional uncertainty in attempting to assist their trauma clients—which has a high potential to trigger countertransference reactions in the process of therapy (Wilson & Lindy, 1994).

In Parts II and III of this volume, the current therapeutic treatment approaches for PTSD are presented; in Part IV, case history analyses are discussed as well as a set of practical considerations for the treatment of PTSD (see in particular Chapters 5 and 15).

Tables 2.1–2.3 present the triad of the core PTSD symptoms which are noted in DSM-IV (American Psychiatric Association, 1994) and its predecessors (DSM-I, 1952; -II, 1968; -III, 1980; and -III-R, 1987—all cited by us in Chapter 1, this volume). Similarly, Tables 2.4 and 2.5 present symptoms related to ego processes and interpersonal relations. Thus, there are five domains of PTSD symptom clusters which are the targets for treatment.

Target I(1). Traumatic Memory and Stress-Reexperiencing Phenomena

Table 2.1 presents 13 distinct but interrelated symptoms or modalities by which a traumatic event is reexperienced. In a general sense, the treatment approaches for PTSD share the objective of reducing the distressing aspects of reliving trauma. In a pragmatic and utilitarian way, the presence of symptoms associated with reexperiencing elements of the traumatic event provides both the client and the therapist trauma-related information to work with in treatment. Understanding the patterns and content of the material allows discovery of how homeostasis was breached and disrupted in the first episodes of trauma and led to allostatic load. As noted by Wilson (1989), intrusive traumatic memories are the *sine qua non* of PTSD; they are the hallmark features which distinguish PTSD from other disorders. Intrusive, traumatic memories and the other forms of reexperiencing trauma are the nodal focal points of treatment. As constructed in the DSM-IV (American Psychiatric Association, 1994), the PTSD C criteria (i.e., avoidance and numbing symptoms) are forms of coping and adaptation manifest after the traumatic event and attempts to remove traumatic memories. The C criteria symptoms are reactions to the various forms of reexperiencing trauma and thus constitute parallel psychological processes which attempt to govern the intensity and severity of distress associated with reliving phenomena.

As a clinical goal, most research and reviews of the literature (e.g., Friedman, 2000; Marmar, Weiss, & Metzler, 1997; Foa et al., 2000; Foa & Meadows, 1997) agree that integration of the traumatic experience within existing cognitive schema is an important objective in the treatment of PTSD. In a

TABLE 2.1. PTSD Triad: The Reexperiencing of Trauma (DSM-IV B Criteria Revised)

1. Involuntary, unbidden, unexpected intrusive thoughts of the trauma with or without distressing emotions
2. Traumatic memory consciously or unconsciously manifest in declarative (visual or verbal memory) or nondeclarative forms (somatic or sensory modalities)
3. Dreams and nightmares associated with the trauma and sleep cycle disruptions which may be fragmented, symbolic, allusory, or accurate visual and emotional recall
4. Emotional flooding states with or without visual imagery (emotional flooding may be disguised in somatic complaints)
5. Conscious or unconscious behavioral reenactments which repeat or parallel behaviors that occurred during the trauma (i.e., peritraumatic and traumatic reenactments)
6. Dissociative and peridissociative episodes which include derealization, depersonalization, amnesia, reduction of awareness, perceptual distortions and reenactment behaviors
7. Trauma-based hallucinatory experiences (i.e., rooted in the experience) as distinct from psychotic hallucinations
8. Anniversary reactions with or without somatic reactions
9. Increased psychological or physiological distress by exposure to "triggering cues" (i.e., trauma-specific cues which have a potential to evoke a cascade of symptoms)
10. Feeling that the traumatic event is, or could be, recurring, or behaving as if it is happening or about to happen
11. Reenactment play in children or expressive behavior in adults, with trauma-specific relevance and psychological meaning
12. Perceptual vigilance, illusions, and similar phenomena triggered by stimuli with trauma-specific information
13. Somatic memories which trigger intrusive or ego-defense processes

Source: Wilson (1989).

basic sense, integration means that the trauma and its emotional aftermath have become part of the life history of the person. Upon successful integration, the client can discuss and recall the trauma without undue distressing or disabling influence. While its effects may change personality, alter meaning and beliefs about life, the deleterious consequences of trauma have been overcome, if not transformed, in a positive direction that energize growth and self-individuation (Lifton, 1993; Wilson, 1989). Unfortunately, this is not always the case, as depressions, alcoholism/drug abuse, suicide, and other forms of self-destructive behavior are sometimes manifest in the absence of treatment.

Table 2.1 is an effort to delineate the diversity of symptoms which constitute the reexperiencing elements of PTSD, listing 13 such symptoms. Further, it notes that the symptoms can be experienced at all levels of awareness (i.e., unconscious, preconscious, conscious, and in nondeclarative memory systems). It recognizes that the symptoms may or may not have associated features of emotional responsiveness. As Table 2.1 indicates, the symptoms involve different forms of cognitive activities: perception, memory, alteration in levels of awareness or behavior, problem-solving activities, dream content, thought processes, and more.

Furthermore, Table 2.1 contains information that reexperiencing phenomena in PTSD are not separable from psychobiological processes. There are distinct somatic components and complex psychophysiological reactions which are associated with the various forms of reliving aspects of the traumatic event. In a different way, there are levels of reenactments of trauma which get "played out" in dissociative processes, including unconscious behavioral acts which parallel the actions at the time of the trauma (i.e., rekindling, peritraumatic, and dissociative-like responses) and painful conscious memories (Marmar et al., 1997). There are also perceptual processes involving stimulus and sensory perceptions, cognitive encoding, and information processing—all of which affect behavioral dispositions. Thus, illusions, hallucinations, stimulus generalization, and sensory sensitivity to trauma-specific cues, reflect elements of the traumatic experience stored in "files" (cognitive domains of memory) consistent with the survivor's capacity to process the experience (Horowitz, 1986). The body stores the records of trauma in declarative and nondeclarative forms of memory (van der Kolk, 1999; Wilson, 1989). Depending on the emotional valence of the memory, the impact on the person may be devastating or lead to forms of avoidance and detachment. For some survivors, being alone in quietude is therapeutic and peaceful. For others, nothing short of extreme stimulation, "action addiction," and risk taking is acceptable as a "normal" part of life (Wilson et al., 1988; Wilson, 1989). Between these extremes are survivors of trauma who show varying degrees of fatigue, malaise, wariness, anger, anxiety states, fears, depressive symptoms, personal vulnerability and a changed sense of psychological well-being.

In regard to the core treatment approaches for PTSD, when we utilize the information from reexperiencing traumatic phenomena, we need to consider that these components of the disorder have their own underlying structure which is discernible through rational, empirical, and statistical factor analyses. The structural components are interrelated aspects of the organism's attempt to master the experience (Freud, 1917, 1920) and restore optimal functioning (Figley, 1985; Wilson, 1989; Horowitz, 1999).

The underlying structural components have several interrelated elements which influence symptom presentation. These core subcomponents are important for therapists because they yield information as to how to decode trauma-specific transference behaviors (i.e., TST projections) and requests for help which are typically shielded by avoidance symptoms. These 10 subcomponents are as follows: (1) intrusive, unbidden, unexpected, and distressing thoughts, feelings, and images associated with the trauma; (2) conscious reflections of traumatic memories which may or may not activate "cascades" of other intrusive processes; (3) dreams, nightmares, and cognitions during the sleep cycle associated with the trauma; (4) emotional flooding associated with the trauma as a form of "somatic intrusive recollection"; (5) physiological symptoms which are linked to the phenomena of sensation (e.g., visual, olfactory, tactile, auditory, kinesthetic) and perception, especially involving perceptual distortions or hallucinations associated with the trauma; (6) dissociative processes; (7) reenactment behaviors with varying levels of personal awareness; (8) somatic memories of the trauma in nondeclarative states (van der Kolk, 1996; Layton & Zonna, 1995); (9) psychophysiological reactivity associated with traumatic information processing; and (10) reenactment of the trauma through play in children or expressive behavior in adults without conscious insight as to the origin or trauma-specific derivation of such behavior. For example, it is relatively easy to see a one-to-one reenactment of a child's or adolescent's reaction to trauma (Pynoos & Nader, 1993), but it is more difficult to discern patterns of reenactment in adults with a history of trauma that has been sealed over or blocked by ego-defensive mechanisms and is symbolic in its behavioral manifestation (Niederland, 1962).

Target I(2). Avoidance, Numbing, Depression, and Coping Adaptations in PTSD

The reexperiencing of trauma is inevitably accompanied by attempts to defend against the pain and distress produced by traumatic memories. In terms of targeting symptom clusters for treatment, assessment should be made of the ways the individual defends against the pervasiveness of distressing intrusive recollections of the traumatic event.

As part of the assessment process, the clinician involved in posttraumatic therapy should evaluate the functionality of symptoms in terms of how they promote positive coping or are associated with problems and conflicts in daily life and personal responsibilities. In extreme cases, the symptoms presented in Table 2.2 are manifestations of human dispiritedness which include helplessness, demoralization, withdrawal, alienation, a lack of ego mastery, detachment, a loss of essential vitality, and a generalized shutting down of organismic functioning. *In severe cases of PTSD, the psychic core, or soul, of the survivor is diminished and attachments to other persons and life itself are lost.* Further, the capacity to experience positive emotions is often enmeshed and lost in a web of depression, despair, and sense of futility. The individual appears to have given up the struggle to remain alive (Wilson et al., 1988; Lifton, 1979, 1993). Such psychological surrender is connected to states of hopelessness and helplessness which are precursors of suicidality or other forms of self-destruction. In the most severe cases of PTSD, clinical interventions target depression, levels of helplessness, despair, and the decompensated downward spiral toward self-destructive behaviors (Wang, Wilson, & Mason, 1996).

TABLE 2.2. PTSD Triad: Avoidance, Numbing, and Detachment—Changes in Coping and Adaptation Not Present before the Trauma (DSM-IV C Criteria Revised)

1. Active or passive avoidance of thoughts, feelings, or conversations associated with the traumatic event
2. Active or passive avoidance of activities, places, or people that are associated with recall of the traumatic event
3. Emotional constriction and psychic numbing (i.e., reductions in emotionality and capacity to express affect)
4. Detachment, estrangement, withdrawal, or alienation
5. Desexualization: loss of sex drive or interest in sexual behavior and physical sensuality in general
6. Amnesia for trauma-related information
7. An inability to recall aspects of the trauma, which may include a loss of chronology or only fragmented and partial memories
8. A sense of a foreshortened future and a negative outlook on life and one's role in it
9. An altered or diminished interest or participation in significant activities
10. Compulsive overactivity as an attempt to avoid thoughts or feelings associated with the trauma (includes action-oriented, high-risk, sensation-seeking behaviors and impulsiveness)
11. Excessive use of alcohol or other substance abuse/dependence as self-medication for allostatic load, hyperarousal states, or depressive moods
12. Social and geographic isolation from others
13. A preference for solitary activities in work, shopping, recreation, and other pursuits

Source: Wilson (1989, 2001).

While it is clear that there are degrees of avoidance and numbing symptoms which range from mild to extremely severe, the 13 symptoms presented in Table 2.2 have an underlying structure which includes the following: (1) active and passive efforts to avoid cues or stimuli that could activate intrusive, distressing, and potentially cascading recollections of the trauma; (2) reduction in emotionality in terms of the capacity to feel or express internal affect; (3) social disengagement and efforts to minimize contact with others in an attempt to control emotional states and levels of arousal; (4) cognitive mechanisms to avoid recall of traumatic memories and feelings by repression, amnesia, dissociation, or frenetic overactivity to "jam" attention (Horowitz, 1986); (5) self-medication with alcohol or drugs to reduce hyperarousal or obliterate reexperiencing phenomena (physical and emotional numbing).

Target I(3). Psychobiological Alterations in Behavior

The three groups of symptom criteria that make up the PTSD algorithm in DSM-IV include psychobiological mechanisms which are part of the disorder (see Friedman, Chapter 4, this volume). The treatment approaches for PTSD recognize the third leg of the core triad as equally important as the other two in terms of target objectives in psychotherapy.

PTSD is a complex pattern of stress response. The psychobiological connection is transparent during treatment of clients with PTSD, as is manifest in their hyperarousal states, sleep disturbance, and problems of concentration. The amelioration or attenuation of the more biologically based symptoms of the disorder is an important part of the treatment plan (van der Kolk & Sapporta, 1993; van der Kolk, 1997). Table 2.3 presents 13 symptoms of psychobiological alterations associated with PTSD. We have made an attempt to expand the five symptoms of the PTSD D criteria in DSM-IV. These symptoms are manifestations of allostatic adaptations which reflect dysregulated neurohormonal processes. As allostatic adaptations, these symptoms can disrupt psychological functioning at varying levels of cognitive, emotional, and interpersonal behavior. The core treatment approaches for PTSD recognize the necessity to reduce physiological hyperarousal through cognitive behavioral therapy, medication, desensitization techniques, meditation, relaxation, exercise, diet, and other forms of deconditioning. *Further, since the triad of PTSD symptoms function synergistically, reduction of physiological alterations will generate changes in the other symptom clusters of PTSD as well* (Yehuda, 1998; DeBellis et al., 1999).

As with the other two core diagnostic legs of the PTSD triad presented in DSM-IV, the persistent symptoms of increased autonomic nervous system arousal have an underlying structure. The four subcomponents are as follows:

TABLE 2.3. PTSD Triad: Psychobiological Alterations Not Present before the Trauma (DSM-IV D Criteria Revised)

1. Sleep disturbances (i.e., early-, middle-, or late-cycle phenomena)
2. Irritability, outbursts of anger or rage, and problems of modulating affect
3. Cognitive processing deficits (e.g., problems of concentration, attention shifts, cognitive "drift" and difficulty encoding and retrieving information)
4. Hypervigilance: excessive perceptual scanning for cues to threat or harm; behavioral readiness to respond and increased emotional arousal
5. Exaggerated startle response
6. Sensory sensitivity to trauma-specific cues, i.e., olfactory, auditory, visual, tactile, and/or kinesthetic—with stimulus generalization to the traumatic event
7. Hyperarousal states: emotional, cognitive, and dispositional
8. Homeostatic dysregulation: emotional lability with variable cycling times and interepisode recovery
9. Chronic fatigue, exhaustion, weariness, and loss of essential vitality as part of PTSD
10. Somatic symptoms which have generalized, symbolic, or trauma-specific significance
11. Endocrine system physiological markers of allostatic load (e.g., thyroid dysfunction)
12. Sensation-seeking, high-risk behaviors, action addiction, impulsive behavior, gambling, sexual acting-out, etc.
13. Generalized existential malaise, ennui, despair, fatigue, loss of vitality, spirit, etc., which may or may not be associated with depressive episodes

Source: Wilson (2001).

1. *Sleep cycle disturbances* (i.e., problems going to sleep, staying asleep, nightmares, dreams of the trauma, early awakening, night sweats, difficulty returning to sleep, etc.)
2. *Hyperarousal phenomena* (i.e., homeostatic dysregulation, hypertension, depression, high risk taking, sensation seeking, action addiction, chronic fatigue, malaise, hypervigilance, startle response, thyroid dysfunction, etc.)
3. *Perceptual and sensory sensitivity* to trauma-specific cues (i.e., olfactory, tactile, visual, auditory, kinesthetic) with stimulus-specific generalization (SSG) to a traumatic event through cognitive associative processes
4. *Cognitive processing deficits* including problems of concentration, attention shifts, cognitive drift, difficulty encoding information, and impaired executive functions

BEYOND THE PTSD TRIAD

Target II(4). PTSD Impact on Attachment, Intimacy, and Interpersonal Relations

The presence of PTSD symptoms impacts a person's psychobiological capacity for attachment, intimacy, and the quality of interpersonal relationships. Table 2.4 presents 13 symptoms associated with traumatic impact on attachment, intimacy, and interpersonal relations. These symptom clusters point to adverse impact to interpersonal and intrapersonal functioning. The impact of PTSD symptoms to interpersonal functioning includes such difficulties as problems with relationship boundaries, sexual intimacy, trust of others, fears of abandonment, repetitive self-defeating relationships, impulsive behavior, and various forms of personal and social alienation. At the individual level, the impact of trauma may be associated with tendencies toward secretive and non-self-disclosing behaviors, object-relation deficits (i.e., interpersonal relations), poor or inadequate self-care, and chronic states of tension and anxiety which make it difficult for the person to accept nurturing from others. A tendency toward guardedness and suspiciousness may underlie difficulties in interacting with others at normal social occasions (e.g., reticence, withdrawal, social isolation, or shyness). Further, if the trauma occurs in the formative years of childhood and adolescence, personality development may be affected and result in features of PTSD in character structure. These features include narcissistic, borderline, dissociative, antisocial, oppositional, schizoid, or other patterns of adaptation (Wilson, 1987). Clearly, trauma can alter the normal trajectory of personality development in the life-course epigenesis (Hyler, 1994; Pynoos & Nader, 1993; Wilson, 1980; Erikson, 1968). Thus, depending on the nature of the traumatic event the

TABLE 2.4. PTSD and Associated Symptoms: Problems in Attachment, Intimacy, and Interpersonal Relations (Not Present before the Trauma)

1. Alienation: social, emotional, personal, cultural, spiritual
2. Mistrust, guardedness, secretive behaviors, non-self-disclosure, reticence towards social encounters
3. Detachment, isolation, withdrawal, estrangement, and feelings of emptiness
4. Anhedonia: loss of pleasure in living; loss of sensuality, sexuality, feeling, capacity for joy, etc.
5. Object relations deficits; loss of capacity for healthy connectedness to others
6. Self-destructive or self-defeating interpersonal relationships which are repetitive in nature
7. Impulsiveness, sudden changes in residence, occupation, or intimate relationships
8. Impaired sensuality, sexual drive, capacity for sexuality or loss of libidinal energy in general
9. Inability to relax; discontent with self-comfort activities and an inability to receive nurturing, affection, or physical touching from others
10. Unstable and intense interpersonal relationships whose origin is in trauma experiences
11. Problems with establishing or maintaining boundaries in relationships based on trauma experiences
12. Anxiety over abandonment or loss of loved ones, which is either conscious or unconscious in nature and based in traumatic experiences
13. Repetitive self-defeating interpersonal relationships which reflect unmetabolized patterns of attachment behavior from abusive developmental experiences

Source. Wilson (2001).

traits of personality transformation which develop (e.g., oppositional features in childhood, narcissistic tendencies in adolescents and adults) reflect damage to the self-structure and ego states. The person protects his or her vulnerability by developing defenses against basic anxiety, vulnerability, and fears of rejection and abuse. The resultant character defenses against inner vulnerability protect traumatized states by developing traits which attempt to optimize functioning while controlling the anxiety, anger, rage, and self-destructive symptoms of PTSD. This process may lead to the development of complex PTSD (Herman, 1992; Wilson, 1994) and alterations in personality functioning and character formation. However, such posttraumatic changes in personality processes are not necessarily the same as "traditional personality disorders" (Wilson et al., 1988; Wilson, 1989).

Traumatic events can cause damage to the fabric of the self at any stage of life-course development (i.e., epigenetic and ontogenetic development; see Wilson, 1980, 1989; Erikson, 1968; Pynoos & Nader, 1993). However, when trauma strikes during formative periods of personality development, it may produce damage to ego states, the sense of personal identity, and the self-concept of the survivor (discussed next). Table 2.5 presents 13 characteristics which reflect forms of damage or changes to the core self-structural dimensions of the traumatized self.

TABLE 2.5. PTSD and the Self-Structure: Problems Associated with Structural Dynamics, Ego States, Personal Identity, and Self (Not Present before the Trauma)

1. Narcissistic and other personality characteristics which reflect damage to the self-structure associated with trauma
2. Demoralization, dispiritedness, dysphoria, and existential doubt as to life's meaning
3. Loss of ego coherence and integration of the self-structure
4. Loss of a sense of sameness and continuity to ego identity or capacity for ego stability
5. Fragmentation of ego identity and identity disturbance (e.g., identity diffusion)
6. Shame, self-doubt, loss of self-esteem, guilt, and self-recrimination
7. Fluctuating ego states; proneness to dissociation and lack of ego mastery
8. Hopelessness, helplessness, and self-recrimination; masochistic, and self-destructive tendencies
9. Suicidality; patterns of self-destructiveness or self-mutilation
10. Chronic feelings of uncertainty and vulnerability; levels of depression, helplessness, and hopelessness
11. Existential personal or spiritual angst; dread, despair, and a sense of futility in living
12. Loss of spirituality, essential vitality, willingness to thrive, loss of religious/cosmic belief systems, etc.
13. Misanthropic beliefs, cynicism, and a view of the world as unsafe, dangerous, untrustworthy, and unpredictable

Source: Wilson (2001).

Target II(5). PTSD Impact on the Self, Identity, and Life-Course Development

To explain adequately the nature of the injury to the self-structure is a difficult task. The self-structure refers to the organization of the ego and inner processes of identity functioning. Thus, there may be several areas of psychic injury. First, there may be a narcissistic injury to the self in which a normal, healthy sense of vitality, integrity, and wholeness is partially lost (Simpson, 1993). Second, repetitive abuse in childhood or adolescence may lead to demoralization and a loss of ego coherence and integration. Third, ego identity may be fragmented and associated with identity diffusion and loss of self-sameness and continuity (Erikson, 1968). The destabilization of core ego processes is frequently associated with feelings of shame, anxiety, panic, doubt, helplessness, hopelessness, guilt, and chronic feelings of uncertainty and vulnerability, as well as obsessive-ruminative thoughts and feelings (Agger & Jensen, 1993). Fourth, assaults on the self-structure are also associated with misanthropic beliefs, existential despair, and a loss of spirituality and faith (Wilson & Moran, 1997). Fifth, single or repetitive abuse may increase the use of dissociation as a defense against pain, humiliation and degradation. Moreover, the internalization of a poor self-image (i.e., PTSD fragmented ego identity) may be expressed as depression and suicidal symptoms. When individuals feel trapped in the trauma *with no foreseeable exit from their distressing symptoms,* they may be at high risk for suicide or repetitive patterns of self-destructive behaviors and personal relationships (Wilson, 1989). The damage to the core ego processes, personality development, and self-structure is one of the least understood aspects of PTSD (Wilson, 1995; Herman, 1992). We believe that this is particularly unfortunate since such damage is injury to the soul—the innermost core of each human being. When a traumatic event breaks a person's spirit, it damages the basis of personhood and the capacity for self-actualization. To restore humanness is to create conditions of acceptance of the spirit. To restore the spirit may require rituals which are organized for collectively shared experiences of pain, stress, and recovery (Manson, 1997; Wilson, 1989). To facilitate the reintegration of psychically traumatized persons may require a collective sense of responsibility and judiciously used rituals for healing that enable transformation of allostatic states of PTSD to new, healthier levels of functioning.

Figure 2.4 presents a summary illustration of PTSD and its organismic impacts. The figure is a simplification of various pathways by which PTSD impacts psychological functioning.

Traumatic events produce organismic impacts which include allostatic load, psychobiological disequilibrium, and effects on life-course development (i.e., epigenesis). Among the direct consequences of a traumatic life event is the development of PTSD in all of its facets.

Traumatic life events have a direct impact on personality processes, ego functions, and the self-structure. Clearly, this encompasses a broad range of psychosocial phenomena including ego identity, ego defenses, cognitive schema, intellectual functions, and psychoformative processes (Lifton, 1993).

Traumatic life events also have an impact on attachment behaviors, capacity for intimacy, and the quality of interpersonal relationships. As Figure 2.4 indicates, this is an important area of psychosocial behavior and encompasses such issues as trust, safety, personal boundaries, sexuality, capacity for self-care, generativity (Erikson, 1968), and alienation from significant others.

In terms of the treatment approaches for PTSD, the 13 specific symptoms for each component of our tetrahedral model are targets for clinical intervention. In this perspective the target symptoms provide clear information to clinicians as to their alternatives for therapeutic interventions.

The core treatment approaches for PTSD recognize that the most profound injuries produced by trauma are located deep within the human psyche. PTSD symptoms are largely surface manifestations of these inner processes which cause allostatic transformations that attempt to restore organismic integrity. The healing transformations are themselves processes which dynamically alter a system dysregulated by overwhelming and painful traumatic experiences. Therapists who treat PTSD in all of its forms need to discover the portals of entry (see Figures 2.2 and 2.3) into traumatized ego states. *The client will, in one way or another, provide the clues to passageways leading to the inner sanctum of traumatization and vulnerability. The portals to traumatized ego states will show the therapist entryways to the path by which to assist in the healing trans-*

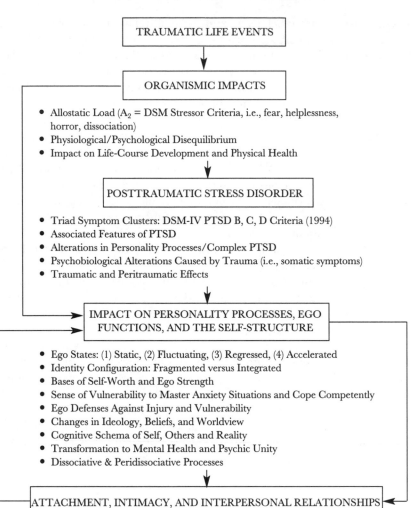

FIGURE 2.4. PTSD and traumatic impact on the self and interpersonal relations (Wilson, 2001).

formations of PTSD. Once discovered, the interactive process becomes a journey of mutually shared transformations: both the healer and patient change in the process. Both persons grow and become wiser and healthier because of their joint journey to overcome the disruption of ego and spiritual continuity in the life of the client.

Toward the end of therapy, healing transformations begin to manifest themselves in reintegration of the survivor's sense of human integrity. For the therapist there may be a sense of enrichment that the efforts to help have been rewarded with more knowledge about trauma, transference, and the client's psychic processes. Healing from PTSD is the transformation of trauma within the self-structure and ego states of the individual. Healing from trauma is self-integration, growth, and the continuance of organismic self-actualization.

In Chapter 3 we identify 60 specific treatment objectives for the five domains of PTSD symptoms. In the present chapter, we have indicated that these five domains of PTSD symptoms have 65 total symptoms, 13 for each cluster: (1) traumatic memory, (2) avoidance/numbing, (3) psychobiological alterations, (4) impacts on ego states, and (5) interpersonal relations. Thus, there is an approximate match between the treatment objectives and the total number of PTSD symptoms identified. The chapters in Parts II and III of this volume illustrate how the treatment approaches are used to ameliorate allostasis and other disruptive and distressing elements of PTSD. The models presented in Chapter 1 and this chapter (i.e., PTSD allostasis; tetrahedral models of PTSD and dissociation; traumatic impact on organismic functioning) can serve as conceptual road maps for therapists and clinicians in their work with traumatized clients.

REFERENCES

Agger, I., & Jensen, S. (1993). The psychosocial trauma of torture. In J. P. Wilson & B. Raphael (Eds.), *International handbook of traumatic stress syndromes* (pp. 703–715). New York: Plenum Press.

American Psychiatric Association. (1994). *Diagnositc and statistical manual of mental disorders* (4th ed.). Washington, DC: Author.

Antonovsky, A. (1979). *Health, stress and coping.* San Francisco: Jossey-Bass.

Aronoff, J., & Wilson, J. P. (1985). *Personality in the social process.* Hillsdale, NJ: Erlbaum.

Bedosky, C., Wilson, J. P., & Iskra, A. (1996). Issues in the diagnosis of PTSD. *Journal of Psychological Process, 2*(4), 1–16.

Bremner, J. D. (1999). Alterations in brain structure and function associated with posttraumatic stress disorder. *Seminars in Clinical Neuropsychiatry, 4,* 249–255.

Breslau, N. (1998). Epidemiology of trauma and posttraumatic stress disorder. In R. Yehuda (Ed.), *Psychological trauma* (pp. 1–27). Washington, DC: American Psychiatric Press.

Dalenberg, C. L. (2000). *Countertransference in the treatment of trauma.* Wshington, DC: American Psychological Association Press.

Danieli, Y. (1988). Confronting the unimaginable: Psychotherapists' reactions to victims of the Nazi Holocaust. In J. P. Wilson, Z. Harel, & B. Kahana (Eds.), *Human adaptation to extreme stress* (pp. 219–239). New York: Plenum Press.

DeBellis, J., Baum, A. S., Birnaber, B., Kesharan, M. S., Eccard, C. H., Boring, A., Jenkins, F. J., & Ryan, N. (1999). Developmental traumatology, Part I: Biological stress symptoms. *Biological Psychiatry, 45,* 1259–1270.

Erikson, E. (1968). *Identity, youth and crisis.* New York: Norton.

Figley, C. (1985). *Trauma and its wake* (Vol. I). New York: Brunner/Mazel.

Flannery, R. B. (1992). *Post-traumatic stress disorder.* New York: Cross-Road Press.

Foa, E. B., Keane, T. M., & Friedman, M. J. (Eds.). (2000). *Effective treatments for PTSD.* New York: Guilford Press.

Foa, E., & Meadows, E. A. (1997). Psychosocial treatments for posttraumatic stress disorder: A critical review. In J. T. Spence, J. M. Dorley, & D. J. Foss (Eds.), *Annual review of psychology* (Vol. 48, pp. 449–480). Palo Alto, CA: Annual Reviews.

Freud, S. (1917). *Introductory lectures on psychoanalysis* (J. Strachey, Trans.). New York: Norton.

Freud, S., & Brewer, J. (1895). *Studies on hysteria.* New York: Avon Press.

Freud, S. (1920). *Beyond the Pleasure Principle.* New York, W.W. Norton.

Friedman, M. J. (1994). Neurobiological sensitization models of post-traumatic stress disorder: Their possible relevance to multiple chemical sensitivity syndrome. *Toxicology and Industrial Health, 10,* 449–462.

Friedman, M. J. (1998). Current and future drug treatments for PTSD. *Psychiatric Annals, 28,* 461–468.

Friedman, M. J. (2000). *Post-traumatic and acute stress disorders.* Kansas , MO: Compact Clinicals.

Green, B., Wilson, J. P., & Lindy, J. (1985). Conceptualizing post-traumatic stress disorder: A psychosocial framework. In C. R. Figley (Ed.), *Trauma and its wake: The study and treatment of post-traumatic stress disorders* (pp. 53–69). New York: Brunner/Mazel.

Haley, S. (1974). When a patient reports an atrocity. *Archives of General Psychiatry, 30,* 191–196.

Harel, Z., Kahana, B., & Wilson, J. P. (1993). War and remembrance: The legacy of Pearl Harbor. In J. P. Wilson & B. Raphael (Eds.), *The international handbook of traumatic stress syndromes* (pp. 263–275). New York: Plenum Press.

Herman, J. (1992). *Trauma and recovery.* New York: Basic Books.

Hoagland, R. (1992). *The monuments of Mars.* Berkeley, CA: North Atlantic Books.

Horowitz, M. (1986). *Stress response syndromes.* Northvale, NJ: Aronson.

Horowitz, M. (1999). *Essential papers on posttraumatic stress disorder.* New York: New York University Press.

Hyler, L. (1994). *Trauma victim: Theoretical issues and practical suggestions.* Muncie, IN: Accelerated Development.

Kinzie, J. D. (1988). The psychiatric effects of massive trauma on Cambodian refugees. In J. P. Wilson, Z. Harel, & B. Kahana (Eds.), *Human adaptation to extreme stress* (pp. 305–319). New York: Plenum Press.

Krystal, H. (1988). *Massive psychic trauma.* New York: International Universties Press.

Laibow, R., & Laue, C. S. (1993). Post-traumatic stress is experienced anomalous trauma. In J. P. Wilson & B. Raphael (Eds.), *International handbook of traumatic stress syndromes* (pp. 93–105). New York: Plenum Press.

Layton, B. S., & Wardi-Zonna, K. (1994). *Posttraumatic stress disorder with neurogenic amnesia for the traumatic event.* Paper presented at the International Neuropsychological Society Meeting, Cincinnati, OH.

Lazarus, R., & Folkman, S. (1984). *Stress, appraisal and coping.* New York: Springer.

Lifton, R. J. (1967). *Death in life: The survivors of Hiroshima.* New York: Simon and Schuster.

Lifton, R. J. (1976). *The life of the self.* New York: Simon & Schuster.

Lifton, R. J. (1979). *The broken connection: On death and the continuity of life.* New York: Basic Books.

Lifton, R. J. (1988). Understanding the traumatized self and images, symbolization and transformation. In J. P. Wilson, Z. Harel, & B. Kahana (Eds.), *Human adaptation to extreme stress* (pp. 1–31). New York: Plenum Press.

Lifton, R. J. (1993). From Hiroshima to the Nazi doctors: The evolution of psychoformative approaches to understanding traumatic stress syndrome. In J. P. Wilson & B. Raphael (Eds.), *International Handbook of Traumatic Stress Syndromes* (pp. 11–25). New York: Plenum Press.

Lindy, J. D. (1987). *Vietnam: A casebook.* New York: Brunner/Mazel.

Mack, J. D. (1999). *Passport to the cosmos.* New York: Crown Books.

Manson, S. (1997). Cross-cultural and multi-ethnic assessment of trauma. In J. P. Wilson & T. M. Keane (Eds.), *Assessing psychological trauma and PTSD* (pp. 239–267). New York: Guilford Press.

Marmar, C. R., Weiss, D. S., & Metzler, T. M. (1997). The Peritraumatic Dissociative Experiences Questionnaire. In J. P. Wilson & T. M. Keane (Eds.), *Assessing psychological trauma and PTSD* (pp. 412–429). New York: Guilford Press.

Maslow, A. H. (1968). *Towards a psychology of being.* New York: Van Nostrand.

Maslow, A. H. (1970). *Motivation and personality.* New York: Harper.

McEwen, B. S. (1998). Protective and damaging effects of stress mediators. *Seminars in Medicine of the Beth Israel Deaconess Medical Center, 338*(3), 171–179.

Niederland, W. G. (1964). Psychiatric disorders among persecution victims—A contribution to understanding concentration camp pathology and its aftermath. *Journal of Nervous and Mental Health Disorders, 139,* 458–474.

Ochberg, F. (1988). *Post traumatic therapy and victims of violence.* New York: Brunner/Mazel.

Ochberg, F. (1993). Posttraumatic therapy. In J. P. Wilson & B. Raphael (Eds.), *International handbook of traumatic stress syndromes* (pp. 773–785). New York: Plenum Press.

Putnam, F. (1997). *Dissociation in children and adolescents.* New York: Guilford Press.

Pynoos, R., & Nader, K. (1993). Issues in the treatment of posttraumatic stress in children. In J. P. Wilson & B. Raphael (Eds.), *International handbook of traumatic stress syndromes* (pp. 527–535). New York: Plenum Press.

Raphael, B., & Wilson, J. P. (2000). *Psychological debriefing: Theory, practice, evidence.* Cambridge, UK: Cambridge University Press.

Simpson, M. (1993). Traumatic stress and the bruising of the soul: The effects of torture coercive interrogation. In J. P. Wilson & B. Raphael (Eds.), *International handbook of traumatic stress syndromes* (pp. 659–667). New York: Plenum Press.

Spiegel, D. (1994). *Dissociation.* Washington, DC: American Psychiatric Association Press.

Steinberg, M. (1997). Assessing post-traumatic dissociation with the structured clinical interview for DSM-IV dissociative disorder. In J. P. Wilson & T. M. Keane (Eds.), *Assessing psychological trauma and PTSD* (pp. 429–448). New York: Guilford Press.

van der Kolk, B. (1996). Trauma and memory. In B. van der Kolk, A. C. McFarlane, & L. Weisaeth (Eds.), *Traumatic stress* (pp. 279–303). New York: Guilford Press.

van der Kolk, B. (1999). The body keeps score: Memory and the evolving psychobiology of posttraumatic stress. In M. Horowitz (Ed.), *Essential papers on posttraumatic stress disorder* (pp. 301–327). New York: New York University Press.

van der Kolk, B. A., McFarlane, A. C., & Weisaeth, L. (1996). *Traumatic stress*. New York: Guilford Press.

van der Kolk, B., & Sapporta, J. (1993). Biological response to psychic trauma. In J. P. Wilson & B. Raphael (Eds.), *International handbook of traumatic stress syndromes* (pp. 25–35). New York: Plenum Press.

Wang, S., Wilson, J. P., & Mason, J. (1996). Stages of decompensation in combat-related PTSD: A new conceptual model. *Integrative Physiological and Behavioral Science, 31*(3), 237–253.

Watkins, J. G., & Watkins, H. H. (1997). *Ego states*. New York: Norton.

Wilson, J. P. (1980). Traumatic events and PTSD prevention. In B. Raphael & G. D. Burrows (Eds.), *The handbook of preventative psychiatry* (pp. 281–299). Amsterdam: Elsevier Press.

Wilson, J. P. (1986). Post-traumatic stress disorder and the disposition to criminal behavior. In C. R. Figley (Ed.), *Trauma and its wake: Vol. II. Theory, research, and intervention*. New York: Brunner/Mazel.

Wilson, J. P. (1987). Understanding the Vietnam veteran. In F. Ochberg (Ed.), *Post-traumatic therapy and victims of violence* (pp. 227–254). New York: Brunner/Mazel.

Wilson, J. P. (1989). *Trauma, transformation and healing: An integrative approach to the research and post-traumatic therapy*. New York: Brunner/Mazel.

Wilson, J. P. (1994, October). Historical evolution of the diagnostic criteria for post-traumatic stress disorder: From Freud to DSM-IV. *Journal of Traumatic Stress, 7*(4), 681–698.

Wilson, J. P. (1995). Traumatic events and PTSD and prevention. In B. Raphael & G. Barrows (Eds.), *The Handbook of studies on preventive psychiatry* (pp. 281–296). Amsterdam: Elsevier.

Wilson, J. P., Harel, Z., & Kahana, B. (Eds.). (1988). *Human adaptation to extreme stress*. New York: Plenum Press.

Wilson, J. P., & Keane, T. M. (Eds.). (1997). *Assisting psychological trauma and PTSD*. New York: Guilford Press.

Wilson, J. P., & Lindy, J. D. (Eds.). (1994). *Countertransference in the treatment of PTSD*. New York: Guilford Press.

Wilson, J. P., & Moran, T. (1997). Psychological trauma: PTSD and spirituality. *Journal of Psychology and Theology, 26*(2), 168–178.

Wilson, J. P., & Raphael, B. (Eds.). (1993). *International handbook of traumatic stress syndromes*. New York: Plenum Press.

Wilson, J. P., & Raphael, B. (2001). *Psychological debriefing*. Cambridge, UK: Cambridge Press.

Yehuda, R. (Ed.). (1998). *Psychological trauma*. Washington, DC: American Psychiatric Press.

II

CLINICAL TREATMENT OF PTSD

3

An Overview of Clinical Considerations and Principles in the Treatment of PTSD

JOHN P. WILSON

The clinical practitioner working with posttraumatic stress disorder (PTSD) clients has a number of considerations and choices to make in terms of assessment and treatment issues. To plan a strategy for effective treatment encompasses a broad domain of questions that require thoughtful decision making. Planning clinical interventions and establishing treatment objectives for PTSD is fundamentally no different than that for other psychiatric disorders. The accumulated empirical, scientific, and clinical data provide information which can facilitate decision making and planning specific decisions, such as that of prescribing medication. As an introduction to chapters in Parts II and III, which describe the core treatment approaches for PTSD (i.e., psychotherapy techniques), in the following sections we highlight some of the important clinical considerations in order to provide an overarching perspective of treatment issues related to PTSD. We also present 30 principles for the treatment of PTSD and 80 specific target goals for the five clusters of symptoms which define PTSD as a psychobiological disorder.

DIAGNOSIS AND CLINICAL ASSESSMENT

It is important that the practitioner have education and training to familiarize him- or herself with the substantial literature on PTSD. The National Center for PTSD (NC-PTSD) houses an international annotated bibliographic database which is readily available through the internet (*www.ncptsd.org*). This database contains nearly 20,000 references and is a good source for published scientific peer-reviewed reports on all facets of PTSD.

As a general rule of thumb, it is useful to make psychological assessments of a client using questionnaires, protocols, checklists, and objective or projective psychometric instruments. There are several reference volumes which review the methods and techniques of assessing psychological trauma and PTSD (e.g., Wilson & Keane, 1997; Carlson, 1997; Friedman, 2000; Wilson & Raphael, 1993). The various assessment tools can be employed for a quick screening of global PTSD symptoms (e.g., the Impact of Event Scale, Revised [IES-R]; Weiss & Marmar, 1997) or can provide a lengthy and detailed protocol record of PTSD and its associated features (Weiss, 1997). Among the advantages of conducting a diagnostic assessment of PTSD is that it provides useful information on the nature and severity of the condition that can be compared to data published on other trauma populations as well as normative data for a particular instrument.

It is a truism that psychological assessment through standardized testing can never "stand alone" when the practitioner is making a diagnosis. The clinical interview is very important as part of a differential diagnosis of PTSD and its common, comorbid conditions (e.g. major depression, alcoholism, generalized anxiety). In the early stages of treatment, the clinical assessment process includes obtaining as detailed a trauma history as possible. It is important to record the chronology as reported by the client and to note discrepancies, inconsistencies, or gaps in the trauma story. Exploring the account of the stressors reported is necessary and important but must be conducted with the safety and comfort level of the client in mind. Ego defenses and protective tendencies are natural and expectable during the initial assessment stages. It is useful to keep in mind that avoidance behaviors, denial, disavowal, amnesia, blocking, forgetting, repression, and mistrust of others are all part of the natural history of PTSD. Clients need to feel safe and that the clinical setting is one of a protective sanctuary rather than a place of interrogation or psychic "disrobing" of some of their most painful, shameful, and difficult life experiences (Wilson & Lindy, 1994). Further, it is important that the trauma story unfold at its own pace and not be forced, pressured, or in any way coerced. The clinician should not ask leading questions or conduct the clinical interview in a judgmental way about the reports of reactions, responses, or failed enactments provided about the client's role in the traumatic event (Lifton, 1993). It is helpful if the clinician can communicate empathy which reflects a genuine concern with how difficult it is for the client to disclose what happened during the trauma. Whenever possible, it is helpful to validate the reality of the experience and offer reassurances that traumatic experiences are abnormal events that have normal, expectable stress response sequelae, which includes the symptoms of PTSD. In some cases, it is also useful to administer instruments that measure (1) exposure to trauma, (2) stressful life events, or (3) specific stressors experienced during the trauma. For example, the life-events checklist (LEC) from the NC-PTSD contains 17 categories of stressful life events that clients can check off, indicating whether they have experienced any of them directly or indirectly and at what age. Friedman (2000), Wilson and Keane (1997), and Carlson (1997) review the various psychometric instruments that are available for assessing exposure to trauma, including such categories as general trauma, childhood trauma, domestic violence, war zone trauma, and torture.

THE TREATMENT APPROACHES FOR PTSD AND THEIR PRIMARY GOALS

Each of the core treatment approaches for PTSD is presented in Parts II and III and summarized in Chapter 16 as a practical set of guidelines for clinicians. Included in that chapter is Table 16.1, which summarizes the following categories of information: (1) 12 distinct treatment approaches for PTSD; (2) the five core dimensions of PTSD as derived from the allostatic organismic model presented in Chapter 2—(a) psychobiological, (b) traumatic memory, (c) avoidance, numbing, denial, and coping, (d) self-structure, ego-states, and identity; and (e) interpersonal relations; and (3) the objectives of the treatment goals.

For convenience, we are reproducing Table 16.1 here as Table 3.1 as a guide and quick overview of the treatment goals of the various clinical approaches. Further, Table 3.1 illustrates the degree of relevance and effectiveness of the core treatment approaches for each of the five dimensions of PTSD discussed in Chapters 1 and 2 and as derived from the organismic models of PTSD and dissociation.

Examination of Table 3.1 reveals the specification of treatment goals. The table also indicates the effectiveness of a particular core treatment approach for PTSD using a 4-point rating scale for each of the five domains of symptom clusters. In this way, Table 3.1 is a reference guide to decision making and information utilization in formulating a treatment plan or a research agenda, or in comparing similarities and differences between the 12 therapeutic approaches summarized by the table. (In Chapter 16, each of these therapies is reviewed in greater detail.)

GENERAL PRINCIPLES OF TREATMENT IN POSTTRAUMATIC THERAPY

The psychological treatment of PTSD involves a core set of general principles that the clinical practitioner can use in posttraumatic therapy. These principles are a list of important considerations which may emerge at any point in the

TABLE 3.1. Treatment Approaches for PTSD and Their Goals

Core treatment approaches for PTSD	Dimensions of PTSD derived from the tetrahedral model					Treatment goals
	I. Psychobiological	II. Traumatic memory	III. Avoidance, numbing, denial, and coping	IV. Self-structure, ego states, and identity	V. Interpersonal relations	
Psychopharmacotherapy	+++	++	+++	0	0	Facilitate normalization toward homeostasis
Psychodynamic	+	+++	+++	+++	++	Restore toward normal intrapsychic functioning
Acute interventions	++	+	++	0	0	Reestablish a normal stress response pattern
Cognitive-behavioral	++	+++	+++	++	+	Gain authority over traumatic memories
Group psychotherapy	0	+++	+++	+	+++	Facilitate normalization of PTSD responses and enhance capacity for healthy relationships
Complex PTSD	0	+++	+++	+++	++	Restore a positive self-schema of effective coping
Dual diagnosis	+++	+++	+++	++	++	Determine treatment that fosters recovery from Axis I and Axis II disorders
Cross-cultural	++	+	+++	+	++	Foster recovery within an embedded cultural framework
Children	++	+++	+++	+	+++	Foster trauma recovery to overcome interruption of normal development
Families and couples	0	++	+++	+	+++	Restore healthy attachments, relationships, and capacity for intimacy
Severe mental illness and PTSD	0	+	++	0	+++	Facilitate social reintegration and support for activities of daily living

Note. +, somewhat relevant; ++, moderately relevant; +++, highly relevant; 0, not applicable.

treatment process. The 30 principles presented below are not intended to be exhaustive but offer a broad spectrum of critical issues which are indigenous to the core treatment approaches discussed in Parts II and III of this book.

Safety and Protection

The treatment setting should be experienced by clients as a place of safety, trust, security, confidentiality, and protection, an emotional sanctuary in which they feel safeguarded and not overwhelmed by personal feelings of vulnerability, fear, anxiety, and uncertainty.

Nonjudgmental Acceptance of the Victim–Client

It is important for the client to feel accepted with unconditional positive regard for their struggle with victimization and PTSD. As a rule, they are reticent to discuss what has happened in the trauma for fear that the therapist will not understand because he or she "was not there." Clients often feel "trapped" within the emotional legacy of their traumatic experience and seek validation and confirmation of the reality of psychic impact to their sense of well-being. The clinician needs to be open minded, flexible, and prepared to hear the trauma story in its full intensity. A nonjudgmental attitude is essential to facilitate disclosure, alliance, therapeutic bonding, and the full range of trauma-specific transference (TST) reactions (Wilson & Lindy, 1994).

Trauma-Specific Transference (TST) and Countertransference in the Treatment of PTSD

The dynamics of PTSD are such that the transference–countertransference reactions are critical and need to be understood in the course of treatment. TST reactions are behaviors which reflect unmetabolized elements of the traumatic event and which involve symbolic parallel reenactments or ego projections as forms of transference behavior with the therapist. In TST, the client reenacts dynamics of the trauma in the context of treatment. TST reactions, in turn, often provoke different types of countertransference behavior in the therapist (e.g., Type I, Type II, and four modes of empathic strain; Wilson & Lindy, 1994). The transference–countertransference matrix creates a dual unfolding process between the client and therapist which evolves and undergoes transformation throughout the course of treatment.

Traumatic Memory

Traumatic memory involves complex forms of information storage in short- and long-term memory. Traumatic memory occurs at different levels of conscious awareness (LCA) and includes declarative and nondeclarative forms of memory storage. Traumatic memories vary in lucidity, detail, form (i.e., complex vs. simple structure), quantity, and chronology, as well as in the extent to which emotion accompanies the memories. Traumatic memories may be intrusive, unexpected, unbidden, and/or involuntary. Such memories may be experienced unconsciously or preconsciously. Traumatic amnesias exist, and such "lost" memories may be retrieved under proper therapeutic conditions. Dissociative and peridissociative processes reflect cognitive mechanisms of alteration in information processing, storage, and retrieval of memory (Marmar & Weiss, 1997). The recovery of traumatic memories is also influenced by ego-defense processes such as repression, denial, disavowal, splitting, and intellectualization. The clinical issue of whether to leave some traumatic memories "sealed over" or uncovered by probing inquiry is an important one.

The Trauma Membrane: Rapid Intervention and the Establishment of Supportive Resources Aids the Stress Recovery Process

Rapid intervention to normalize the stress response sequence (i.e., acute stress disorder, ASD) helps to restore disrupted psychobiological processes at work in PTSD. A supportive trauma membrane protects and buffers against secondary stressors following a traumatic event (Lindy, 1993). However, the creation of a "trauma membrane" to cushion the effects of the stress response sequelae must be carefully applied so as to not prematurely aggravate the fresh psychological wound incurred from the traumatic experience.

Vulnerability, Fear, and Uncertainty in PTSD

Traumatization leads to states of personal vulnerability, fear, and uncertainty which vary in severity, frequency, and intensity. States of vulnerability reflect the perceived threat to organismic well-being, personal integrity, self-esteem, and psychological intactness. The greater the degree of experienced vulnerability, the stronger will be defensive measures which include preemptive aggressiveness and hostility; isolation, withdrawal, and emotional numbing; or "frozen states" characterized by nonresponsiveness and inaction. Clinical interventions or treatments which supply nurturance and support while reducing perceived threat to organismic well-being will facilitate healthy coping and mastery behaviors. In cases of PTSD resulting from acts of interpersonal violence or abuse, personal states of vulnerability are experienced as narcissistic injuries to the self. In PTSD, narcissistic scarring is protected by ego defenses whose function is to guard against further injury to ego states (Watkins & Watkins, 1997).

Psychoeducational Materials about PTSD Promote the Stress Recovery Process

It is useful therapeutically to provide the PTSD client with psychoeducational materials about PTSD and its associated conditions, especially proneness to self-medication with alcohol or drugs (prescribed or illicit). Also, it is often reassuring for the client to learn that PTSD is the normal response to abnormal traumatic life events. Placing the human stress response in the context of normal psychobiological processes is not only supportive but allows for positive, constructive decision making in the same way that a diabetic needs to understand that sugar intolerance is detrimental to health and perhaps life itself. We encourage clients to access the internet to discover the vast amount of available literature on posttraumatic stress syndromes (*www.ncptsd.org*).

Alteration in Psychoformative Processes, Self-Schemas, and Beliefs about Human Nature, Justice, Authority, and Life's Meaning

Trauma can alter every aspect of organismic functioning. A holistic–dynamic approach to the treatment of PTSD recognizes that a change in one component of organismic functioning produces changes in other psychological processes and organ systems.

Trauma often produces changes in basic cognitive processes: memory, concentration, executive function, short- and long-term retrieval capacities, analytical and logical reasoning, and more. Traumatic experiences which generate narcissistic injuries to the self often also violate a person's assumptions about equity, fairness, justice, decency, and the goodness of human nature. Traumatic stress may produce profound changes in beliefs, attitudes, values, and ideological systems.

In the treatment of PTSD states, the practitioner should be alert to such cues as cynical comments and overt, occasionally dramatic outbursts of rage at the circumstances or persons that led to the client's victimization. Fantasies of "retaliation," "payback," "revenge," "reparation," "evening the score," and "balancing the scales of justice" are normal PTSD processes for clients who are attempting to understand how or why their particular experiences occured (Horowitz, 1986). Moreover, when traumatic events violate that which is held to be sacrosanct, inviolable, anchored in unshakable religious beliefs, nonchallengeable ideological values, etc., the magnitude of cognitive disequilibrium and accompanying emotional distress will be greater and have farther-reaching consequences for coping, adaptation, and recovery.

As Viktor Frankl (1959) so poignantly expressed it, humankind's search for meaning is part of its spirit essence and survivorship. Trauma survivors instinctively understand that the search for meaning is not an elective existential choice. Rather, as Robert J. Lifton (1993) noted, it is a protean task in which the cards of fate were dealt by God.

The PTSD Landscape: Boundaries Make for Good Relations

Clinical wisdom dictates that in the treatment of PTSD it is imperative that clients understand that no matter what the cause of their injury (e.g., natural or technological disaster, child abuse, war trauma, domestic violence, torture, rape) there are posttraumatic consequences in the maintenance of healthy ego boundaries.

Practitioners working with trauma clients, may observe a wide range of difficulties in the clients' capacity for effective boundary management in interpersonal relations. At one extreme, such boundaries may be nonfunctional, weak, insufficient, "thin," and readily permeable, often resulting in trauma victims being trammeled by others who exploit their inability to erect reasonable and proper barriers against intrusions into their lives and fragile ego states. At the other extreme are trauma clients with fortified, rigid, "reinforced concrete," nonpermeable boundaries that shut out anyone and anything that might potentially threaten their vulnerable inner psychic core. Such persons typically overuse ego defenses of denial, repression, disavowal, and avoidance behaviors.

Obviously, in terms of the PTSD landscape, there are qualitative and quantitative differences in how PTSD clients protect themselves. Ego vulnerability has extremes which are functionally equivalent to the degree to which ego defenses are used to contain states of emotional distress. Clients who lack the capacity for adequate boundary maintenance are malleable and prone to engage in self-ingratiating, subservient, masochistic, obsequious, conforming and nonassertive behavior. Such ego-defensive, safety-oriented adaptive strategies seek to minimize anxiety associated with personal vulnerability caused by traumatic injury. Whether they are overdefended by "Great Walls of China" or underdefended by permeable and tattered "fishnets," it is important to help clients learn how to manage their personal boundaries during the course of treatment.

Self-Care, Meditation, Exercise, Diet, and Health Monitoring as Basic Maintenance in the Recovery Process

Recovery from trauma does not occur in a vacuum. There are many therapeutic foundations which underpin the recovery process from PTSD. Stated simply, none are more important than self-care which serves to bolster the psychological movement toward allostatic homeostasis, that is, the return to healthy, optimal levels of organismic functioning.

The process of recovery from PTSD requires the ability of the client to access multiple modes of physical exercise that have antianxiety effects associated with PTSD. It is known that psychological well-being increases with regular physical exercise, no matter what the psychiatric disorder or stress-related condition. The practitioner should encourage regular cardiovascular exercise and other forms of somatic focus (e.g., Tai Chi, yoga, meditation, walking) that have a wide range of palliative, health promotive, or healing effects on psychiatric trauma.

Triggers or Trauma-Specific Cues (TSCs) for PTSD Symptom Intensification

A wide range of stressors can occur in traumatic events. The stressors (stimuli, actions, events, interpersonal dynamics, etc.) have specific physical and psychological properties (e.g., particular sights, sounds, smells, or weather conditions; certian voices or movements or times of the year) with the potential to evoke trauma-specific symptoms or generalized emotional states of anxiety, depression, or anger. In the course of treatment, it is important to identify and inventory the specific triggers (situations, anniversaries, and the like) that have the power to activate, aggravate, or intensify existing PTSD symptom clusters as well as reactivate (i.e., rekindle) latent PTSD phenomena leading to an episode of behavioral reenactment or reexperiencing of traumatic events. Such triggering events are most often trauma specific in nature; a stimulus cue may well lead to an association with a distressing element of the traumatic experience. Trauma specific cues (TSCs) may activate either declarative or nondeclarative memory. The client may experience different levels of conscious awareness (LCA) generated by the trauma-specific informational cue. On the one end, TSCs may lead to emotionally overwhelming memories of the precipitating trauma. At the other end, TSC may evoke unconscious mechanisms, including flashbacks (Blank, 1985), and create less discernible forms of reenactment behaviors. The unconscious expression of PTSD invariably has an underlying structure to it which can be identified through careful linkage to the history of the traumatic experience. Moreover, conscious and unconscious forms of reliving traumatic experiences triggered by TSCs may lead to the overuse of maladaptive defensive and coping behaviors, such as excessive drinking, anger, withdrawal, geographic isolation, escape activities, overwork, or loss of adequate ego boundaries. It is important that the clinician help the client understand the nature of TSCs and their relationship to PTSD symptoms, patterns of defense, coping behaviors, and the disposition to experience states of vulnerability associated with the disorder.

Anger and Depression Management

It is a truism that many survivors of trauma feel angry at the circumstances that led to their victimization. Outbursts of irritability, anger, and external-ized hostility are also a component of the psychobiology of PTSD. Anger states are indications of allostatic functioning and are part of hyperarousal which reflects altered thresholds of functioning. Anger management is im-portant in the treatment of PTSD. It is useful if the client can identify specif-ic triggers for anger responses and link them to cognitive appraisal that oc-curred during the traumatic event (i.e., peritraumatic emotional states) and the cognitive expectancies, beliefs, and assumptions that developed after the event.

In a similar way, depressive responses are also part of posttraumatic phenomenology. Depressed moods, feelings of helplessness, hopelessness, de-jection, despair, ennui, desolation, psychological surrender, and thoughts of suicide all fall along this continuum. Depressive mood states reflect the psy-chobiology of trauma and may require medical treatment (Friedman, 2000) to alleviate the primary symptoms of depression (e.g., sleep disturbance, sui-cidality, loss of concentration and attention, weight fluctuations, loss of ener-gy and motivation). Depressive mood states are also manifestations of ego vulnerability and feelings of inadequacy in trying to defend against perceived threats or to meet the everyday demands of life. In PTSD-related depression, survivor guilt or having a sense of a failed enactment (i.e., the failure to act effectively during the trauma) is associated with self-recrimination, shame, and guilt.

The presence of depressive symptoms must be managed during the treatment process. In severe cases of PTSD and major depressive disorder, clients may be at risk for attempted suicide, especially if prior efforts at treat-ment and recovery have failed and they perceive that there is no escaping their current fate of living in a "black hole" of trauma-related misery. When clients feel "trapped in the trauma," they are especially vulnerable to ineffec-tive coping efforts which include alcohol and drug abuse and other high-risk-taking behaviors (e.g., action addiction, adrenalized sensation and thrill seek-ing, impulsive gambling or spending, and sexual acting-out).

The core therapeutic approaches recognize that anxiety, anger, and de-pression are interrelated processes in PTSD that require clinical intervention and management. Anger and depression in PTSD have TSCs that can trig-ger intense affective states which become manifest in cognition, motivation, and orientation to self and others.

Alcohol and Drug Dependence in PTSD

The comorbidity of alcohol and drug abuse/dependency varies among trau-ma populations (Breslau, 1999). Nevertheless, alcohol and drug use is often a common form of self-medication for the distressing emotions which are part of the disorder. Alcohol abuse/dependence is more common that other substance dependence in PTSD, primarily because it is legal, readily available, and relatively inexpensive.

Alcohol and drug use as self-medication in PTSD is an attempt to reduce hyperarousal states or, in cases of PTSD/major depression, to enhance feelings of well-being and alleviate depressive moods. If the clients' use of chemical substances is severely impairing, they may require a period of detoxification prior to PTSD treatment. However, it should be noted that chronic PTSD which involves frequent alcohol use presents a complex clinical picture. It may not be advisable to remove the "crutch" of self-medication until other supportive resources are in place to facilitate the transition from dependence on the substance to withdrawal and nonuse. In some cases, it may be imperative to tailor a treatment program so that the chemical dependence and PTSD are treated simultaneously through a dual-diagnosis approach. In severe, chronic, and complex forms of PTSD, self-medication with alcohol and drugs may be a form of numbing to control anxiety and suppressed fears associated with states of vulnerability. Thus, the achievement of detoxification may intensify states of vulnerability and produce a significant increase in traumatic memories, flashbacks, hyperarousal, anxiety, hypervigilance, and proneness to defensive avoidance. It is important to explain to the patient the dynamics of PTSD and alcohol/drug abuse and commonly experienced effects of detoxification during the treatment process. Stated metaphorically, a sedated lion will sleep in his cage and growl when in bad moods whereas a nonsedated lion will pace around the cage and seek freedom to roam; if frightened, threatened, or provoked, it is likely to attack.

As part of the psychoeducational process concerning PTSD and substance abuse, it is helpful to explain the psychobiology of addiction to the client. First, chronic substance abuse/dependence results in changes in the neurotransmitter functions in the brain, especially in opioid receptor sites. Increased tolerance for alcohol/drugs is associated with addiction cycles of intoxication and withdrawal since larger doses of substances are required to achieve a pleasurable "high" from the substance. Second, chronic stress will alter neurotransmitter functions and influence a person's capacity to tolerate alcohol or drugs (Blum, 1991). Similarly, chronic use of alcohol or drugs will adversely influence serotonergic and dopaminergic neurotransmitter functions, leading to depletions in receptor functions, thus influencing cognition, mood, anxiety, depression, and capacity for pleasure (Fromme & D'Amico, 1999).

Chronic alcohol use and withdrawal effects associated with abuse/dependence effect neurochemical functioning in the following ways: dopamine (DA), decrease associated with craving, feelings of vulnerability, and dysphoria; norepinephrine (NE), decrease associated with cognitive deficits (e.g., memory, depression, detachment); serotonin, or 5-hydroxytryptamine (5-HT), decrease associated with depression and cognitive processing defects; opioid peptides, decrease associated with depression, anxiety, and anhedonia; and γ-aminobutyric acid (GABA), decrease associated with anxiety and agitation. Chronic alcohol abuse/dependence creates an addictive trap because prolonged use and increased tolerance damages reward centers in the brain, reducing the biological capacity for coping with the allostatic effects of PTSD. Further, as Blum (1991) notes, even in persons with nonalcoholic genetics, chronic stress can cause a deficiency of internal opioids leading to stress-related alcoholism. Thus, clients with chronic PTSD are doubly at risk for problems of substance abuse due to (1) the effects of chronic hyperarousal states (i.e., the allostatic chronic stress-related processes) and (2) the effects of wear and tear of substance abuse on central nervous functioning, which likewise alters opioid and other receptor sites in the brain. Treatment of a PTSD client with a dual diagnosis of substance abuse/dependence thus requires care for the whole person which establishes clear objectives for a successful outcome.

Sleep Disturbance, Nightmares, and Physiological Hyperarousal

Sleep disturbance is almost universal in PTSD case histories. Disruptions can occur at the beginning, middle, or terminal phases of the sleep cycle. Clients who report difficulties going to sleep may self-medicate with alcohol/drugs to reduce arousal and facilitate relaxation. Nightmares of trauma typically disrupt the middle of the sleep cycle (e.g., 2:00–3:00 A.M.) and may or may not be accompanied by sweating. Some clients are aware of their trauma-related dream content, whereas others do not recall their anxiety dreams or trauma-related nightmares. Significant others who sleep with their partners are often reliable sources of information regarding the frequency of nightmares, vocalizations, sleep agitation, bodily movements, sweating, and somnambulism. It is informative to inquire as to what happens after the client awakens from a nightmare. The context of what PTSD patients are dreaming reflects unmetabolized aspects of traumatic memory. Many report that it is difficult to return to sleep and therefore find activities to occupy their attention, including alcohol/drug use.

Sleep disturbances in PTSD tend to cause physical and psychological fatigue, malaise, and loss of motivation for work, sexual relations, sports, and social activities. The recall of traumatic material from the nightmare state may trigger cascades of distressing intrusive recollections of the traumatic event, which in turn may give rise to ego-defense processes (see Lindy & Wilson, Chapter 5, this volume). If sleep disturbances persist, consideration should be given to sleep medication or the use of relaxation techniques to facilitate healthy sleep patterns.

Dissociation, Psychic Numbing, Emotional Anesthesia, Denial/Disavowal, and Splitting Are Common Ego-Defensive Processes in PTSD

There are many forms of individual subjective responses to trauma during the experience (i.e., peritraumatic) or after the event (i.e., posttraumatic). In terms of cognitive processes, Wilson (1989) classified five categories of individual subjective response to trauma: (1) denial, disavowal, and/or avoidance; (2) perceptual and cognitive disturbances; (3) dissociation; (4) intrusive processes associated with traumatic memories; and (5) accurate appraisal and information processing. The treatment approaches for PTSD recognize that there are different forms of peridissociative and dissociative mechanisms (Marmar & Weiss, 1997). Similarly, there are degrees of psychic numbing which range from maladaptive to highly adaptive and functional (Lifton, 1979). Various ego-protective mechanisms in PTSD include forms of disavowal, denial, splitting, and emotional anesthesia (or loss of capacity to identify feelings, i.e., alexithymia). In functional terms, dissociation, numbing, splitting, etc. are all mental processes in the service of coping with threat appraisal, information overload, and incongruities in self-esteem, identity, and values.

Self-Recrimination, Survivor Guilt, Shame, and Victim Thinking

The terms "guilt" or "survivor guilt" do not appear in the formal diagnostic criteria in the DSM-IV. It is assumed that if a person is experiencing survivor guilt in one form or another (e.g., a failed enactment), he or she is reliving an aspect of the trauma which is a form of "persistently re-experiencing the traumatic event" (American Psychiatric Association, 1994, p. 428).

Self-recrimination is commonly associated with shame, guilt, and tendencies toward self-punishment and self-destructive behaviors. In some rarer cases, such as that depicted in the novel and movie *Sophie's Choice* (Styron, 1979), self-recrimination leads to self-destructiveness and suicide through drugs, alcohol, or masochistic relationships. Similarly, self-recrimination and shame are interrelated processes. Posttraumatic shame is a state of vulnerability combined with attributions that one deserves a bad fate, ill treatment, punishment, humiliation, or degradation because one has "caused it to happen" and therefore deserves the adverse consequences. Clearly, such attributions are usually irrational and distort the causal circumstances of the client's role in a traumatic event. Furthermore, self-recrimination, shame, self-blame, and survivor guilt are inextricably linked to "victim thinking," which permeates decision making and activities in all areas of psychosocial functioning. In victim thinking, the client maintains ego states and sets of beliefs about the outcome of events which parallel and reflect that which occurred at the time of interpersonal abuse or traumatization. At an uncon-scious level, victim thinking sets up self-fulfilling prophecies and outcomes which serve to confirm the client's negative self-image, self-recrimination, guilt, and sense of unworthiness as a person. In some cases, victim thinking may perpetuate episodic cycles of PTSD and be associated with secondary gain phenomena.

Traumatic Events and Their Impact on Life-Stage Development

Traumatic events can occur anywhere in the life cycle between birth and death. Any stage of human development can be impacted by trauma: infan-cy, childhood, adolescence, and middle and later adulthood years. No one is immune from a traumatic life experience. As Lifton (1979) noted, humans have an inborn propensity for having an "illusion of invulnerability." Trau-matic events shatter such illusions and make the sense of human frailty and mortality all too salient.

Trauma produces differential impacts and consequences to the stages of epigenetic development (Pynoos & Nader, 1993; Wilson, 1980; Erikson, 1968). Traumatic events may cause fixations, regressions, and accelerated de-velopment, depending on the type of event, age, and biological/genetic dis-position of the person. Trauma will also impact the predominate state of ego identity, which is the "central processing" unit of the self-structure. Traumat-ic injury to ego identity, especially in the formative years, may result in deep psychological injuries associated with dissociation, ego fragmentation, and narcissistic wounds to the self.

The Processing, Integration, and Transformation of Trauma

The core treatment approaches for PTSD share the common objective of healing states of traumatization. As noted in Table 3.1, each of the 11 treat-ment approaches has as its goal descriptive words such as "normalize," "re-store," "reestablish," "integrate," and "foster recovery." These treatment goals indicate that the resolution of PTSD requires transformation of the ego-alien, self-incongruent, distressing components of the traumatic experi-ence into a different cognitive schema.

Transformation of PTSD may be a lifelong task, despite successful reso-lution and healthy adaptation after the trauma. We have found that histori-cally profound traumatic events (e.g., Hiroshima and Nagasaki; other major happenings in World War II such as the Pearl Harbor attack, D. Day, and the Holocaust; or the Vietnam War) leave a psychic legacy that undergoes a transformative set of revisions. The reflective appraisal processes and views of the traumatic event may be recast, revisited, and reprocessed in different ways as the aging process unfolds throughout the life cycle (Wilson, 1989; Harel, Kahana, & Wilson, 1993; Wilson, Harel, & Kahana, 1989). Furthermore, various triggers, TSCs, societal events, personal life transitions, and the aging process itself may rekindle new episodes of PTSD as well as nonpathological reflections on the traumatic experience. Thus, the transformation of trauma is a lifelong process in which the ego identity of the survivor turns and twists the kaleidoscope of memory.

Recovery from PTSD Occurs in Client-Directed Dose Rates

PTSD is an episodic disorder which waxes and wanes in the frequency, severity, and intensity of symptom manifestation. Recovery from PTSD goes through early, middle, and later phases reflecting degrees of integration of the traumatic experience. The nature of the intrusion and avoidance/numbing cycles in PTSD are variable in their ratio to each other and impact the rate of processing and integration of the traumatic experience. There is a range of capacity for the client's ability to tolerate treatment. The pattern of processing and integrating traumatic memory may take place in client-directed dose rates rather than in continuous or time-limited therapy.

Medical Treatments for PTSD Require Clinical Trials

Medical treatments for PTSD should be tailored to the psychobiology of the patient's symptom presentation (see Friedman, Chapter 4, this volume). Clinical trials may be necessary to evaluate the effects of medications on PTSD symptoms and to determine which medications are most useful for the patient (e.g., antiadrenergic agents, selective serotonin reuptake inhibitors [SSRIs], trycyclic antidepressants [TCAs], monoamine oxidase inhibitors [MAOIs], or antianxiety agents). In posttraumatic therapy, it is imperative that the therapist work closely with the primary care physician to monitor the efficacy of medical treatment, especially if the patient has a history of alcohol or drug abuse/dependency.

Limits of Group Psychotherapy for PTSD

Group psychotherapy is often a useful form of treatment for PTSD. As discussed by Wilson, Friedman, and Lindy in Chapter 16, this volume, the benefits of group treatment include the following: (1) reinforcement of survivor identity and validation of the traumatic experience; (2) appropriate and contained self-disclosure of trauma-related information; (3) acceptance and social support for recovery; (4) learning by the client of effective ways to cope with PTSD from other survivors; (5) shared information about the progression and dynamics of the disorder; and (6) mechanisms of support which counter tendencies toward isolation, detachment, withdrawal, and relapse. Group therapy is not for all PTSD clients however and careful screening to assess personality, psychopathology, PTSD, the type of trauma exposure, and fitness for the group is critical to avoid problems associated with faulty group processes which impede recovery and healing.

Traumatic Bereavement and PTSD

Traumatic bereavement often results in complex forms of prolonged stress response syndromes that contain features of bereavement (e.g., loss, mourning, yearning, and increased arousal) and PTSD (e.g., intrusion, avoidance/denial, and hyperarousal). The treatment of traumatic bereavement requires decision making as to which objectives are of primary concern. In some cases, immediate demands posed by the loss of a partner or other loved ones will require bereavement counseling prior to posttraumatic therapy for PTSD. On the other hand, the nature of traumatic bereavement may be of such intensity and immediacy in terms of PTSD processes (i.e., especially distressing traumatic memories in which the death and the stressors associated with the events are vividly reexperienced) that they take priority in treatment (Raphael & Martinek, 1997).

PTSD and Comorbidity with Other Axis I and Axis II Diagnoses

The issue of comorbidity with PTSD is a complex one (see Chapter 10, this volume, by McFarlane). The clinician treating PTSD must determine treatment strategies based on accurate psychological assessment and diagnosis. Several considerations are central to the formulation of a treatment plan. First, is there any psychiatric history prior to the traumatic event that would suggest an Axis I or Axis II disorder? Second, is there any history of drug or alcohol abuse/dependence prior to the traumatic event? Third, are there discernible, observable and independently verifiable changes in personality processes (i.e., traits, styles, characteristics, behaviors) that are present after the trauma but were not present before it occurred? If so, do the changes reflect alterations in ego states and personality functioning caused by the trauma? Fourth, are there posttraumatic adaptations which may be temporary or permanent in nature? Fifth, if there is a preexisting Axis I or Axis II disorder, to what extent does it contribute to the current PTSD symptom manifestation? Theoretically, a pre-PTSD history of psychiatric disorder may or may not influence how the individual processes trauma. However, an active Axis I or Axis II disorder at the time of a trauma will likely affect the PTSD symptom presentation and make the treatment process more complex in focus since multiple disorders may interact with each other (e.g., PTSD + major depression + alcoholism; PTSD + bipolar disorder; PTSD + antisocial personality disorder + cocaine dependence) Clearly, there are many combinations and permeations possible which create a matrix of options in terms of posttraumatic therapy (Wilson, 1989).

Hyperarousal States Reflect Allostatic Changes in PTSD

As noted in Chapter 1, this volume, allostasis refers to the organism's effort to maintain stability through change when stressors tax the normal levels of functioning and adaptation. Traumatic events have the strong potential to dysregulate homeostatic functioning. Traumatic events trigger human stress response and mobilize the sympathetic nervous system with the flight-or-fight response pattern. One component of the flight-or-fight pattern is persistent hyperarousal which, if prolonged, may lead to the general adaptation syndrome (Selye, 1980) and the various forms of allostasis: (1) repeated hits, (2) lack of adaptation, (3) prolonged stress, (4) inadequate system response, and (5) the combined-fusion form. The treatment of PTSD should recognize that there are at least seven distinct allostatic processes which reflect psychobiological alterations associated with hyperarousal mechanisms and their specific relation to PTSD symptom manifestation (see Chapter 1, Table 1.1).

Acute Interventions for Stress Response Syndromes

After a trauma, acute interventions for stress response syndromes include a variety of techniques such as short-term cognitive behavioral treatments, critical incident stress debriefings, supportive counseling, community-based crisis interventions, as well as relief efforts and/or deployment of trauma action teams to major disasters. The goal of all acute interventions is to reestablish the normal (i.e., healthy) stress response sequence and provide adequate social, economic, medical, and psychological resources to aid in the restoration of homeostasis and effective coping (Raphael & Wilson, 2000).

Victimization in Childhood and Adolescence

Early victimization in childhood and adolescence may permanently shape psychosocial development, attachment behaviors, and cognitive expectancies about the self, interpersonal relationships, and the world. Repeated episodes of childhood abuse (i.e., sexual, physical, and emotional) may be associated with how the individual perceives, understands, and experiences what is "normal" in human relationships. Victims of repetitive childhood trauma of an interpersonal nature may have an inverted sense of normality versus abnormality. Specifically, adaptation to abusive, threatening, chaotic, and unpredictable environments may become the "normal" baseline of functioning. As such, the child who grows up in an unstable, abusive environment is likely to have problems in the following areas: (1) attachment behaviors, (2) impulse control, (3) high-risk-taking behaviors, (4) ego and moral development, (5) stimulus seeking, (6) proneness to act out conflicts, (7) beliefs about human nature, and (8) boundary management.

PTSD and Reenactment Behaviors in Children

PTSD symptom presentation will vary in children depending on their age, developmental stage, level of ego and intellectual development, and predominant stage of epigenetic identity formation. Reenactment behaviors in young children who have been traumatized often are expressed in play, fantasies (e.g., revenge, reversal of outcome, or denial), dreams, and symbolic forms of acting-out which parallel what they experienced in the traumatic event (see Nader, Chapter 12, this volume). In preverbal children, reenactment behavior may be expressed in somatic forms which reflect generalized distress, anxiety, or hyperarousal states.

PTSD and Spirituality: Transformation of Trauma May Result in Higher Spirituality

The struggle to overcome the nature and injustice of certain forms of trauma may result in the evolution and development of higher spirituality (Wilson & Moran, 1997). The process of healing and overcoming the pain caused by trauma may result in personal struggles with the meaning of life, justice, the existence of God, and the search for a purpose in living. The resolution of trauma's impact to the self may lead to a deeper understanding in clients sense of a Higher Power and their mission in life. As a result of this process, new character qualities may emerge along with a greater capacity for self-actualization.

Self-Disclosure, Altruism, Prosocial Behavior, and Caring for Others Facilitate the Stress Recovery Process

Clinical and empirical research confirms that prosocial behavior, altruism, and caring for others facilitates recovery from trauma and PTSD (Wilson et al., 1989; Wilson & Raphael, 1993). Similarly, judicious and proper self-disclosure of trauma history is also correlated with healing, resilience, and growth. The capacity to reach out to other trauma survivors enhances feelings of self-efficacy and is associated with psychological processes of acceptance, surrender, and realistic appreciation of how a trauma impacted the self and others with a commonly shared fate.

PTSD and Organismic Functioning

PTSD is a complex psychobiological disorder which affects all levels of organismic functioning in synergistic ways. The core triad of PTSD symptoms impacts ego states which include personality processes, identity, and the self-structure. The principle of holistic dynamic functioning implies that changes in one system will affect changes in the others. In this regard, psychobiological dysregulation, cognitive thought processes, unconscious ego defenses, personality processes, and core ego-identity mechanisms codetermine how PTSD gets transformed through the different approaches to treatment.

In summary, the 30 principles just discussed provide considerations for the treatment of PTSD. Healing and recovery from PTSD is a gradual process of integration within the fabric of the self. The process of treatment may be short or long term and employ different therapeutic strategies and experiences. PTSD is a multidimensional psychobiological process with its own structure and mechanisms. The 30 principles of treatment reflect the need to appreciate that PTSD requires a holistic–dynamic approach to clinical intervention and the creation of opportunities that facilitate organismically based healing.

TREATMENT GOALS FOR TRAUMATIC MEMORY, REEXPERIENCING, AND RELIVING PHENOMENA

Table 3.2 presents 20 specific objectives for the treatment of the ways that persons relive or reexperience traumatic events associated with PTSD.

As a primary treatment goal, the therapies for PTSD seek to reduce the debilitating aspects of reexperiencing phenomena and help the client reframe, reappraise, and understand what occurred so that it becomes integrated in the life story of epigenetic development. In this regard, treatment goals may include identifying cues or triggering mechanisms for flashbacks; repeated episodes of desensitization to threatening and emotionally overwhelming emotions or memories; identifying stimulus precursors to dissociative episodes; graduated retrieval of fragmented, partial, or forgotten memories; identifying perceptual distortions, denial, avoidance, or other cognitive information processing mechanisms that occurred during the trauma (i.e., peritraumatic cognitive encoding) or afterward (Marmar, Weiss, & Metzler, 1997). *Since traumatic memories have the power to elicit strong emotions, the linkage between reexperiencing phenomena, subjective vulnerability, and affective states must be evaluated, explained, and reprocessed in ways that do not amplify or activate allostatic load mechanisms.* What makes the treatment of this cluster so important, as noted by Marmar et al. (1997) is that PTSD can coexist with other Axis I or Axis II mental disorders or problems in living (e.g., depression, substance abuse,

TABLE 3.2. Treatment Goals for PTSD: Traumatic Memory Symptoms

1. To identify trigger mechanisms (trauma specific cues, TSCs) which produce recurring distressing recollections of the traumatic event (i.e., stimuli, situations, perceptions, etc.)

2. To facilitate positive coping and the reduction of hyperarousal by cognitive reappraisal which regulates the intensity of affect associated with threat appraisal and intrusive, distressing recollections of trauma

3. To facilitate learning to integrate traumatic memories within a life-cycle perspective of epigenetic, life-course development

4. To facilitate learning to use information from intrusive traumatic memories, nightmares, dissociative episodes, trauma-based hallucinations and other forms of cognitive disruptions so as to identify patterns of psychobiological dysregulation

5. To facilitate the accurate recall of traumatic stressors and experiences; this includes learning the relevance and significance of amnesia, or gaps in memory and the chronology of experience, in order to reconstruct a relatively complete memory for the traumatic event

6. To facilitate learning ways to reduce unrealistic threat appraisal, hypervigilance, hyperarousal states, and overdriven behavioral activities which are epiphenomenal of traumatic memories

7. To identify patterns of high-risk behaviors that have either a short- or long-term potential as self-destructive actions; such high-risk behaviors reflect unmetabolized traumatic memories which are reenacted (acted-out behaviorally)

8. To encourage self-disclosure of aspects of the trauma story within the context of a good working alliance and a safe, nurturing therapeutic sanctuary to move from allostasis to a normal stress response pattern

9. To facilitate the development of insight and awareness of the relationship between traumatic memory and somatic expressions of PTSD (e.g., fatigue, tension, bowel symptoms, headaches, irritability, restlessness, sleep disturbance)

10. To facilitate awareness and understanding of dissociation (i.e., depersonalization, derealization, dissociative amnesia, dissociative identity disorder, dissociative fugue states, etc.) as a mechanism in PTSD which reflects psychic attempts to ward off perceived threat; this includes learning to identify episodes of unconscious flashbacks, or behavioral reenactments of traumatic episodes

11. To facilitate learning to differentiate the integrated memory of trauma from distressing intrusive recollections triggered by external or internal cues

12. To facilitate the understanding of comorbidity, especially the risks for major depression and alcohol and drug use during the lifetime and their relation to traumatic memories

13. To facilitate the appreciation for negatively viewed behaviors during the traumatic event which are related to survivor guilt and its many forms which are associated with shame, self-recrimination, despair, and suicidal ideation

14. To facilitate the process of reestablishing the normal stress response, life-course development, healthy attachments, relationships, and capacity for intimacy; to achieve a resolution of traumatic memory that leads to a sense of self-efficacy

15. To facilitate normal intrapsychic functioning and to restore a positive self-schema for effective coping with unmetabolized elements of traumatic memories

(continued)

TABLE 3.2. *cont.*

16. To facilitate differentiating pre- and posttraumatic personality functioning and behavioral traits and trauma-influenced personality dimensions and adaptation

17. To facilitate awareness of the need for social reintegration and support for activities of daily living

18. To restore integration of the self and facilitate the transformation of cognitive schema from victim identity to survivor identity with a sense of coherence and continuity in time, space, and culture

19. To foster recovery within an embedded cultural framework which allows for congruence and unity in the self, the integration of traumatic memory, and a sense of the culture in which the trauma occurred

20. To encourage awareness that the nature of traumatic memories will change over the lifetime as part of the aging process

traumatic bereavement, adjustment disorders, psychosis, dissociation, and premorbid medical problems). Nevertheless, the core objective of treating traumatic memories is to assist clients in finding ways to integrate the trauma into their daily living without deleterious, maladaptive, or disruptive consequences. The transformation of trauma is healing and the restoration of vitality—establishing a sense of well-being and a sense that life is worth living. As noted earlier, according to Lifton (1993), reformulation of trauma is a protean task which may occur with or without the restoration of a sense of self-sameness in time, space, and culture. In healing, some survivors experience a restoration of self-sameness and continuity. For other survivors, a void exists between two psychological realities created by the advent of trauma. This discontinuity is typically experienced as the "old self" and its replacement after trauma by a "different self." The incongruities within the self may motivate creativity, drama, or self-destruction.[1]

TREATMENT GOALS FOR THE AVOIDANCE AND NUMBING COMPONENTS OF PTSD

Table 3.3 lists 20 specific treatment goals for clinical work with the avoidance and numbing component of PTSD. These objectives of treatment are discussed in this section.

Traumatic events leave their imprint in memories which are disturbing and often difficult to process cognitively and emotionally. Horowitz (1986) in his seminal contribution to the study of PTSD, developed an elaborate model of the denial/numbing phase of stress response syndromes. Horowitz's work was a synthesis of psychodynamic and psychological insights; experimental psychology, and information processing theory, especial-

TABLE 3.3. Treatment Goals for PTSD: Avoidance, Numbing, Denial, and Maladaptive Coping Symptoms

1. To facilitate the identification of and insight into ego defenses associated with patterns of avoidance, denial, detachment, and emotional constriction

2. To facilitate recall of fragmented, amnestic, repressed, or blocked memories associated with the trauma

3. To treat alcohol and substance abuse as avoidant/numbing behaviors that must be managed concurrently with PTSD

4. To facilitate the reduction of anxiety and fear responses associated with traumatic memory

5. To identify patterns of interpersonal disengagement, withdrawal, isolation, alienation, and estrangement

6. To facilitate a reduction of psychic numbing and emotional constriction by pharmacological and therapeutic techniques

7. To facilitate understanding of how avoidance patterns were learned in response to fear, anxiety, vulnerability, extreme emotional distress, and helplessness

8. To facilitate cognitive reappraisal of irrational or faulty beliefs associated with avoidance behaviors

9. To facilitate the capacity to respond competently to perceived threat with accurate appraisal rather than irrational fear, denial, minimization, or avoidance behaviors

10. To facilitate the capacity to tolerate painful affects associated with distressing traumatic memories

11. To identify areas of previously enjoyed significant activities that have been given up or disengaged; to facilitate the resumption of self-directed activities that are gratifying and enhance a sense of affective motivation

12. To facilitate fear and anxiety reduction associated with active or passive avoidance of thoughts, feelings, conversations, activities, places, or people associated with recall of the trauma

13. To facilitate cognitive behavioral modification of irrational beliefs, including a sense of an ominous foreshortened future as part of maladaptive avoidance responses

14. To identify patterns of work and daily living in which there is a compulsive (i.e., driven) overactivity to block attention and awareness of intrusive recollections of the trauma

15. To identify cognitive patterns which reflect disavowal or denial of stimuli with trauma-specific significance for behavior

16. To identify counterphobic behaviors which reflect unconscious unmetabolized aspects of traumatic memory and affect

17. To identify preferences for solitary activities in work, shopping, recreation, or other pursuits which are learned avoidance patterns to minimize social contact and enhance a false sense of personal control

18. To facilitate understanding and insight into desexualized behaviors following trauma; to identify loss of sex drive and capacity for intimacy, reflecting states of vulnerability and fear of loss

19. To facilitate insight and understanding between defenses against affect related to PTSD and somatic expressions of internal conflict (e.g., headaches, bowel symptoms, hypertension, fatigue, muscle tension)

20. To facilitate a reduction in obsessive thinking, brooding, and other forms of rigid thought as inhibitory controls to ward off the contents of traumatic memory

ly the research of Richard S. Lazarus (1966), George Klein (1967), and Irv-ing L. Janis (1969). In his theoretical model, Horowitz (1986) notes that trau-matic events involve incongruities between existing cognitive schemas and the sequence of events in a trauma. When such incongruities exist, a drive to-ward cognitive completion occurs (i.e., a mechanism is created to assimilate the information encoded during the traumatic event into the existing cogni-tive framework). To quote Horowitz:

> The simple model leads to oscillatory states of high and low anxiety, high and low degrees of representation, and continuation and cessation of cog-nitive processing. The oscillation continues because of the intrinsic tenden-cy of active memory towards repeated representation until the point of completion. Only startle controls or absent controls would lead to a steady state[,] a situation seldom encountered in human psychology. . . . [W]ith relative completion of cognitive processing the cycle terminates because the relevant contents are cleared from active memory storage. The new in-formation has now been integrated with internal sources of information, that is, with inactive memory. Put another way, schemata have been re-vised so that they are now congruent with new information about the self and world. (1986, p. 96)

Horowitz's (1986) theoretical model is congruent with the concept of al-lostasis as part of the stress response process in PTSD. Allostatic stress in-cludes cognitive overload or insufficiencies in the mechanisms to process the impact of the trauma. Indeed, in Freud's original model of neurosis (i.e., his 1895 seduction theory), repression and denial were considered to be the core ego-defense mechanisms by which a person avoids the anxiety produced by a trauma, leading to neurotic symptoms (Wilson, 1994). From the perspective of the stress response, or what the DSM-IV refers to as "persistent avoidance of stimuli associated with the trauma and numbing of general responsiveness (not present before the trauma" (American Psychiatric Society, 1994; p. 428), such symptoms are variations in styles of coping with trauma.

The DSM-IV C criteria for PTSD detail several symptom groups which involve avoidance and numbing behaviors of various types, including loss of recall of aspects of the trauma, changes in interpersonal relations, and changes in emotional expressiveness and views of the future. In Chapter 2, we presented an expanded list (see Table 2.2) of 13 avoidance, numbing, de-tachment, and other such coping mechanisms.

In terms of allostatic processes, these treatment goals include the devel-opment of insight as to the functions of avoidance mechanisms as an attempt to reduce allostatic load. The treatment goals also include the facilitation and processing of fragmented, amnestic, or repressed memories. Moreover, since coping often involves active and passive forms of avoidance and problems in interpersonal relationships, treatment attempts to restore self-esteem and the capacity to actively process the painful and unbidden intrusive recollections of the trauma. Where substance dependence or abuse is a form of self-medication in PTSD and allostatic dysregulation (Friedman, 2000), multimodal approaches may be required in which treatment of the chemical dependence is part of the overall plan.

The cyclical or episodic nature of PTSD has been recognized by practitioners and researchers alike (Horowitz, 1986; Friedman, 2000; Marmar et al., 1993). The avoidance and numbing cluster of PTSD symptoms reflects the tendency toward completion noted by Horowitz (1986), who states:

> If fear or anxiety are likely to increase beyond limits of toleration, controls are activated which will modify the cognitive processes. For example, the path from active memory storage to representation and cognitive processing can be inhibited. This reduction in cognitive processing reduces anxiety and, in turn, reduces motivation for control operations. With the reduction in control, the tendency of active memory towards representation reasserts itself. . . . [C]ognitive processing of the stress-related information resumes, anxiety increases, control increases, and the cycle continues. (pp. 94–95)

Thus, from the perspective of allostatic processes, the DSM-IV C criteria for avoidance and numbing of "general responsiveness" can be viewed as attempts to offset the psychobiological nature of PTSD as a stress response syndrome. *As coping behaviors, all of the symptom variations in the C cluster of the PTSD triad are reactive mechanisms of trauma's impact on the person, altering his or her psychobiological baseline of adaptive functioning.* Whereas among the treatment goals for the reexperiencing cluster of PTSD are attempts to identify techniques that can assist in the cognitive processing of the trauma in an integrative manner congruent with self-schemas and life-course development, the treatment of the avoidance and numbing cluster is primarily that of finding ways to strengthen positive coping which attempts to reduce allostatic load by restoring the normalization of functioning and the elimination of ineffective coping that perpetuates the cycle described by Horowitz. In this way, it becomes possible to target the specific avoidance and numbing symptoms to reduce those behaviors that perpetuate the episodic cycle between reexperiencing phenomena and avoidance, denial, numbing, and ineffective coping processes.

TREATMENT GOALS FOR PSYCHOBIOLOGICAL ALTERATIONS IN PTSD

Table 3.4 presents 15 specific treatment objectives for the psychobiological components of PTSD and associated disorders.

The core treatments for PTSD recognize that trauma has the potential to alter neural, hormonal, and immune systems within the body (DeBellis et al., 1999; Friedman, 2000; van der Kolk & Sapporta, 1993). In Chapter 2,

TABLE 3.4. Treatment Goals for PTSD: Psychobiological Symptoms

1. To identify trigger mechanisms for hypervigilance and exaggerated startle response

2. To identify areas of psychobiological sensitivity to TSCs

3. To identify and understand factors that are associated with hyperreactivity and dysregulated emotional states

4. To identify and understand somatic symptoms as part of PTSD dynamics

5. To identify and inventory types of impulsive and/or high-risk behaviors that have a potential for self-destructive consequences (e.g., high sensation seeking; action-addict syndromes)

6. To facilitate positive self-care and lifestyle activities (i.e., exercise, diet, stress management, absence of drug and alcohol use) to effectively manage allostatic dysregulations

7. To facilitate the management of anger, rage, and impulsive and explosive behaviors as manifestations of hyperarousal phenomena

8. To facilitate education about PTSD and its psychobiological manifestations (e.g., sleep disturbance, hypervigilance, problems of concentration, exaggerated startle response, irritability, outbursts of anger)

9. To identify areas of vulnerability to TSCs which trigger hyperarousal states and ego-defensive behavior

10. To facilitate normalization toward homeostatic functioning

11. To identify and understand somatic expressions of chronic hyperarousal (e.g., fatigue, malaise, dysphoria, physical complaints, depressive states, loss of initiative, tension states, irritability, loss of concentration, and attention)

12. To facilitate the use of medications that treat psychobiological symptoms which cause maladaptive behaviors and impair psychosocial functioning (i.e., SSRIs, TCAs, MAOIs, propranolol, antianxiety agents)

13. To facilitate proper concurrent treatment for patients with PTSD and alcohol/drug abuse

14. To facilitate and design a treatment plan for patients with PTSD and comorbidity with another Axis I or Axis II diagnosis, including severe mental illness

15. To facilitate, coordinate, and monitor medical care for PTSD-related problems of hypertension, thyroid dysfunctioning, and drug interaction effects, including those with alcohol and substance abuse

---

Tables 2.2 and 2.3 summarize the psychobiological changes associated with PTSD. More specifically, the primary psychobiological changes present in PTSD include the following: (1) sleep cycle disturbances; (2) the spectrum of hyperarousal phenomena ranging from startle responses to hypervigilance to homeostatic dysregulation; (3) sensory and perceptual sensitivity to TSCs; and (4) cognitive processing deficits such as problems of concentration, encoding difficulties in information processing, and attentional shifts. The core treatment goals include reestablishing the normal stress response pattern. From the point of view of allostatic load, this refers to reestablishing "switch-off" mechanisms so that prolonged states of hyperarousal and stress response do not continue to operate when it is not necessary to deal with current life stressors. As many clinicians have noted (e.g., Ochberg, 1988; Matsakis, 1994; Marmar et al., 1997), it is often useful to educate patients about PTSD symptoms as being the normal response to abnormal events which includes hyperarousal mechanisms as part of the syndrome dynamics.

A wide range of therapeutic techniques may be necessary to help the client understand how hyperarousal states are manifest (e.g., sleep disturbance, hypervigilance, frenetic activities, compulsive overwork at the job or overexertion in leisure activities, high-risk behaviors, sensation seeking, selfmedication with alcohol or drugs, emotional depletion [fatigue, depressed states, dysphoria], and/or preference for solitary activities). Clearly, the techniques to treat these symptoms can be targeted and tailored to the individual and may include the following: (1) medications (e.g., antidepressants, antiadrenergic agents, anticonvulsants); (2) meditation; (3) relaxation and deconditioning techniques of various types; (4) exercise; and (5) the creation of social support mechanisms.

In Chapter 2, Table 2.3 details 13 specific symptoms of psychobiological alteration in PTSD as an allostatic load phenomenon. As will be discussed in the chapters that follow, these 13 symptoms can be thought of as potential target objectives of the core treatment approaches. Nevertheless, while research has demonstrated changes in brain function (DeBellis et al., 1999) and the potential for neurotoxicity associated with allostasis as a prolonged stress response, it is not known at present to what extent clinical interventions can reverse or attenuate the cascade of psychobiological changes described by McEwen (1998). A holistic–dynamic approach to organismic healing assumes that synergistic interactions can promote health and the restoration of vitality. In this regard, future research should be designed to measure such synergistic effects of positive therapeutic treatments.

TREATMENT GOALS FOR TRAUMATIC INJURY TO SELF-CONCEPT, EGO STATES, PERSONAL IDENTITY, AND SELF-STRUCTURE

Table 3.5 lists 15 specific treatment goals that address traumatic impact on ego states, the self-structure, and the configuration of personal identity.

It is important to note here that the treatment approaches for PTSD recognize that traumatic events can produce profound alterations to personality, psychoformative processes (Lifton, 1976, 1979), ego-adaptive capacities, personal identity, and the perspective of the future self (Watkins & Watkins, 1997). Such alterations in ego processes are referred to as narcissistic injuries to the self.

In Chapter 2, Table 2.5 presents 13 symptom clusters reflecting what has become known as "complex PTSD," a term which simply expands the

TABLE 3.5. Treatment Goals for PTSD: Self-Structure, Ego States, and Personal Identity

1. To empower self-esteem, trauma mastery, and the capacity to overcome and integrate the traumatic experience into a self-reference schema

2. To facilitate integration of the self (i.e., dissociated, fragmented, or diffuse ego identity and components of the self)

3. To facilitate the development of a positive self-schema of effective coping; to achieve effective motivation in social and career endeavors

4. To facilitate normal intrapsychic functioning with a minimum of maladaptive ego defenses for traumatic memory and allostatic processes

5. To facilitate the assimilation of the traumatic experience into cognitive schemas in ways that contravene ego-alien dimensions of the stressful life event

6. To restore a sense of self-sameness and continuity in ego functioning, despite potential changes in life-course development, career goals, and other aspirations

7. To facilitate a reduction of shame, doubt, guilt, self-recrimination, and self-destructive behaviors

8. To facilitate awareness of triggering mechanisms for dissociative episodes, alterations in awareness, and disruptions in cognitive information processing

9. To facilitate positive coping that counteracts hopelessness, helplessness, and negative emotional states as personality states or traits

10. To identify and intervene to minimize suicidal ideation, self-inflicted injuries, or other patterns of self-destructiveness

11. To facilitate the personal growth of spirituality and the creation of meaning which overcomes the pain produced by trauma

12. To identify angst, dread, existential despair and loss of selfhood caused by the trauma and facilitate cognitive behavioral reappraisals to restore self-activation

13. To facilitate the restoration of ego coherency and the healing of narcissistic injury to the fabric of the self

14. To facilitate a sense of the self as existentially grounded, centered, and capable of creating a meaningful future with vitality, meaning, and purpose

15. To facilitate understanding of pre- and posttrauma changes to ego states, the structure of the inner self, and the sense of personal identity

---

phenomenology of PTSD beyond the DSM-IV diagnostic criteria. Complex PTSD encompasses what is absent conceptually in the differential algorithm in the DSM-IV. Damage to inner-core processes of the individual's sense of self-worth, self-esteem, and coherency in the organization of the self-structure is a part of traumatic injury for many victims. Indeed, one of Lifton's (1976) pioneering contributions to understanding trauma and its impact to the self was his report that the survivors of the atomic bomb at Hiroshima experienced a radical discontinuity in their self-structure, belief systems, and views of time, space, culture, and reality. To the Japanese survivors of the atomic bomb, their sense of self and the world was profoundly altered. The very sense of life and death as a conceptual framework became murky, confused, and without a meaningful reference point.

Research supports the idea that it is psychologically easier to endure a traumatic event which is an "act of God," such as a natural disaster, than those which reflect premeditation and purposeful harm (Wilson & Raphael, 1993). As Table 3.5 illustrates, a psychodynamic perspective views trauma inflicted on the self as potentially the most psychologically lethal. Traumatic injury to core ego processes is clearly an assault to ego functioning and its dynamic relatedness to other components of coping and adaptation inherent to the processing of PTSD (Horowitz, 1986). Acts of interpersonal violence (Goodwin, 1993; Breslau & Davis, 1992) have higher risk for comorbidity, especially depression, substance abuse, and self-destructive behavior. Repeated tears at the fabric of the human tapestry eventually will mar the design, whether it is simple or complex. Thus, trauma victims may lose their capacity to stay internally integrated and coherent. To attempt to maintain some degree of ego mastery and self-coherency, survivors may need to protect their perceived areas of vulnerability. Simpson (1993) has described "soul murder," in which the most basic foundations of humanness are degraded, denigrated, or undermined with a ruthlessness designed to bring about physical and psychological breakdown, abject surrender, false confessions, or other forms of desperate, distraught behavior in order just to survive. The disintegration of a culture is one form of trauma, and the fragmentation of persons through acts of interpersonal violence is yet another. In that regard, PTSD as a core injury to internal ego processes is of a different type than, for example, that which results from enduring an earthquake, a car accident, or an unexpected severe medical illness. When trauma damages the core of an individual's selfhood, the expressions in allostasis are diverse but discernible and allow us to identify the portals of entry into core phenomenology of PTSD for that particular client (see Chapter 2, this volume, Figure 2.2). Damage to core ego processes and the fabric of the self is one of the important portals of entry to PTSD phenomena, especially for psychodynamic approaches to treatment.

The treatments for PTSD recognize the need to restore adaptive functioning and wellness to the highest possible level. At present, we do not have enough data to suggest which of the various treatment modalities (some yet to be developed) can best treat complex PTSD and psychological damage to the self-structure (see Lindy & Wilson, Chapter 5, this volume). As far as we can discern at this time, there are not enough comparative clinical trials with "Gold Standard" criteria to suggest any single or combined approach to treatment and healing of profoundly damaged ego states. It is our view that the treatment of PTSD, especially in cases involving an assault on the ego and self-structure of the person, must address how the event impacted subsequent behavioral adaptations which may range from depression and suicidal ideation to complex forms of achievement, compensatory behaviors, lifestyle patterns, and daily coping behaviors and personality processes.

In examining this issue from a different perspective, the publishing and entertainment industries over the years have produced books, films, and plays that have attempted to confront the realities of events which are traumatic in nature and produce human suffering. For example, a partial list of such cinematic productions would include *Sophie's Choice, Schindler's List, Platoon, Coming Home, The Pawnbroker, Nuts, Ordinary People, Jacob's Ladder, Full-Metal Jacket, Distant Thunder, Saving Private Ryan, The Prince of Tides, The Color Purple, Beloved, The Best Years of Our Lives, Key Largo, Fearless, The Accused, Au Revoir, Les Enfants,* and *Dead Presidents.* It is not by chance that creative cinematic artists and writers have attempted to capture major traumatic events that changed the world in so many ways. Yet, from a purely psychological perspective, these various attempts by the media only mirror the reality of the impact of trauma on the particular cultures or nations affected by such historical events. In this regard historical events of global dimensions change the psyche of those who survive, and they in turn impact the generations that follow (Danieli, 1998).

The core issues concerning the treatment of PTSD can now be expanded further. As the research of Dalenberg (2000) and Wilson and Lindy (1994) found, delving into the areas of damage to the self-structure of a trauma victim is a source of significant risk to a clinician's empathic ability and the development of countertransference reactions in the treatment of PTSD. However, without the willingness or ability of practitioners to probe trauma-specific transference (TST) in the treatment of PTSD, the clinical capacity to treat the disorder may be not only limited but counterproductive to the well-being of the client.

PTSD AND INTERPERSONAL RELATIONS: TREATMENT GOALS FOR PROBLEMS IN ATTACHMENT, INTIMACY, AND SOCIAL RELATIONS

The power of trauma to alter the fabric of human social attachments is well documented in the scientific literature (Wilson & Raphael, 1993). Robert J. Lifton (1983) used the metaphor of the "broken connection" to characterize the ways in which traumatic events may sever both a personal and interpersonal sense of continuity in life. Traumatic experiences may shatter individual integrity, family cohesiveness, marital intimacy, and one's capacity for attachment, bonding, and integration into groups and organizations. From the perspective of complex PTSD, the treatment goals recognize that it is important to assess how the disorder impacts areas of psychosocial functioning, including the nature of interpersonal relationships. In Chapters 1 and 2, above, Tables 1.2 and 2.4 summarize these effects; Table 2.4 lists 13 PTSD symptoms and associated behaviors that impact various domains of social relations. Here, more specifically, Table 3.6 lists 10 primary treatment goals pertaining to PTSD's impact on interpersonal relationships.

TABLE 3.6. Treatment Goals for PTSD: Attachment, Intimacy, and Interpersonal Relations

1. To facilitate the restoration of healthy attachments, relationships, and capacity for intimacy

2. To reduce detachment, estrangement, alienation, and emotional isolation from others

3. To facilitate and encourage the capacity for healthy self-awareness of the trauma's impact upon interpersonal functioning

4. To facilitate learning to relate to others without undue worry as to personal vulnerability in relationships

5. To facilitate understanding and insight into trauma-related repetitive patterns of relationships which are self-destructive

6. To facilitate establishing and maintaining healthy boundaries in relationships

7. To facilitate cognitive reappraisals which reduce anxiety and fear over abandonment and the loss of loved ones

8. To facilitate self-acceptance and empower self-esteem and a positive schema of the self as effective in social encounters

9. To facilitate learning healthy sensuality, and sexuality unburdened by unbidden memories of prior abuse or trauma

10. To facilitate self-acceptance so as to be capable of receiving nurturance, affection, and physical touching

The impact of trauma on the nature and quality of social relations needs to be placed into epigenetic and ontological perspectives:

First, when does the traumatic experience occur in the life cycle? As Pynoos and Nader (1993) have discussed, trauma may strike at any developmental stage in the life cycle, producing different consequences to organismic functioning ranging from neurological disturbances to impairments in object relations, self-concept, cognitive processing (e.g., use of denial in children), adolescent dispositions to "act-out," and more (see Nader, Chapter 12, this volume, for a discussion). The power of trauma to influence the quality and trajectory of epigenetic or life-span development, while not yet fully understood, cannot be underestimated (Laufer, 1988). For example, in a recent study Bremner et al. (1999) demonstrated neurobiological differences between adult women with a history of sexual abuse from a control sample without such experiences. Among the women with a history of sexual abuse prior to adulthood, positron emission tomography imaging of the brain (PET scans) showed abnormal brain function following exposure to narratives about their sexual trauma. This study thus showed traumatic impact at the biological level of organismic functioning associated with a specific period of psychosocial development. In summary, traumatic stressors may impact any stage of life-course development and generate allostatic processes whose nature may vary considerably depending on the person's age and the nature of prior life experiences in coping with stress, trauma, and abuse (Pynoos & Nader, 1993).

Second, the effects of collectively experienced traumatic events may have impacts on many individuals and families (e.g., the Holocaust, political internment, or a natural disaster such as a major earthquake). The consequent family breakdown and loss of connection to society and culture, viewed as meaningful sources of relatedness (i.e., communal relations), may result in alienation, anomie, isolation, detachment, estrangement, or other maladaptive patterns of behavior, including aggressive–defensive attacks on those perceived as responsible for the loss of connection and meaning (Lifton, 1979; Ochberg, 1988; Horowitz, 1999; Raphael, 1983). In the broadest sense, alienation generated by traumatic events sets up a continuum of responsiveness, with forms of detachment and withdrawal at one end of the spectrum and impulsive, erratic, aggressive, and risk-taking behavioral tendencies at the other end. In psychodynamic terms, this continuum embraces such phenomena as borderline personality disorder, dissociative processes, depressive states, object relations and attachment concerns, interpersonal boundary management, and narcissistic self-injuries, personality processes, and styles of interpersonal behavior (Aronoff & Wilson, 1985; Herman, 1992).

Third, the impact of trauma and the development of PTSD impacts ego functioning, self-structure configuration, the style of personal identity, and cognitive processes.[2] As Tables 1.1 and 1.2 in Chapter 1 illustrate, these are also allostatic processes at the organismic level, reflecting respectively: (1) altered initial response patterns, (2) altered capacity of internal monitoring, (3) altered feedback based on distorted information, and (4) altered continuous response capacity. The clinical treatment protocols recognize the necessity to assess the manner in which trauma has shaped or determined the manner in which PTSD and associated psychological phenomena have influenced the individual's capacity for attachment, intimacy, and interpersonal relationships. The treatment goals include the following: (1) learning to modulate affect which reflects allostatic dysregulation, that is, to a healthier, more adaptive emotional responsiveness to self and others; (2) learning to control, maintain, and monitor boundaries between healthy and potentially disruptive, maladaptive interpersonal relationships; (3) learning to accept, identify, and—to the extent possible—transform areas of personal vulnerability; (4) learning to modulate (i.e., understand allostasis) biological states (e.g., hyperarousal, withdrawal, anhedonia, psychic numbing, anger/rage) and develop positive coping skills that result in a sense of self-efficacy, self-worth and the freedom to choose freely the degree of emotional closeness to others and societal involvement. The transformation of trauma by one of the core treatment approaches increases individual consciousness, autonomy, spiritual awareness, genuine self-directed freedom of choice, and satisfaction with the trajectory of the self within the society and culture or from a larger worldview perspective (i.e., what the existentialists sometimes refer to as the "self-in-the-world").

We can think of PTSD as a rich tapestry woven from thousands of fibers spun from unique lines of discovery by the therapist and the client. The transformation of trauma by one of the core treatment techniques allows the traumatized individual to sit before his or her own loom and weave fabrics of color to create the most exquisite design that imagination, vision, and sense of purpose can create. The treatment and recovery from PTSD are processes of subtle complexities. Transformation, growth, and the reduction of negative allostatic processes in PTSD require a holistic–dynamic, organismic model of such changes. In this chapter, we have presented 80 specific treatment goals for the five interrelated components that reflect allostatic processes in PTSD. In Part IV, Chapter 16 presents a comparative analysis of the 11 treatment approaches presented in Parts II and III of this book.

NOTES

1. See Wilson and Lindy (1994) for a discussion of the difficulties in analyzing, interpreting, and using trauma-specific transference (TST) projections during the course of psychotherapy.
2. Erik Erikson (1968), in discussing the impact of trauma on the ego, made the following comment in reference to World War II veterans: "most of our patients . . . had neither been shell shocked nor become malingerers, but through the exigencies of war lost a sense of personal sameness and historical continuity. . . . I spoke of a loss of ego-identity" (p. 17). He continued: "we may formulate the ego's task (and maybe, the ego) by recognizing it as one of three indispensable and ceaseless processes by which man's existence becomes and remains continuous in form. The first of these . . . is the *biological processes*, by which an organism comes to be a hierarchic organization of organ systems living out its life-cycle. The second is the *social process*, by which organisms come to be organized in groups which are geographically, historically, and culturally defined. What maybe called the *ego-process* is the organizational principle by which the individual maintains himself as a coherent personality with a sameness and continuity both in his self-experience and in his actuality for others" (p. 73; emphases in original).

REFERENCES

American Psychiatric Association (1994). *Diagnostic and statistical manual of mental disorders* (4th ed.). Washington, DC: Author.

Aronoff, J., & Wilson, J. P. (1985). *Personality in the social process*. Hillsdale, NJ: Erlbaum.

Blank, A. S., Jr. (1985). The unconscious flashback to the war in Vietnam Veterans: Clinical mystery, legal defense, and community problem. In S. M. Sonnenberg, A. S. Blank, Jr., & J. A. Talbott (Eds.), *The trauma of war: Stress and recovery in Vietnam veterans*. Washington, DC: American Psychiatric Press.

Blum, K. (1991). *Alcohol and the addictive brain.* New York: Face Press.

Bremner, J. D. (1999). Alterations in brain structure and function associated with posttraumatic stress disorder. *Seminars in Clinical Neuropsychiatry, 4*(4), 249–255.

Breslau, N. (1999). Epidemiology of trauma and PTSD. In R. Yehuda (Ed.), *Psychological trauma* (pp. 9–27). Washington, DC: American Psychiatric Press.

Breslau, N., & Davis, G. C. (1992). Post-traumatic stress disorder in an urban population of young adults: Risk factors for chronicity. *American Journal of Psychiatry, 2,* 671–675.

Carlson, E. (1997). *Trauma assessments.* New York: Guilford Press.

Dalenberg, E. L. (2000). *Countertransference in the treatment of trauma.* Washington, DC.

Danieli, Y. (Ed.). (1998). *International handbook of multigenerational legacies of trauma.* New York: Plenum Press.

DeBellis, J., Baum, A. S., Birnaber, B., Kesharau, M. S., Eckard, C. H., Boring, A., Jenkins, F. J, & Ryan, N. (1999). Developmental traumatology, Part 1: Biological stress symptoms. *Biological Psychiatry, 45,* 1259–1270.

Erikson, E. (1968). *Identity, youth and crisis.* New York: Norton.

Frankl, V. (1959). *From death camp to existent lives.* New York: Beacon Press.

Freud, S., & Brewer, J. (1895). *Studies on hysteria.* New York: Avon Press.

Friedman, M. F. (2000). *Post-traumatic stress disorders.* Kansas City, MO: Compact Clinicals.

Fromme, K., & D'Amico, E. (1999). Neurological bases of alcohol's effects. In K. E. Leonard & H. T. Blane (Eds.), *Psychological theories of drinking and alcoholism* (2nd ed., pp. 232–276). New York: Guilford Press.

Goodwin, J. M. (1993). *Rediscovering childhood trauma.* Washington, DC: American Psychiatric Association.

Harel, Z., Kahana, B., & Wilson, J. (1993). War and remembrance: The legacy of Pearl Harbor. In J. P. Wilson & B. Raphael (Eds.), *International handbook of traumatic stress syndromes* (pp. 263–275). New York: Plenum Press.

Herman, J. (1992). *Trauma and recovery.* New York: Basic Books.

Horowitz, M. (1999). *Essential papers on post-traumatic stress disorder.* New York: New York University Press.

Horowitz, M. (1986). *Stress response syndromes* (2nd. ed.). Northvale, NJ: Aronson.

Janes, I. L. (1969). *Stress and frustration.* New York: Harcourt, Brace, Jovanovich.

Klein, G. (1967). *Peremptory ideation: Structure and force in motivated ideas.* New York: Holt.

Laufer, R. S. (1988). The serial self: War trauma, identity and adult development. In J. P. Wilson, Z. Harel, & B. Kahane (Eds.), *Human adaptation to extreme stress: From the Holocaust to Vietnam* (pp. 33–56). New York: Plenum Press.

Lazarus, R. S. (1966). *Psychological stress and the coping process.* New York: McGraw-Hill.

Lifton, R. J. (1967). *Death in life: The survivors of Hiroshima.* New York: Simon and Schuster.

Lifton, R. J. (1976). *The life of the self.* New York: Simon & Schuster.

Lifton, R. J. (1983). *The broken connection: On death and the continuity of life.* New York: Basic Books.

Lifton, R. J. (1993). From Hiroshima to the Nazi doctors: The evolution of psychoformative approaches to understand traumatic stress syndromes. In J. P. Wilson & B. Raphael (Eds.), *International handbook of traumatic stress syndromes* (pp. 11–25). New York: Plenum Press.

Lindy, J. (1993). Focal psychoanalytical psychotherapy of post-traumatic stress disorder. In J. P. Wilson & B. Raphael (Eds.), *International handbook of traumatic stress syndrome* (pp. 803–811). New York: Plenum Press.

Marmar, C., Weiss, D., & Metzler, T. M. (1997). The Peritraumatic Dissociative Experiences Questionnaire. In J. P. Wilson & T. M. Keane (Eds.), *Assessing psychological trauma and PTSD* (pp. 412–425). New York: Guilford Press.

Matsakis, A. (1994). *Post-traumatic stress disorder.* Oakland, CA: New Harbinger Press.

McEwen, B. S. (1998). Protective and damaging effects of stress mediators. *Seminars in Medicine of the Beth Israel Deaconess Medical Center, 338*(3), 171–179.

Ochberg, F. (1988). *Post-traumatic therapy and victims of violence.* New York: Brunner/Mazel.

Pynoos, R., & Nader, K. (1993). Issues in the treatment of post-traumatic stress in children and adolescents. In J. P. Wilson & B. Raphael (Eds.), *International handbook of traumatic stress syndromes* (pp. 535–551). New York: Plenum Press.

Raphael, B. (1983). *When disaster strikes.* New York: Basic Books.

Raphael, B., & Martinek, T. (1997). Assessing traumatic bereavement and PTSD. In J. P. Wilson & T. M. Keane (Eds.), *Assessing psychological trauma and PTSD* (pp. 373–399). New York: Guilford Press.

Raphael, B., & Wilson, J. P. (2000). *Psychological debriefing: Theory, practice, evidence.* Cambridge, UK: Cambridge University Press.

Selye, H. (1980). The stress concept today. In I. L. Kutash & L. B. Schlesinger (Eds.), *Handbook on stress and anxiety* (pp. 19–31). San Francisco: Jossey-Bass.

Simpson, M. (1993). Traumatic stress and the bruising of the soul: The effects of torture and coercive interrogation. In J. P. Wilson & B. Raphael (Eds.), *International handbook of traumatic stress syndromes* (pp. 659–667). New York: Plenum Press.

Styron, W. (1979). *Sophie's choice.* New York: Random House.

van der Kolk, B., & Sapporta, J. (1993). *Biological response to psychic trauma.* In J. P. Wilson & B. Raphael (Eds.), *International handbook of traumatic stress syndromes* (pp. 25–35). New York: Plenum Press.

Watkins, J. G., & Watkins, H. H. (1997). *Ego states.* New York: Norton.

Weiss, D. (1997). Structural clinical interview techniques. In J. P. Wilson & T. M. Keane (Eds.), *Assessing psychological trauma and PTSD* (pp. 493–512). New York: Guilford Press.

Weiss, D., & Marmar, C. (1997). The Impact of Event Scale, Revised. In J. P. Wilson & T. M. Keane (Eds.), *Assessing psychological trauma and PTSD.* New York: Guilford Press.

Wilson, J. P. (1980). Conflict, stress and growth: The effects of war on psychosocial development among Vietnam veterans. In C. H. Figley & K. S. Levertman (Eds.), *Strangers at home: Vietnam veterans since the war* (pp. 123–165). New York: Preegar.

Wilson, J. P. (1989). *Trauma, transference and healing.* New York: Brunner/Mazel, Inc.

Wilson, J. P., Harel, Z., & Kahana, B. (1988). *Human adaptation to extreme stress.* New York: Plenum Press.

Wilson, J. P., Harel, Z., & Kahana, B. (1989). War and remembrance: The legacy of Pearl Harbor. In J. P. Wilson (Ed.), *Trauma, transformation and healing* (pp. 129–159). New York: Brunner/Mazel.

Wilson, J. P., & Keane, T. M. (Eds.). (1997). *Assessing psychological trauma and PTSD.* New York: Guilford Press.

Wilson, J. P., & Moran, T. (1997). Psychological trauma: PTSD and spirituality. *Journal of Psychology and Theology, 26*(2), 168–178.

Wilson, J. P., & Lindy, J. (1994). *Countertransference in the treatment of PTSD.* New York: Guilford Press.

Wilson, J. P., & Raphael, B. (Eds.). (1993). *International Handbook of Traumatic Stress Syndromes.* New York: Plenum Press.

4

Allostatic versus Empirical Perspectives on Pharmacotherapy for PTSD

MATTHEW J. FRIEDMAN

The concept of allostatic load, as originally proposed (McEwen & Steller, 1993; McEwen, 1998) is a biological model of stability through change. In this book we have expanded that context to include intrapsychic, interpersonal, and social as well as biological domains, because allostasis is such a rich heuristic model through which to seek to understand the many complex biopsychosocial manifestations of posttraumatic stress disorder (PTSD). It is also a useful context in which to consider the specific treatments that have been tested and proposed for ameliorating the symptoms and general distress associated with this disorder. In this chapter, the focus is specifically on the many psychobiological mechanisms that are disrupted in PTSD and on the various medications that have been tested and proposed for reversing such abnormalities.

When considering allostatic load models, it is important to keep in mind that there are a number of ways in which a system can overshoot, undershoot, fail to recover, or become otherwise dysregulated because it is incapable of accurately titrating its adaptive repertoire to environmental demands (McEwen, 1998). Furthermore, even if the organism's overall response capability has remained intact, it may become encumbered by allostatic load because its antennae are not well calibrated to accurately assess the challenge at hand. Here the problem lies with signal detection rather than response potential so that the organism either fails to recognize all the stressors to which it must respond (e.g., false negatives) or it tends to misperceive harmless stimuli as threats to survival (e.g., false positives). In PTSD, it is well recognized that the appraisal process is biased toward perceiving danger rather than safety (e.g., false positives) and hence the response bias is toward over rather than underreaction. Such a hypervigilant, hyperreactive posture for engaging the environment is a prescription for shifting from a homeostatic to an allostatic steady state.

From an allostatic perspective, PTSD is extremely complex. As has been stated elsewhere (Friedman, Charney, & Deutch, 1995, pp. xix–xx), this is because humans who fail to meet the demands of traumatic stressors utilize and perturb the many psychobiological mechanisms that have evolved through evolution for coping, adaptation, and preservation of the species. This is why it should come as no surprise that people with PTSD exhibit abnormalities in almost every psychobiological system that has been investigated. Indeed, in the same way that many different pathological circumstances may produce the same clinical abnormality (e.g., fever or edema), many different psychobiological abnormalities may lead to PTSD. Furthermore, it is not too far fetched to anticipate that a spectrum of posttraumatic syndromes may be elucidated by future research and that each syndrome will be associated with a unique allostatic configuration. Furthermore, each syndrome may respond optimally to a different medication. But we are getting ahead of ourselves. First, we must consider current evidence that allostatic load is present in PTSD by reviewing the many different psychobiological abnormalities associated with this disorder. Next we consider a rational pharmacotherapeutic strategy based on this analysis. Then we consider how such an allostatic perspective compares with the current empirical approach to pharmacotherapy. And finally we review the decision process in pharmacotherapy and the many factors by which it is influenced.

WHAT IS THE CURRENT EVIDENCE FOR ALLOSTATIC LOAD IN PTSD?

The best evidence for allostatic load in PTSD comes from research with the two systems that have been most associated with the human stress response: the adrenergic and hypothalamic–pituitary–adrenocortical (HPA) systems. There is also evidence for allostasis in the serotonergic, opioid, and other systems.

Allostasis and the Adrenergic System

It is well recognized that adrenergic reactivity is enhanced in PTSD patients. This conclusion is based on psychophysiological research on the sympathetic nervous system (SNS), which consistently shows heightened cardiovascular and acoustic startle responsivity (see the review by Pitman, Orr, Shalev, Metzger, & Mellman, 1999). Likewise, research on the adrenergic nervous system consistently indicates elevated catecholamine levels and heightened sensitivity to the adrenergic alpha-2 receptor antagonist yohimbine (see the review by Southwick et al., 1999)

Despite the heightened adrenergic reactivity observed in PSD, resting SNS and adrenergic activity is not elevated. For example, PTSD patients do not show elevated blood pressures or heart rates at rest; it is only when they are challenged by some psychological probe (e.g., trauma-related stimuli) or pharmacological probe (e.g., yohimbine) that such adrenergic abnormalities can be unmasked. In short, at rest the PTSD patient exhibits adrenergic and SNS stability. But such stability comes at a price. This price is what McEwen (1998) has termed allostatic load. With respect to PTSD, the adrenergic price of stability appears to be a reduction (or downregulation) of alpha-2 adrenergic receptors (Perry, 1994). The potential impact to the person with PTSD of excessive adrenergic stimulation is blunted by an adaptive reduction in the number of receptor sites available to react to such increased neurotransmitter levels. During the relative "quiet" of baseline function, a physiological stability is apparent that is indistinguishable from the homeostatic steady state seen in individuals without PTSD. During a stressful episode or some other provocation, however, the downregulation of adrenergic receptors is unequal to the task and therefore unable to maintain stability. Hence, under such circumstances, PTSD patients exhibit the heightened reactivity mentioned above. This is another aspect of allostatic load, another price that must be paid because the adrenergic systems of PTSD patients are inadequately equipped to cope with the demands of stress, in contrast to the systems of people without this disorder.

Allostasis and the Hypothalamic–Pituitary–Adrenocortical Systems

The case for allostasis in PTSD is easier to make with resect to the HPA system because of elegant research that has investigated the different components of HPA function more thoroughly than has been the case with the adrenergic system (see the review by Yehuda, 1999). Here the allostatic balance appears to be the reverse of that seen with adrenergic mechanisms. Whereas excessive adrenergic reactivity is partially offset by downregulation of alpha-2 receptors, in the HPA system reduced serum cortisol levels are offset by upregulation and increased sensitivity of glucocorticoid receptors. The principle is the same—only the direction of change is different. The price of stability is an adaptive change at the receptor level that can be unmasked by psychological or pharmacological probes. I have suggested elsewhere (Friedman, 1998) that, behaviorally speaking, the price of such stability is stress intolerance because people with PTSD appear less able to cope with the normal hassles and vicissitudes of life. Pharmacologically, allostatic load is evident because people with PTSD (in comparison to those without PTSD) exhibit supersensitivity or supersuppression of HPA function in response to the glucocorticoid dexamethasone (Yehuda et al., 1993).

Allostasis and the Serotonergic System

The third example of psychobiological allostasis in PTSD is admittedly much more speculative. It is worth discussing, however, because of the importance of serotonin (5-hydroxytryptamine, or 5-HT) in the human stress response and because of the recently demonstrated efficacy of drugs that modify 5-HT function in PTSD. Southwick and associates (1997) have shown that some Vietnam veterans with PTSD are especially sensitive to the 5-HT agonist m-chlorophenylpiperazine (mCPP) which interacts primarily with 5-HT_2 and 5-HT_{1c} receptors.

One interpretation of these results is that those veterans who exhibited a panic/flashback response to MCPP did so because of upregulation or supersensitivity of 5-HT receptors. If that were the case, one would predict that administering a drug that could downregulate 5-HT receptors might be an effective treatment for PTSD. Indeed, sertraline, a selective serotonic reuptake inhibitor (SSRI), does downregulate postsynaptic 5-HT receptors. Sertraline is also an effective treatment for PTSD (see below). Is this a coincidence? Or is this circumstantial evidence in support of the allostatic load hypothesis?

This speculative example is also a good place to illustrate how a rational approach to pharmacotherapy could be based on an understanding of allostasis. The pharmacological agent of choice would be a medication that reduces allostatic load by pushing the system back toward a homeostatic steady state. Thus SSRI-mediated downregulation of allostatically upregulated 5-HT receptors is definitely a therapeutic step in the correct homeostatic direction.

The presumption that selective reduction of allostatic load will produce clinical improvement is the guiding principle for the subsequent discussion of rational pharmacotherapy for PTSD.

Before leaving the 5-HT system, it is instructive to consider an additional finding in the MCPP study (Southwick et al., 1997). Whereas some veterans with PTSD exhibited panic and flashback reactions following administration of MCPP, others did not. Among those who did not were many who displayed panic and flashback reactions to the adrenergic agent yohimbine. Thus some veterans were MCPP (but not yohimbine) responders, indicating excessive serotonergic sensitivity, whereas others were yohimbine (but not MCPP) responders, indicating excessive adrenergic reactivity. Veterans without PTSD did not react to either drug. Therefore, this provocative study suggests that different people may implement different psychobiological adaptive strategies for coping with chronic stress. For some veterans allostatic load was best understood as an adrenergic abnormality, whereas for others allostatic load was best understood as a serotonergic adaptation.

Allostasis and the Opioid System

Although there is little clinical research on the opioid system in PTSD, there is abundant evidence that endogenous opioids (endorphins, dynorphins, and enkephalins) play an important role in the stress response of animals. A well-established laboratory phenomenon, stress-induced analgesia (SIA), occurs when experimental animals are exposed to stressful stimuli such as electric shock, forced swimming, or restraint. Under such circumstances, laboratory animals exhibit a reduced responsiveness to pain (e.g., SIA) that can be reversed by narcotic antagonists, thus indicating that SIA is an opioid response to stress (Stout, Kilts, & Nemeroff, 1995). There is one experiment suggesting that SIA can also be produced in humans with PTSD (Pitman, van der Kolk, Orr, & Greenberg, 1990), although these findings have never been replicated. Other studies have shown additional abnormalities in opioid function among PTSD patients (reviewed in Friedman & Southwick, 1995).

With respect to allostasis, there is one very interesting report concerning an open-label trial with a narcotic antagonist that was administered to Vietnam veterans with PTSD (Glover, 1993). The guiding hypothesis was that emotional numbing in PTSD is mediated by opioids. It was expected that by reversing opioid activity the narcotic antagonist would reduce numbing symptoms and thereby diminish PTSD severity. Indeed, several veterans responded as predicted and reported that they felt more alive, less numb, and less constricted emotionally. Unfortunately, other veterans reported that their PTSD became dramatically worse because of intolerable anxiety, panic, arousal, and even flashbacks, in some cases.

How can we understand such diametrically opposite effects among a cohort of apparently similar people (male Vietnam veterans) who all received the same medication? One explanation is that opioid-related allostatic load was balanced differently in different veterans. If we accept the hypothesis that opioid activity is an adaptive (allostatic) response to blunt/numb the excessive (adrenergic) arousal associated with this disorder, we can propose that individuals may differ in their capacity to mobilize opioid mechanisms to achieve allostatic stability. Thus, we might expect that those veterans who exhibited excessive emotional numbing (hypothetically because of excessive opioid activity) experienced relief from the narcotic antagonist because their elevated opioid function was reduced toward homeostatic levels. We might suggest that, in contrast to their "numbed out" colleagues, those veterans who had a severe anxiety reaction were those whose allostatic steady state consisted of a much smaller opioid component. They were at high risk to experience a severe anxiety reaction because the narcotic antagonist blocked what little opioid activity they had been able to mobilize to antagonize adrenergic hyperarousal.

There are several points to underscore here regarding how adaptive psychobiological strategies may differ from one individual to the next. In some cases, the difference may be (quantitatively) related to the capacity to mobilize one particular (e.g., opioid) mechanism to achieve stability. On the other hand, the yohimbine versus MCPP example suggests that different people with PTSD may utilize (qualitatively) different psychobiological allostatic strategies (e.g., adrenergic vs. serotonergic) to achieve stability. Finally, if different quantitative and/or qualitative adaptations can underlie PTSD, then different medications may be indicated for different people even though they appear to have the same DSM-IV disorder.

Allostasis and Corticotropin-Releasing Factor

Corticotropin-releasing factor (CRF) is a neuropeptide that ignites the complex cascade of adrenergic, HPA, immunological, and other psychobiological systems that participate in the human stress response. As a neurotransmitter, CRF activates adrenergic neurons in the locus coeruleus (Aston-Jones, Valentino, Van Bockstaele, & Meyerson, 1994) while as a neurohormone, CRF promotes the HPA response by releasing adrenocorticotropic hormone (ACTH) from the pituitary gland. Two studies indicate that CRF activity is increased in PTSD. CRF levels are elevated in the cerebrospinal fluid (CSF) (Bremner et al., 1997), and hypothalamic release of CRF is apparently enhanced (Yehuda et al., 1996) in people with PTSD. It would be impossible at this time to calculate the total allostatic load produced by excessive CRF activity because it has such far-reaching direct and indirect effects on so many psychobiological systems. Certainly adrenergic, HPA, 5-HT, and opioid abnormalities (described above) are important parts of this picture but there are many other elements as well.

Allostasis and Neuropeptide Y

Neuropeptide Y (NPY) is heavily concentrated in brain structures that mediate the human stress response. Clinical trials suggest that it is an anxiolytic, and laboratory research suggests that it antagonizes the actions of CRF and other stress-released neuropeptides. Recent evidence with military personnel exposed to the intense rigors of extremely stressful training exercises indicate that those individuals with the highest NPY levels tolerated this experience better than those with lower levels (Morgan, Wang, Southwick, Rasmusson, Hazlett, Hauger, & Charney, 2000).

Such findings suggest that allostasis does not always promote vulnerability. Indeed, achieving an allostatic stability characterized by higher NPY levels might be a psychobiological signature for resilience rather than vulnerability. Hence, rather than allostatic load, we may need to think in terms of allostatic support. From this perspective, homeostatic stability may not always be optimal. Improved coping with stress may be achieved through psychobiological strategies that promote resilience. Enhancing NPY function to achieve allostatic support may turn out to be such a strategy.

Another implication of these findings is that NPY activity might be reduced in people with PTSD. A deficiency in NPY function would mean the loss of a major system that can buffer the intense impact of the human stress response. Since NPY can attenuate the actions of CRF (Stout et al., 1995), it might be expected to lighten the allostatic load in PTSD through allostatic support. Given that CRF plays such a decisive role in the human stress response, the potential salutary actions of NPY may be of enormous significance.

Allostasis and Thyroid Function

Thyroid function is enhanced in PTSD, as indicated by elevated levels of both active thyroid hormones triiodothyronine (T3) and thyroxine (T4). In fact, PTSD symptom severity was positively associated with such increases in thyroid function (Mason et al., 1995; Wang & Mason, 1999).

Since glucocorticoids (e.g., cortisol) normally suppress thyroid activity (Michelson, Licinio, & Gold, 1995) and since cortisol levels are reduced in PTSD, it appears that elevated thyroid function in PTSD may be a secondary effect caused by the lower cortisol levels due to the disturbance in HPA function described earlier. Thus the allostatic load due to altered thyroid activity appears to be a downstream component of HPA-related allostasis. This is a good example of how disturbed function in one system can produce additional abnormalities in other systems.

Allostasis and Sensitization

Sensitization is a well-established laboratory phenomenon concerning progressive alterations in neuronal reactivity, especially in the limbic system and cerebral cortex. In a typical sensitization experiment, neurons are repeatedly (e.g., once a day) exposed to a subthreshold dose of a stimulant drug such as cocaine (or electrical stimulation). Initially the subthreshold dose of cocaine produces no effects. With the passage of time, the single daily dose of cocaine begins to produce prominent behavior or neurophysiological effects. This is called "sensitization." If there is continued daily administration beyond the sensitization phase, the same dose of cocaine can produce seizures. This is called "kindling" (as if a neuronal fire has slowly been building up until it erupts into the flames of a seizure). Sensitization/kindling models have been proposed for a variety of neurological and psychiatric disorders including epilepsy, recurrent psychosis, and PTSD (Post, Weiss, & Smith, 1995; Post, Weiss, Li, Leverich, & Pert, 1999).

In certain respects, sensitization is a highly dramatic example of allostatic load. A potentially explosive steady state is produced that may be very difficult to reverse. It is also an extremely complicated process that is mediated through profound alterations in a wide spectrum of synaptic (first, second, third, etc.) messenger systems and in regulator genes that control neuronal reactivity (Post et al., 1995, 1999).

To summarize, we have described eight psychobiological examples of allostatic load in PTSD. They illustrate that allostatic load may be expressed in a number of interrelated manifestations:

1. Allostatic stability may not be apparent in the baseline state (e.g., normal blood pressure). During stressful stimulation, however, the adaptation may be unable to preserve normal function, as in the adrenergic system, which is hyperreactive in PTSD.
2. Allostasis may be unmasked by psychological probes (e.g., stress, trauma-related stimuli) or pharmacological probes (e.g., yohimbine, MCPP, dexamethasone).
3. Qualitatively different allostatic adaptations may be detected in different people with PTSD as shown in excessive serotonergic (e.g., MCPP but not yohimbine responders) versus excessive adrenergic (e.g., yohimbine but not MCPP responders) sensitivity.
4. Quantitative differences may be detected in allostatic adaptation, as in PTSD patients who found a narcotic antagonist therapeutic in comparison to those who found that the same drug produced severe anxiety and distress.
5. Allostatic load detectable in one system may have far reaching consequences affecting other systems, as shown by downstream effects produced by CRF-induced allostatic load which clearly affects adrenergic, HPA, serotonergic, opioid, and thyroid hormone (T3 and T4) systems.
6. Allostatic alterations are not always deleterious; hence excessive NPY may actually provide allostatic support (e.g., resilience) rather than allostatic load (e.g., vulnerability).
7. Some allostatic changes may be easier to ameliorate than others. Altered neuronal excitability as in sensitization/kindling may be much more resistant to reversal than allostatic load in neurotransmitter, neuropeptide, and neurohormonal systems.

RATIONAL PHARMACOTHERAPY BASED ON ALLOSTATIC LOAD

Table 4.1 summarizes the previous discussion and shows the kinds of allostatic load proposed to occur in people with PTSD. The findings on adrenergic

TABLE 4.1. Rational Pharmacotherapy Based on Allostatic Load

Psychobiological system	Allostatic load	Clinical manifestations	Proposed treatment
Adrenergic	Hyperreactivity, downregulation of alpha-2 receptors	Hyperarousal, hypervigilance, hyperreactivity, panic/anxiety, intrusion/dissociation	Adrenergic antagonists (clonidine, propranolol)
HPA	Enhanced negative feedback, upregulation of glucocorticoid receptors, reduced cortisol levels	Stress intolerance	Glucocorticoids? SSRIs?
5-HT	Systemic dysregulation, upregulation of 5-HT$_2$ receptors?	Intrusion/avoidant/numbing/arousal, impulsivity, rage, aggression, depression, panic, obsessional thoughts alcoholism/chemical dependency	SSRIs, nefazodone
Opioid	Sytemic dysregulation	Numbing, chemical dependency	Opioid agonists/antagonists?
CRF	Elevated activity, enhancement of stress response	Hyperarousal, hypervigilance, hyperreactivity, intrusion/dissociation, stress intolerance, numbing	CRF antagonists
NPY	Reduced activity, enhancement of stress response	Same as CRF	NPY agonists
Thyroid	Elevated activity, secondary to reduced cortisol	Hyperarousal, anxiety	Normalization of HPA function
Sensitization/kindling	Neuronal excitability (limbic/cortical)	Hyperarousal, intrusion	Anticonvulsants

and HPA function have reasonably secure empirical support. The rest of this table is highly speculative, based on my own interpretations of a relatively sparse literature—although these speculations are consistent with most of the published research in this field.

The third column presents my suggestions as to the clinical implications of allostatic load in each system and is modified from earlier speculations of this sort (Friedman, 1998).

The fourth column is most relevant to the present discussion. It illustrates the kind of pharmacological agent that might be selected to normalize each specific allostatic abnormality. As will be shown later, very few of these agents have been systematically tested in empirical medication trials. Indeed, the lion's share of attention has been devoted to drugs affecting 5-HT mechanisms such as SSRIs. There have only been a few (nonrandomized trials) with antiadrenergic agents and anticonvulsants. We can expect that CRF antagonists will be tested once the pharmaceutical companies have developed safe and effective medications in that category.

Had the knowledge about allostatic load influenced research on the clinical pharmacology for PTSD, there would have been many more trials of antiadrenergic (and possibly anticonvulsant) medications. We shall consider why this has not been the case below as we consider the empirical approach to pharmacotherapy that has been the dominant research strategy up to this time.

EMPIRICAL FINDINGS
ON PHARMACOTHERAPY IN PTSD

Selective Serotonin Reuptake Inhibitors

Without doubt, the most important new development in the clinical pharmacology of PTSD is the recent decision by the U.S. Food and Drug Administration (FDA) to designate the SSRI sertraline as a drug indicated for treatment of PTSD. This decision was based on findings from two large clinical trials in which approximately 400 men and women (approximately 200 in each trial) were randomly assigned to receive either sertraline or a placebo (Brady et al., 2000; Davidson, Malik, & Sutherland, 1996). There are a number of notable findings to report from these studies. First, sertraline effectively reduced symptoms in all three PTSD diagnostic clusters (e.g., intrusion, avoidant/numbing and hyperarousal). This was a surprising and welcome result, since previous studies had suggested that there was not a broad spectrum drug (e.g., a "magic bullet") for PTSD. Indeed, a few years ago Friedman and Southwick (1995) seriously questioned whether there was a single drug that could ameliorate all three clusters of PTSD symptoms, and suggested that optimal pharmacotherapy might consist of one class of drug for intrusion symptoms, another class for avoidant/numbing symptoms, and a third class for arousal symptoms.

Another important finding from the sertraline trials is that the SSRI's efficacy is not due to its potency as an antidepressant. When subjects who had PTSD plus a history of major depressive disorder (MDD) were compared to PTSD subjects without MDD, there was no difference. Both groups exhibited an equal reduction in PTSD symptoms, suggesting that sertraline is an effective and specific treatment for PTSD.

A final set of results from these important studies raise provocative questions about gender and type of trauma. First, women appeared to be much more responsive to medication than men. Second, people with sexual trauma appeared to be more responsive than those with other types of trauma. Indeed, men with a history of sexual trauma appeared to respond well to sertraline, suggesting that it is not simply a matter of gender but something much more complicated that determines responsivity to sertraline that needs to be clarified in future research. After considering this evidence very carefully, the FDA concluded that sertraline is definitely effective for women with PTSD and that its efficacy for men has not been demonstrated conclusively. It is important to recognize that the FDA *did not* conclude that sertraline is ineffective in men.

There are other studies with SSRIs that must be mentioned. Two randomized clinical trials with fluoxetine of van der Kolk et al. (1994) and Davidson et al. (1997) showed marked improvement in PTSD symptoms and the Clinical Global Improvement (CGI) Scale, respectively, in mostly female cohorts with a history of sexual trauma. On the other hand, Vietnam veterans with PTSD were largely unresponsive to fluoxetine (van der Kolk et al., 1994). I have argued elsewhere (Friedman, 1997) that poor results with Vietnam veterans may have less to do with either male gender or combat trauma and much more to do with the fact that these veterans have much more severe, chronic, and treatment-refractory PTSD than do nonveteran subjects enrolled in similar treatment protocols.

Recent open-label trials with sertraline in rape trauma survivors (Rothbaum, Ninan, & Thomas, 1996), fluvoxamine in Vietnam combat veterans (Marmar et al., 1996), and paroxetine in subjects previously traumatized by rape, criminal assault, or accidents (Marshall et al., 1998) have all had positive results. In fact, the data from randomized and open trials all show effectiveness of SSRIs in reducing all three PTSD symptom clusters. Data from trials with fluoxetine, fluvoxamine, and paroxetine are consistent with the sertraline data detailed previously, although they have all been small single-site studies as compared to the large multisite sertraline trials.

At the present time, SSRIs are the treatment of choice as first-line drugs in PTSD. Two recent large-scale initiatives to assess the effectiveness and efficacy of current PTSD treatments have confirmed this conclusion. In the first, an extensive survey by mail in which 57 international experts in PTSD pharmacotherapy were asked a variety of questions about treatment, SSRIs were clearly selected as the top choice by this expert consensus panel (Foa, Davidson, & Frances, 1999). In the second, a treatment guideline developed by the International Society for Traumatic Stress Studies (ISTSS), it was concluded that the empirical literature strongly supports that SSRIs are the most effective medication for PTSD at the present time (Friedman, Davidson, Mellman, & Southwick, 2000).

There are several other reasons why SSRIs have emerged as first-line treatments for PTSD. First, they have proven efficacy against disorders that are frequently comorbid with PTSD. These include depression, panic disorder, social phobia, and obsessive–compulsive disorder. SSRIs also effectively reduce a number of clinically significant symptoms that are frequently associated with PTSD such as rage, impulsivity, suicidal intent, and misuse of alcohol or drugs (Friedman, 1990). Brady, Sonne, and Roberts (1995) reported that sertraline effectively reduced both PTSD and alcohol-related symptoms in patients with comorbid PTSD and alcohol dependence. Finally, SSRIs generally produce fewer disturbing side effects than other medications that have been prescribed for this disorder.

Other Serotonergic Agents

Nefazodone

Nefazodone is an effective antidepressant that combines SSRI activity with postsynaptic 5-HT_2 blockade. Although there is a little evidence from one open trial (Hertzberg, Feldman, Beckham, Moore, & Davidson, 1998) and no published randomized clinical trial, nefazodone was strongly endorsed as a second choice (after SSRIs) by the aforementioned expert consensus panel (Foa et al., 1999). It is curious that nefazodone should be so strongly favored by experts in the absence of a convincing proof of efficacy. I can only understand this as the result of the following: clinician awareness of nefazodone's effectiveness against MDD, with which PTSD is frequently comorbid; its lack of side effects; its conspicuousness to practitioners because of aggressive marketing strategies by pharmaceutical companies; and the expectation among clinicians that it will prove to have the same spectrum of action as SSRIs. There are multisite trials with nefazodone currently in progress, and we await their results with interest.

Trazodone

Trazodone, like nefazodone, is an SSRI plus 5-HT_2 antagonist. It has shown only modest effectiveness in one small open trial with PTSD patients (Hertzberg, Feldman, Beckham, & Davidson, 1996). It differs from nefazodone in that it is less potent as an antidepressant but much more sedating as a hypnotic. Trazodone has been rediscovered by clinicians in recent years because its serotonergic action is synergistic with SSRIs and its sedative action often overcomes the insomnia produced by SSRIs (Cook & Conner, 1995).

Venlafaxine

Venlafaxine is a potent antidepressant that, in addition to possessing an SSRI action, is a strong reuptake inhibitor of norepinephrine and a weak reuptake inhibitor of dopamine. There are no published randomized or open trials with venlafaxine in PTSD. Despite the lack of evidence for efficacy, it was selected as the third-most-favored drug by the expert consensus panel, after SSRIs and nefazodone (Foa et al., 1999). One can only guess that the reasons for its popularity with experts are similar to those cited above concerning nefazodone. It is important to keep this in mind, and to recognize that evidence supporting the use of venlafaxine in PTSD has yet to make an appearance.

Cyproheptadine

Cyproheptadine is a 5-HT antagonist that has been suggested as an effective treatment for traumatic nightmares. Evidence for this claim was based on two brief reports on a total of six patients, although there are unpublished reports supporting these results (reviewed in Friedman & Southwick, 1995). A recent two-site randomized clinical trial with veterans has not confirmed these findings. It was found that cyproheptadine was no better than placebo in reducing PTSD symptoms, preventing traumatic nightmares, or improving sleep (Jacobs-Rebhun, Schnurr, Friedman, Peck, Brophy, & Fuller, 2000). Based on these latter findings, cyproheptadine cannot be recommended for PTSD treatment.

Buspirone

Buspirone is an anxiolytic that acts as a 5-HT$_{1A}$ partial agonist. One published case report on three veterans indicated that buspirone ameliorated anxiety, insomnia, flashbacks, and depression (see Friedman & Southwick, 1995). As yet, no further data are available on the usefulness of this drug.

Antiadrenergic Agents

Perhaps the best evidence that clinical pharmacological research in PTSD has been driven by the empirical rather than the allostatic perspective can be found by perusing the published findings regarding antiadrenergic agents. Since we have known about elevated urinary catecholamines, downregulation of alpha-2 receptors, yohimbine sensitivity, and SNS hyperreactivity for many years (see Southwick et al., 1999), one would have expected the literature to be full of reports on the effectiveness of antiadrenergic agents such as postsynaptic antagonists (e.g., propranolol) or presynaptic alpha-2 agonists (e.g., clonidine and guanfacine). Surprisingly, this is not the case.

An open trial with both propranolol and clonidine in Vietnam veterans with PTSD, conducted by Kolb, Burris, and Griffiths (1984), reported marked symptom reduction with both medications. Patients reported diminution of intrusive recollections, traumatic nightmares, hypervigilance, startle reactions, insomnia, and angry outbursts. An A-B-A designed study (6 weeks off—6 weeks on—6 weeks off) of propranolol in 11 children with PTSD due to sexual and/or physical abuse was likewise successful, with significant reductions observed in reexperiencing and arousal (but not avoidant/numbing) symptoms during the active treatment phase which rebounded to predrug severity after propranolol was discontinued (Famularo, Kinscherff, & Fenton, 1988).

Despite such promising data, there have been no randomized clinical trials with any antiadrenergic agent and very few open trials (see Friedman, 1998). In general, clonidine has been more successful than propranolol (in trials with abused children, Cambodian refugees, and Vietnam veterans), but the data are much too sparse to enable us to draw any conclusions with confidence.

I use antiadrenergic agents, especially alpha-2 agonists, extensively in my practice. This enthusiasm is clearly based on my allostatic perspective, since there is very little empirical support for prescribing such drugs. In addition to selecting antiadrenergic agents to reduce allostatic load from hyperarousal and hyperreactive symptoms, I use such agents to treat dissociation and flashbacks. I formulated such a strategy by extrapolation from the previously mentioned studies in which yohimbine produced dissociation/PTSD flashbacks in Vietnam veterans. It seemed to me that if an alpha-2 antagonist such as yohimbine could produce such symptoms, a drug with the opposite action, an alpha-2 agonist such as clonidine, should be an effective antidote.

Case 1: KM

KM was a 42-year-old divorced mother of two school-aged children who had become unable to maintain employment at the large banking firm where she had previously been functioning very well at an executive level. She was totally incapacitated by a resurgence of traumatic memories (of childhood sexual abuse) and other PTSD avoidant/numbing and hyperarousal symptoms. Most distressing, by far, were the dissociative episodes that could disrupt any activity at any time and which consisted of complex behavioral sequences over which she had no control and about which she had no recollection. An incisive and thorough historian regarding information that was accessible to her memory, KM recalled that amnestic episodes were usually preceded by escalating levels of arousal and anxiety.

When prescribed clonidine 0.2 mg twice daily, KM reported marked reduction in dissociative episodes within the first week of treatment. She also reported reduced anxiety, improved concentration, and better sleep. Three weeks later the dose had to be increased to 0.2 mg thrice daily because her dissociative symptoms started to return. This dosage adjustment was also effective for several weeks until she again began to become tolerant to the medication as evidenced by a return of dissociative symptoms.

At this point, I was hesitant to increase the clonidine any further for fear that it might provoke a reduction in blood pressure (since clonidine is used clinically in the treatment of hypertension). Therefore, I switched KM to guanfacine 1 mg twice daily because that drug has the same pharmacological actions as clonidine but is less likely to produce tolerance because of its longer half-life (Horrigan, 1996). This was quite successful, and KM remained on the same dose of guanfacine for 4 years. Not only were her dissociative and other PTSD symptoms well controlled, but she was able to resume her previous duties at the bank.

Recently, KM had to undergo treatment for cancer. Her oncologist discontinued the guanfacine because of concerns about drug interactions with some of the powerful antineoplastic drugs that needed to be prescribed. Within a week's time, dissociative symptoms that had been well controlled for years returned with alarming intensity. Resumption of guanfacine once again negated the dissociative symptoms and restored her psychiatric remission.

This vignette illustrates the successful treatment of dissociative symptoms that had failed to respond to SSRIs, nefazodone, or other medications. It shows how a treatment strategy based on allostatic concerns may produce clinical success. I should note that I have had many patients like KM who have had good responses to antiadrenergic agents. I make this statement with full knowledge that proof of efficacy must await a conclusive randomized clinical trial. KM's case also illustrates the not uncommon occurrence that clonidine responders may become tolerant to this agent. It shows that clonidine-tolerant patients may subsequently be stabilized indefinitely on guanfacine. Finally, beta blockers such as propranolol are often as effective as alpha-2 agonists such as clonidine or guanfacine, although I hesitate to prescribe them for patients who have MDD in addition to PTSD.

Tricyclic Antidepressants

The first reports on effective pharmacotherapy for PTSD concerned tricyclic antidepressants (TCAs) (see the extensive review of this literature by ver Ellen & van Kammen, 1990). Clinicians found TCAs to be useful agents for reducing reexperiencing and hyperarousal (but not avoidant/numbing) symptoms. Three randomized clinical trials, all with Vietnam veterans, had mixed results. Imipramine produced moderate reduction in reexperiencing symptoms and clinically significant global improvement (Kosten et al., 1991). Amitriptyline produced global improvement and modest reduction in avoidant/numbing symptoms (Davidson et al., 1990). In the third randomized clinical trial, which lasted only 4 weeks in contrast to the 8-week duration of the other studies, desipramine was no better than placebo (Reist et al., 1989). Finally, in a quantitative review of all randomized and open trials with tricyclics, Southwick and associates (1994) concluded that 45% of patients (mostly Vietnam veterans with PTSD) showed global improvement in PTSD that was mostly due to amelioration of intrusion symptoms.

Based on the above reports, TCAs have largely fallen out of favor as first-line treatment for PTSD. Reasons for this are as follows: (1) they have a more complicated spectrum of side effects than newer agents such as SSRIs, nefazodone, and venlafaxine; (2) the newer agents are equipotent to TCAs as antidepressants, so TCAs are prescribed much less frequently, in general, by practicing psychiatrists; (3) no new clinical trials with TCAs have been published in almost 10 years; and (4) aggressive strategies have been engaged in by pharmaceutical companies to promote SSRIs and other new antidepressants, both through the launching of multisite clinical trials and through promotion of their use for comorbid disorders (e.g., depression, panic disorder, social phobia, and obsessive–compulsive disorder). For all these reasons, TCAs have faded from the short list of medications most favored by prescribing clinicians in the treatment of PTSD (and other psychiatric disorders).

It is useful to ask ourselves whether the verdict against the usefulness of TCAs was declared prematurely. Certainly their array of side effects would place them behind SSRIs, but is there evidence that they might actually exhibit greater efficacy against PTSD symptoms under certain circumstances? First, their pharmacological action—to block reuptake of both 5-HT and norepinephrine—suggests, from an allostatic load perspective, that they may still have a place in PTSD treatment. Second, the randomized trials that produced mixed results were all conducted on Vietnam veterans seeking treatment in VA (Veterans Administration) hospital-based PTSD programs. As I have argued elsewhere (Friedman, 1997), these patients appear to be a severe, chronic, and treatment-refractory cohort who have also failed to respond to SSRIs (van der Kolk et al., 1994). Perhaps TCAs have more to offer than both the empirical literature and PTSD experts (Foa et al., 1999) would suggest. They may well deserve reconsideration either with less chronic cohorts or with SSRI-refractory patients.

In this regard, the first publication in several years on TCA treatment for traumatized patients recently appeared concerning the prospective use of imipramine for pediatric burn patients (aged 2–19 years) who suffered from acute stress disorder (ASD) in addition to their burn injuries (Robert, Blakeney, Villarreal, Rosenberg, & Mayer, 1999). Twenty-five children with a mean total-burn surface of 45% were randomly assigned to 7 days of treatment with either imipramine or chloral hydrate (a sleeping medication currently used extensively in burn units to ameliorate insomnia and traumatic nightmares). Imipramine produced marked symptom relief to complete symptom relief in 83% of the children in contrast to chloral hydrate, which was only effective for 38% of the children. Furthermore, after completion of the 7-day trial, 20% of the 25 children and their parents elected to continue imipramine treatment for approximately the next 6 months. Intrusion, avoidant/numbing, arousal, and dissociative symptoms were well controlled during that period, and there was no rebound of PTSD symptoms when imipramine was discontinued.

Obviously larger and additional studies are needed to confirm these results, but there are two important points raised by this study: first, TCAs may have an important role in treatment of ASD and prevention of PTSD; second, TCAs may be worth reconsidering for treatment of PTSD.

Monoamine Oxidase Inhibitors

The story with monoamine oxidase inhibitors (MAOIs) is similar to that with TCAs except that MAOIs have been used much less extensively than TCAs and their performance against PTSD symptoms has generally been better. As with TCAs, however, they have been largely replaced by SSRIs and other new antidepressants in PTSD treatment.

From an allostatic perspective, MAOIs also foster downregulation of 5-HT and adrenergic receptors through a metabolic action that blocks destruction of these neurotransmitters by the intracellular enzyme, MAO. Psychiatrists have generally not been predisposed to prescribe MAOIs as first-line treatments (despite their powerful efficacy as antidepressants and antipanic agents) because patients must be extremely compliant and reliable; they must adhere to strict dietary restrictions, avoid a number of medications (including illicit drugs), and abstain from alcohol. Failure to adhere to such dietary, drug, and alcohol restrictions can result in a sudden large-scale elevation in blood pressure that precipitates a hypertensive crisis that is a medical emergency.

In two published randomized trials with the MAOI phenelzine, excellent global improvement and reduction of intrusion symptoms was found in one study (Kosten et al., 1991) whereas the second, a methodologically flawed investigation, demonstrated no efficacy of the MAOI in reducing PTSD severity (Shestatzky, Greenberg, & Lerer, 1988). In addition, a number of successful open trials and positive case reports concerning MAOI (usually phenelzine) treatment for PTSD have been reported (see the review by De Martino, Mollica, & Wilk, 1995).

In recent years, there have been trials with RIMAs, reversible inhibitors of monoamine oxidase A (MAO-A) that appear to share the pharmacological action of traditional MAOIs without the serious side effects. Results with RIMAs have not been as impressive as with traditional MAOIs but have not been without promise. An open trial with 20 patients who received moclobemide (a RIMA not available in the United States) produced clinically significant improvement in reexperiencing and avoidant symptoms (Neal, Shapland, & Fox, 1997). Two randomized multisite clinical trials with the experimental RIMA/SSRI agent brofaramine had mixed results. Patients in both studies exhibited 52–60% reduction in PTSD severity, but high response rates in the placebo group (Baker et al., 1995) nullified any treatment effect whereas a lower placebo response in the second study suggested moderate efficacy in PTSD (Katz et al., 1994/95). Unfortunately, the manufacturers have discontinued testing of brofaramine, so there is presently no possibility that it will be used in PTSD or any other treatment.

Finally, in the same quantitative review of TCAs mentioned earlier (Southwick et al., 1994), MAOIs appeared to be more effective than TCAs, having produced moderate-to-good global improvement in 82% of all patients, primarily due to amelioration of reexperiencing symptoms, in contrast to only 45% improvement with TCAs.

Benzodiazepines

Benzodiazepines are proven anxiolytic agents for which there is no proof of efficacy in PTSD. In the only published randomized clinical trial, alprazolam reduced insomnia, general anxiety, and irritability but was without effect on PTSD intrusion, avoidant/numbing, startle response, or hypervigilance symptoms (Braun et al., 1990). A prospective study in which clonazepam was given to recently traumatized emergency room patients did not demonstrate that such a prophylactic approach prevented the later development of PTSD (Gelpin, Bonne, Peri, Brandes, & Shalev, 1996). Other open trials have yielded similarly negative results (see Friedman & Southwick, 1995). The only positive finding was a pilot study in which temazepam (a hypnotic benzodiazepine) prescribed at bedtime specifically to improve insomnia among trauma survivors with ASD, was associated with a marked reduction in PTSD symptoms subsequently (Mellman, Byers, & Augenstein, 1998).

Current evidence suggests that benzodiazepines exhibit no efficacy against PTSD intrusion, avoidant numbing, hypervigilant, or startle symptoms. Furthermore, there is a report of exacerbation of such symptoms marked by intense arousal and flashbacks among PTSD patients undergoing abrupt discontinuation of alprazolam (Risse et al., 1990). In short, there is no empirical justification for prescribing benzodiazepines to PTSD patients.

Anticonvulsants

The anticonvulsants carbamazepine and valproate have been prescribed in open trials with PTSD patients because such drugs have exhibited antikindling actions in research protocols with laboratory animals. Results have been mixed but generally favorable in small open trials. Carbamazepine appears effective in reducing intrusion and arousal symptoms, while valproate has reduced avoidant/numbing and arousal (but not intrusion) symptoms (see Friedman & Southwick, 1995, for references). Based on the theoretical importance of sensitization/kindling models in PTSD, discussed earlier, it is hoped that there will be more extensive and rigorous research with anticonvulsants in the future. Both carbamazepine and valproate have an extensive side effect profile, although the latter medication is used widely in current pharmacotherapy for bipolar affective disorder. Given current interest in the usefulness of newer anticonvulsants such as lamotrigine and gabapentine in affective disorders, there will most likely be research in the future on the effectiveness of old and new anticonvulsants for PTSD.

Antipsychotics

The final class of medications to be considered here are antipsychotics. Both conventional and newer atypical antipsychotic agents are potent dopamine antagonists. There are a few studies suggesting allostatic load in the dopaminergic system of PTSD patients, although this has received little attention (see Friedman & Southwick, 1995, for references). Indeed, one might propose that dopaminergic abnormalities contribute to the hypervigilance/paranoia, social withdrawal, and trauma-related hallucinations seen in the most severely affected PTSD patients. Indeed, PTSD syndromes associated with auditory hallucinations (Mueser & Butler, 1987) and comorbid with psychotic disorders (Mueser et al., 1998) have been described. Finally, given favorable properties of newer, atypical antipsychotics including 5-HT_2 antagonism, safety, and lack of toxicity (with respect to tardive dyskinesia and extrapyramidal symptoms), we can expect that such agents will be investigated as PTSD treatments in the near future. Clinicians have already begun to use them with severely affected, treatment-refractory patients, and anecdotal reports have begun to appear in the literature regarding their successful use (Hamner, 1996).

Summary of Empirical Findings

The results of clinical trials are summarized in Table 4.2.

1. In general, empirical research with PTSD has consisted of a small number of randomized clinical trials with medications that, for the most part, were initially designed as antidepressants and later shown to be effective in treating panic disorder, social phobia, and obsessive–compulsive disorder. No drugs specifically designed to target the allostatic load in PTSD have been tested.
2. Testing of older drugs (e.g., TCAs, MAOIs, older anticonvulsants) has largely been abandoned in favor of new antidepressants (e.g., SSRIs, nefazodone) and possibly new anticonvulsants (e.g., lamotrigine, gabapentine). This is especially unfortunate since older medications such as antiadrenergic (clonidine, guanfacine, and propranolol) and anticonvulsants (carbamazepine and valproate) may yet prove effective.
3. Many older trials were conducted on Vietnam veterans with severe, chronic, and treatment-refractory PTSD. Lack of demonstrable efficacy in such trials may be related to the specific responsivity of the

TABLE 4.2. Summary of Empirical Literature on Pharmacotherapy for PTSD

Medication class	Mechanism of action	Specific medication	Dose	No. RCTs	PTSD symptoms				Remarks
					B	C	D		
SSRI	SSRI	Sertraline	50–200 mg	2	X	X	X		• Sertraline has FDA approval as an indicated treatment for PTSD
		Fluoxetine	20–80 mg	3	X	X	X		• SSRIs are effective for comorbid disorders such as depression, panic disorder, social phobia, and obses-sive–compulsive disorder; They've also been used effectively for alco-hol/drug abuse/dependence
		Paroxetine	20–50 mg	0	X	X	X		• They may also reduce symptoms associated with PTSD such as rage, impulsivity, suicidal thoughts, agres-sion, panic/anxiety, obsessional thoughts, chemical abuse/depen-dency
		Fluvoxamine	100–300 mg	0	X	X	X		
Antidepressant	SSRI/5-HT$_2$ blockage	Nefazodone	300–00 mg	0	x/?	x/?	x/?		• Very few data: one small open trial; despite this, nefazodone is greatly favored by "expert consensus" as an excellent antidepressant
		Trazodone	25–500 mg	0	x/?	x/?	x/?		• Results from one small open trial: effective sleeping medication for patients with SSRI-induced insom-nia; moderately effective as an anti-depressant

(continued)

TABLE 4.2. cont.

Medication class	Mechanism of action	Specific medication	Dose	No. RCTs	PTSD symptoms B	C	D	Remarks
	Strong reuptake inhibitor of 5-HT and NE Weak DA reuptake inhibitor	Venlafaxine	75–225 mg	0	?	?	?	• Never tested in PTSD; despite this, is third choice of expert consensus panel, after SSRIs and nefazodone
Serotonin antagonist	Postsynaptic 5-HT blockade	Cyproheptadine	4–28 mg	1	0	0	0	• Without effect on PTSD flashbacks and nightmares, despite early favorable anecdotal reports
Serotonin partial	5HT$_{1A}$ partial agonist	Buspirone	30–60 mg	0	x/?	0	x/?	• Few data—just a few case reports
Antiadrenergic	Alpha-2 agonist	Clonidine Guanfacine	0.2–0.6 mg 1–3 mg	0 0	X X	0 0	X X	• Few trials to date; patients tolerant to clonidine are often responsive to guanfacine
	Beta blocker	Propranolol	40–160 mg	A-B-A (see text)	X	0	X	• Few trials—mixed results in some; may exacerbate major depressive disorders
TCA	Inhibit reuptake of	Imipramine	150–300 mg	1	X	0	x/?	• Major effect on global improvement and B symptoms • Effective in prospective trial with pediatric burn patients with ASD
		Amitriptyline	150–300 mg	1	x/?	X	0	• Most effective on avoidant/numbing

Class	Agent	Dose					Comments
	Desipramine	150–300 mg	1	0	0	0	• Ineffective in brief RCT • All TCAs have clinically significant cardiovascular, anticholinergic, and other side effects; they are good antidepressants and effective in panic disorder
MAOI Irreversible MAOI	Phenelzine	45–75 mg	2	X	0	X	• One very postive RCT, and one methodologically flawed RCT with negative results • Cliniciant are reluctant to prescribe MAOIs because of dietary restrictions and serious side effects • Good antidepressants and antipanic agents
Reversible MAO-A inhibitor (RIMA)	Moclobemide		0	0		0	• Promising medication but few data • Free of MAOI dietary restrictions and side effects.
Benzodiazepines BZD-GAA agonist	Alprazolam	0.5–6 mg	1	0	0	X	• Good general anxiolytic (reduce insomnia anxiety and irritability) but not effective against core PTSD symptoms • Serious withdrawal syndrome with exacerbation of PTSD symptoms
	Clonazepam	1–6 mg	0	0	0	X	• Ineffective in prospective trial of emergency rcom patients with ASD

(continued)

115

TABLE 4.2. *cont.*

Medication class	Mechanism of action	Specific medication	Dose	No. RCTs	PTSD symptoms			Remarks
					B	C	D	
Anticonvulsants	Antikindling action	Carbamazepine	600–1,000 mg	0	X	0	X	• Many side effects • Few studies • Good mood stabilizer
		Valproate	750–1,750 mg	0	0	X	X	• Few studies • Used widely as mood stabilizer
Antipsychotics	D-2 receptor antagonist	Thioridazine	200–800 mg	0	x/?	0	x/?	• Effective conventional antipsychotic • May produce tardive dyskinesia; also extrapyramidal and other side effects • Case reports only
	5-HT$_2$/D$_2$ receptor antagonist	Clozapine	300–900 mg	0	x/?	0	x/?	• Effective • Atypical antipsychotics—fewer motor side effects but other potential toxicities • May have mood-stabilizing properties • Case reports only
		Risperidone	4–12 mg	0	x/?	0	x/?	

Note. RCT, randomized clinical trial; PTSD B symptoms, intrusive recollections; PTSD C symptoms, avoidant/numbing; PTSD D symptoms, hyperarousal; 5-HT, serotonin; NE, norepinephrine; DA, dopamine; BZD, benzodiazepine; GABA, γ-aminobutric acid; D$_2$, dopamine-2 receptor; SSRI, selective serotonin reuptake inhibitor; TCA, Tricyclic antidepressant; MAOI, monoamine oxidase inhibitor; RIMA, reversible MAO-A inhibitor. Statistical significance in PTSD Symptoms column (column 6): X, definite positive effect; x, possible positive effect; 0, nonsignificant effect; ?, no data (never tested).

116

veteran cohort tested rather than the efficacy of the drugs themselves.

4. It is impossible to disentangle gender from trauma type in attempts to understand factors predicting a favorable response to medication, since most women tested have had sexual trauma while most men tested have been Vietnam veterans with chronic PTSD who are neither representative of males in general or of veterans in general.

5. Prospective studies are a very high priority. Two such trials have been reported: positive results in pediatric burn patients with ASD treated with imipramine, and negative findings with emergency room trauma survivors treated with clonazepam.

6. Recent FDA approval of sertraline as an indicated drug for treatment for PTSD is an important milestone in pharmacotherapy for this disorder that should affect current practice patterns and stimulate new research.

PSYCHOBIOLOGICAL VERSUS PSYCHOLOGICAL ALLOSTASIS IN PTSD

The following case example is a sober reminder that PTSD is not only a complicated disorder to treat from a psychobiological perspective but that psychological factors may sometimes overwhelm the most thoughtful allostatically conceptualized pharmacological approach.

Case 2: DG

DG was a 55-year-old married man without children who had been horribly abused, both physically and sexually, by his father and mother from early childhood through adolescence, when he ran away from home. He got married in his early 20s and functioned reasonably well as a manual laborer despite recurrent traumatic nightmares, avoidant behaviors, problems with intimacy, and startle/hypervigilant symptoms. At age 25 he suffered a severe back injury while logging in the woods. In addition to pain and movement restrictions, this injury precipitated an overwhelming sense of vulnerability and helplessness that produced severe intensification of PTSD symptoms with which he had coped prior to the accident. In fact, although his back recovered during the next 6 months, his PTSD symptoms worsened to such an extent that he was unable to resume work because of his psychiatric disability. He remained incapacitated because of PTSD for the next 30 years.

He was referred by his primary care practitioner, who was currently prescribing an adrenergic beta receptor antagonist, metoprolol (similar to propranolol), for his elevated blood pressure, which was partially effective, and a sleeping medication for his insomnia, which was completely ineffective.

DG was an intense, agitated, unhappy man who was extremely jumpy, mistrustful, and hopeless. He thought constantly about his childhood trauma and had distressing nightmares of such events on a daily basis that were so intense that he was afraid to go to sleep. In fact, his wife reported that he was so jumpy and apprehensive at night that she had reluctantly decided to sleep in another room since she felt that she needed her nocturnal rest to attend to his many emotional needs and physical complaints during the day. Other prominent PTSD symptoms were avoidance of thoughts, feelings, stimuli or situations that might evoke traumatic memories, social withdrawal, arousal symptoms, and psychic numbing that was easily and frequently overwhelmed by trauma-related feelings and memories.

Since he was already receiving a beta blocker, metoprolol, for hypertension, I increased the dose (rather than prescribe clonidine) with the expectation that it would take the edge off his arousal symptoms and might attenuate the re-experiencing symptoms as well. When DG reported some daytime benefit from metoprolol in the predicted direction, I suggested that he take it at bedtime with the hope that it might reduce his nocturnal anxiety sufficiently so that he might get some sleep. Two days later he phoned to announce that "that medication made me worse, Doc. It makes me so nervous that I won't take it anymore."

On careful questioning, he reported that the exact same dose of metoprolol that reduced anxiety and other symptoms during the day made him much worse at night. Given his refusal to try it at bedtime again, I suggested that he once again take the metoprolol twice a day, in the morning and at noon. He did so, with the same benefit as before, although he complained that he was so drowsy during the day that he sometimes couldn't get out of his chair.

Given his bitter distress about persistent insomnia, I then prescribed a small dose of trazodone at bedtime. Again he phoned within a few days with the same complaint—that trazodone made him unbearably anxious and wakeful at night. Again, when trazodone was rescheduled for daytime administration, it made him drowsy.

From a pharmacological perspective, it was impossible for me to explain how the same dose of the same drugs (both metoprolol and trazodone) had diametrically opposite effects depending on whether they were taken at bedtime or during daylight hours. I concluded that, since all of his sexual and physical abuse had occurred at night, it was too dangerous from a PTSD perspective for DG to make himself vulnerable at night, lest he be assaulted once again. In short, I concluded that DG could not respond to any medication that would blunt his hypervigilance or make him lose consciousness at night because of persistent trauma-related fears from childhood.

I believe that this vignette illustrates the difference between clinical pharmacology and therapeutics in PTSD treatment: DG's paradoxical response to two different medications cannot be understood pharmacologically. His response is not paradoxical, however, when the difference between his daytime and nighttime psychological states are taken into consideration. Medications that during the day successfully reduced his PTSD symptoms blunted his ability to protect himself at night. Even though the medications were the same, DG was not the same person at these two different times of day. This may show that psychological allostasis (e.g., a steady state promoting hypervigilance and a defensive posture) was more salient than psychobiological allostasis with regard to alterations in key neurotransmitter/neurohormonal systems. On the other hand, it may also suggest that allostatic load may itself sometimes have a diurnal variation, so that psychobiological as well as psychological steady states may exhibit crucial differences at different times of day. Whatever the explanation, from a therapeutics perspective it made no sense to prescribe an antiadrenergic or sleeping medication at night. I told this to DG and gave him my reasons for this decision. He agreed that that made sense. Hence, my current attempts to help him are focused entirely on efforts to improve his PTSD symptoms during the day.

PHARMACOTHERAPY AS A PSYCHOTHERAPEUTIC INTERACTION

Pharmacotherapy is much more than clinical assessment and writing prescriptions. The patient and psychiatrist participate in a relationship which has therapeutic potential beyond the normalization of psychobiological abnormalities.

My own technique is a Rogerian approach (Rogers, 1951) in which the patient and I are in an active collaboration to reduce his or her distress. I am the expert on medications, while the patient is the expert on him- or herself. We both must share information and observations that each of us is uniquely positioned to provide. Although we speak about thoughts, feelings, behaviors, symptoms, interpersonal relationships, and side effects, the implicit communication is about acceptance and promotion of self-efficacy. In short, therapeutic momentum is always toward empowerment to help the patient acquire more control over his or her life.

Since an important aspect of PTSD is a pervasive sense of helplessness and personal incompetence, I believe that any treatment that promotes empowerment is an effective therapeutic approach. In other words, pharmacotherapy can also be an effective psychotherapeutic intervention.

Therefore, this approach not only provides a more efficient and accurate strategy for selecting the correct drug and finding the optimal dose, it also provides a context in which promotion of empowerment clearly enhances the benefits achieved with medication.

CONCLUSIONS

It is an exciting time. New discoveries about the psychobiology of the human stress response and about the pathophysiology of PTSD continue to expand our understanding of this complex disorder. At the same time, renewed interest in testing recently developed medications holds great promise that more effective treatments will be discovered in the foreseeable future. My hope is that these two initiatives will not continue to proceed on parallel paths, as has been the case to date, but will soon intersect. As we begin the new century, it is heartening to realize that new classes of drugs currently under development may more effectively target stress-related mechanisms in general and PTSD allostasis in particular. I have suggested elsewhere some specific classes of new pharmacological agents that might address the unique pathophysiology of PTSD. Among such medications are the following: CRF antagonists; NPY agonists; substance P (a peptide neurotransmitter) antagonists; anticonvulsants with antikindling/antisensitization properties; agents that can downregulate glucocorticoid receptors; more specific serotonergic agents; medications to normalize opioid function; and agents affecting glutamatergic mechanisms that might ameliorate dissociation, memory, and information processing problems associated with PTSD (Friedman, 2000). We can certainly look to the future with anticipation and with the hope that we will not have to wait too much longer for the development of more effective medications for PTSD.

REFERENCES

Aston-Jones, G., Valentino, R. J., Van Bockstaele, E. J., & Meyerson, A. T. (1994). Locus coeruleus, stress, and PTSD: Neurobiological and clinical parallels. In M. Murburg (Ed.), *Catecholamine functions in post-traumatic stress disorder: Emerging concepts* (pp. 17–62). Washington, DC: American Psychiatric Press.

Baker, D. G., Diamond, B. I., & Gillette, G., et al. (1995). A double-blind, randomized placebo-controlled multi-center study of brofaromine in the treatment of post-traumatic stress disorder. *Psychopharmacology, 122*, 386–389.

Brady, K., Pearlstein, T., Asnis, G. M., Baker, D., Rothbaum, B., Sikes, C. R., & Farfel, G. M. (2000). Efficacy and safety of sertraline treatment of posttraumatic stress disorder: A randomized controlled trial. *Journal of the American Medical Association, 283*, 1837–1844.

Brady, K. T., Sonne, S. C., & Roberts, J. M. (1995). Sertraline treatment of comorbid posttraumatic stress disorder and alcohol dependence. *Journal of Clinical Psychiatry, 56*, 502–505.

Braun, P., Greenberg, D., Dasberg, H., et al. (1990). Core symptoms of posttraumatic stress disorder unimproved by alprazolam treatment. *Journal of Clinical Psychiatry, 51*, 236–238.

Bremner, J. D., Licino, J., Darnell, A., et al. (1997). Elevated CSF corticotropin-releasing factor concentrations in posttraumatic stress disorders. *American Journal of Psychiatry, 154*, 624–629.

Cook, M. D., & Conner, J. (1995). Retrospective review of hypnotic use in combination with fluoxetine or sertraline. *Clinical Drug Investigations, 9*, 212–216.

Davidson, J., Kudler, H., Smith, R., et al. (1990). Treatment of post-traumatic stress disorder with amitriptyline and placebo. *Archives of General Psychiatry, 47,* 259–266.

Davidson, J., Landburg, P. D., Pearlstein, T., et al. (1997). *Double-blind comparison of sertraline and placebo in patients with posttraumatic stress disorder (PTSD).* Abstract of paper presented at the 36th annual meeting of the American College of Neuropsychopharmacology, San Juan, Puerto Rico.

Davidson, J. R. T., Malik, M. L., & Sutherland, S. M. (1996). Response characteristics to antidepressants and placebo in post-traumatic stress disorder. *International Clinical Psychopharmacology, 12,* 291–296.

DeMartino, R., Mollica, R. F., & Wilk, V. (1995). Monoamine oxidase inhibitors in posttraumatic stress disorder. *Journal of Nervous and Mental Diseases, 183,* 510–515.

Famularo, R., Kinscherff, R., & Fenton, T. (1988). Propranolol treatment for childhood post-traumatic stress disorder, acute type: A pilot study. *American Journal of Diseases of Childhood, 142,* 1244–1247.

Foa, E. B., Davidson, J. R. T., & Frances, A. (Eds.). (1999). The expert consensus guideline series: Treatment of posttraumatic stress disorder. *Journal of Clinical Psychiatry, 60*(Suppl. 16), 1–18.

Friedman, M. J. (1997). Drug treatment for PTSD: Answers and questions. *Annals of the New York Academy of Sciences, 821,* 359–371.

Friedman, M. J. (1998). Current and future drug treatment for post-traumatic stress disorder patients. *Psychiatric Annals, 28,* 461–468.

Friedman, M. J. (1990). Interrelationships between biological mechanisms and pharmacotherapy of post-traumatic stress disorder. In M. E. Wolfe & A. D. Mosnaim (Eds.), *Post-traumatic stress disorder: Etiology, phenomenology, and treatment* (pp. 204–225). Washington, DC: American Psychiatric Press.

Friedman, M. J. (2000). What might the psychobiology of PTSD teach us about future approaches to pharmacotherapy? *Journal of Clinical Psychiatry, 61*(Suppl. 7), 44–51.

Friedman, M. J., Charney, D. S., & Deutch, A. Y. (1995). *Neurobiological and clinical consequences of stress: From normal adaptation to post-traumatic stress disorder.* Philadelphia: Lippincott-Raven Press.

Friedman, M. J., Davidson, J. R. T., Mellman, T. A., & Southwick, S. M. (2000). Pharmacotherapy. In E. B. Foa, T. M. Keane, & M. J. Friedman (Eds.), *Effective treatments for PTSD: Practice guidelines from the International Society for Traumatic Stress Studies* (pp. 84–105). New York: Guilford Press.

Friedman, M. J., & Southwick, S. M. (1995). Towards pharmacotherapy for PTSD. In M. J. Friedman, D. S. Charney, & A. Y. Deutch (Eds.), *Neurobiological and clinical consequences of stress: From normal adaptation to post-traumatic stress disorder* (pp. 465–481). Philadelphia: Lippincott-Raven Press.

Gelpin, E., Bonne, O., Peri, T., Brandes, D., & Shalev, A. (1996). Treatment of recent trauma survivors with benzodiazepines: A prospective study. *Journal of Clinical Psychiatry, 57,* 390–394.

Glover, H. (1993). A preliminary trial of nalmefane for the treatment of emotional numbing in combat veterans with post-traumatic stress disorder. *Israel Journal of Psychiatry and Related Sciences, 30,* 255–263.

Hamner, M. B. (1996). Clozapine treatment for a veteran with comorbid psychosis and PTSD [Letter]. *American Journal of Psychiatry, 153,* 841.

Hertzberg, M. A., Feldman, M. E., Beckham, J. C., & Davidson, J. R. T. (1996). Trial of trazodone for posttraumatic stress disorder using a multiple baseline group design. *Journal of Clinical Psychopharmacology, 16,* 294–298.

Hertzberg, M. A., Feldman, M. E., Beckham, J. C., Moore, S. D., & Davidson, J. R. T. (1998). Open trial of nefazodone for combat-related posttraumatic stress disorder. *Journal of Clinical Psychiatry, 59,* 460–464.

Horrigan, J. P. (1996). Guanfacine for PTSD nightmares [Letter]. *Journal of the American Academy of Child and Adolescent Psychiatry, 35,* 975–976.

Jacobs-Rebhun, S., Schnurr, P. P., Friedman, M. J., Peck, R., Brophy, M., & Fuller, D. (2000). Cyproheptadine for treating PTSD [Letter to the editor]. *American Journal of Psychiatry, 157,* 1525–1526.

Katz, R. J., Lott, M. H., Arbus, P., et al. (1994/95). Pharmacotherapy of post-traumatic stress disorder with a novel psychotropic. *Anxiety, 1,* 169–174.

Kolb, L. C., Burris, B. C., & Griffiths, S. (1984). Propranolol and clonidine in the treatment of the chronic post-traumatic stress disorders of war. In B. A. van der Kolk (Ed.), *Post-traumatic stress disorder: Psychological and biological sequelae* (pp. 97–107). Washington, DC: American Psychiatric Press.

Kosten, T. R., Frank, J. B., Dan, E., et al. (1991). Pharmacotherapy for post-traumatic stress disorder using phenelzine or imipramine. *Journal of Nervous and Mental Diseases, 179,* 366–370.

Marmar, C. R., Schoenfeld, F., Weiss, D. S., et al. (1996). Open trial of fluvoxamine treatment for combat-related posttraumatic stress disorder. *Journal of Clinical Psychiatry, 57*(Suppl. 8), 66–72.

Marshall, R. D., Schneier, F. R., Fallon, B. A., et al. (1998). An open trial of paroxetine in patients with noncombat-related, chronic posttraumatic stress disorder. *Journal of Clinical Psychopharmacology, 18,* 10–18.

Mason, J. W., Wang, S., Yehuda, R., Bremner, J. D., Riney, S. J., Lubin, H., Johnson, D. R., Southwick, S. M., & Charney, D. S. (1995). Some approaches to the study of the clinical implications of thyroid alterations in post-traumatic stress disorder. In M. J. Friedman, D. S. Charney, & A. Y. Deutch (Eds.), *Neurobiological and clinical consequences of stress: From normal adaptation to post-traumatic stress disorder* (pp. 367–379). Philadelphia: Lippincott-Raven Press.

McEwen, B. S. (1998). Protective and damaging effects of stress mediators. *New England Journal of Medicine, 338,* 171–179.

McEwen, B. S., & Stellar, E. (1993). Stress and the individual: Mechanisms leading to disease. *Archives of Internal Medicine, 153,* 2093–2101.

Mellman, T. A., Byers, P. M., & Augenstein, J. S. (1998). Pilot evaluation of hypnotic medication during acute traumatic stress response. *Journal of Traumatic Stress, 11,* 563–569.

Michelson, D., Licinio, J., & Gold, P. W. (1995). Mediation of the stress response by the hypothalamic–pituitary–adrenal axis. In M. J. Friedman, D. S. Charney, & A. Y. Deutch (Eds.), *Neurobiological and clinical consequences of stress: From normal adaptation to post-traumatic stress disorder* (pp. 225–238). Philadelphia: Lippincott-Raven Press.

Morgan, C. A., Wang, S., Southwick, S. M., Rasmusson, A., Hazlett, G., Hauger, R. L., & Charney, D. S. (2000). Plasma neuropeptide-Y concentrations in humans exposed to highly intense uncontrollable stress. *Biological Psychiatry, 47,* 902–909.

Mueser, K. T., & Butler, R. W. (1987). Auditory hallucinations in combat-related chronic post-traumatic stress disorder. *American Journal of Psychiatry, 144*, 299–302.

Mueser, K. T., Goodman, L. A., Trumbetta, S. L., Rosenberg, S. D., Osher, F. C., Vidaver, R., Auciello, P., & Foy, D. W. (1998). Trauma and posttraumatic stress disorder in severe mental illness. *Journal of Consulting and Clinical Psychology, 66*, 493–499.

Neal, L. A., Shapland, W., & Fox, C. (1997). An open trial of moclobemide in the treatment of post-traumatic stress disorder. *International Clinical Psychopharmacology, 12*, 231–237.

Perry, B. D. (1994). Neurobiological sequelae of childhood trauma: PTSD in children. In M. Murburg (Ed.), *Catecholamine function in posttraumatic stress disorder: Emerging concepts* (pp. 233–255). Washington, DC: American Psychiatric Press.

Pitman, R. K., Orr, S. P., Shalev, A. Y., Metzger, L. J., & Mellman, T. A. (1999). Psychophysiological alterations in post-traumatic stress disorder. *Seminars in Clinical Neuropsychiatry, 4*, 234–241.

Pitman, R. K., van der Kolk, B. A., Orr, S. P., & Greenberg, M. S. (1990). Naloxone-reversible analgesic response to combat-related stimuli in post traumatic stress disorder. *Archives of General Psychiatry, 47*, 541–544.

Post, R. M., Weiss, S. R. B., Li, H., Leverich, G. S., & Pert, A. (1999). Sensitization components of post-traumatic stress disorder: Implications for therapeutics. *Seminars in Clinical Neuropsychiatry, 4*, 282–294.

Post, R. M., Weiss, S. R. B., & Smith, M. A. (1995). Sensitization and kindling: Implications for the evolving neural substrate of PTSD. In M. J. Friedman, D. S. Charney, & A. Y. Deutch (Eds.), *Neurobiological and clinical consequences of stress: From normal adaptation to post-traumatic stress disorder* (pp. 203–204). Philadelphia: Lippincott-Raven Press.

Reist, C., Kauffman, C. D., Haier, R. J., et al. (1989). A controlled trial of desipramine in 18 men with post-traumatic stress disorder. *American Journal of Psychiatry, 146*, 513–516.

Risse, S. C., Whitters, A., Burke, J., Chen, S., Scurfield, R. M., & Raskind, M. A. (1990). Severe withdrawal symptoms after discontinuation of alprazolam in eight patients with combat-induced post-traumatic stress disorder. *Journal of Clinical Psychiatry, 51*, 206–209.

Robert, R., Blakeney, P. E., Villarreal, C., Rosenberg, L., & Mayer, W. J. (1999). Imipramine treatment in pediatric burn patients with symptoms of acute stress disorder: A pilot study. *Journal of the American Academy of Child and Adolescent Psychiatry, 38*, 873–878.

Rogers, C. R. (1951). *Client-centered therapy.* Boston: Houghton Mifflin.

Rothbaum, B. O., Ninan, P. T., & Thomas, L. (1996). Sertraline in the treatment of rape victims with posttraumatic stress disorder. *Journal of Traumatic Stress, 9*, 865–871.

Shestatzky, M., Greenberg, D., & Lerer, B. (1988). A controlled trial of phenelzine in post-traumatic stress disorder. *Psychiatry Research, 24*, 149–155.

Southwick, S. M., Krystal, J. H., Bremner, J. D., et al. (1997). Noradrenergic and serotonergic function in posttraumatic stress disorder. *Archives of General Psychiatry, 54*, 749–758.

Southwick, S. M., Paige, S., Morgan, C. A., Bremner, J. D., Krystal, J. H., & Charney, D. S. (1999). Neurotransmitter alterations in PTSD: Catecholamines and serotonin. *Seminars in Clinical Neuropsychiatry, 4,* 242–248.

Southwick, S. M., Yehuda, R., Giller, E. L., et al. (1994). Use of tricyclics and monoamine oxidase inhibitors in the treatment of PTSD: A quantitative review. In M. M. Murburg (Ed.), *Catecholamine function in post-traumatic stress disorder: Emerging concepts* (pp. 293–305). Washington, DC: American Psychiatric Press.

Stout, S. C., Kilts, C. D., & Nemeroff, C. B. (1995). Neuropeptides and stress: Preclinical findings and implications for pathophysiology. In M. J. Friedman, D. S. Charney, & A. Y. Deutch (Eds.), *Neurobiological and clinical consequences of stress: From normal adaptation to post-traumatic stress disorder* (pp. 103–123). Philadelphia: Lippincott-Raven Press.

van der Kolk, B. A., Dryfuss, D., Michaels, M., et al. (1994). Fluoxetine in post-traumatic stress disorder. *Journal of Clinical Psychiatry, 55,* 517–522.

ver Ellen, P., & van Kammen, D. P. (1990). The biological findings in post-traumatic stress disorder: A review. *Journal of Applied Social Psychology, 20*(21, Pt. 1), 1789–1821.

Wang, S., & Mason, J. (1999). Elevations of serum T3 levels and their association with symptoms in World War II veterans with combat-related post-traumatic stress disorder: Replication of findings in Vietnam combat veterans. *Psychosomatic Medicine, 61,* 131–138.

Yehuda, R. (1999). Linking the neuroendocrinology of post-traumatic stress disorder with recent neuroanatomic findings. *Seminars in Clinical Neuropsychiatry, 4,* 256–265.

Yehuda, R., Levengood, R. A., Schmeidler, J., Wilson, S., Guo, L. S., & Gerber, D. K. (1996). Increased pituitary activation following metyrapone administration in post-traumatic stress disorder. *Psychoneuroendocrinology, 21,* 1–16.

Yehuda, R., Southwick, S. M., Krystal, J. H., Bremner, J. D., Charney, D. S., & Mason, J. W. (1993). Enhanced suppression of cortisol following dexamethasone administration in posttraumatic stress disorder. *American Journal of Psychiatry, 150,* 83–86.

5

An Allostatic Approach to the Psychodynamic Understanding of PTSD

JACOB D. LINDY and JOHN P. WILSON

One of the thematic underpinnings of this book is to examine posttraumatic stress disorder (PTSD) from the vantage point of allostasis, that is, complex and interrelated systems which in response to severe stress keeps the organism in an altered but more or less steady state of adaptation. Earlier chapters of this book have addressed allostasis in PTSD from the points of view of neuroendocrine and neuroanatomical systems (Chapter 2 by Wilson, Friedman, and Lindy) and psychological systems (Chapter 4 by Friedman), considering the ways in which these different perspectives alter treatment approaches. In the present chapter, we discuss how a psychodynamic understanding of allostasis enables clinicians to address stable patterns of interrelated maladaptation. Further, psychodynamic therapy is more empathic and effective when the defensive purposes of allostasis are understood.

FROM THE TERMINOLOGY OF DEFENSE TO ALLOSTASIS

The terminology of traditional psychoanalytic (i.e., dynamic) psychotherapy owes its origins to 19th-century theories of thermodynamics in the physical sciences. Sigmund Freud was, like his *fin de siècle* scientific colleagues, intrigued with advances in the understanding of thermodynamic forces, of flow of energy (emergence, pressure, and breakthrough) and resistance to that flow (friction, repression, turbulence, and countercurrents). While he hypothesized first a positive unconscious energy (libido) and later a negative entropy-seeking energy (destrudo), he was of a mind that these dynamic forces operated according to scientific laws and that some day the neuroanatomical and physiological underpinnings of these forces would be known.

In general he presumed these laws would be consistent with Hegelian dialectical principles holding that both human history and natural evolution were unfolding in a continuing process in which opposing forces, theses and antitheses, compromised and coalesced to form new syntheses along an infinite series. He thought of the regulating or homeostatic state as one conforming to both a "pleasure principle" and a "reality principle" in which the organism's ego compromised between the opposing forces of unconscious drives and the demands of civilization. In his prepsychoanalytic days (Freud, 1895/1966) he saw these principles at work in the interaction of actual physical substances in the nervous system. Even later, he would return from time to time to his roots as a neurologist, envisioning an era in which his law-oriented, dialectical metaphoric language might become rooted in neurophysiology.

As just noted, in Freud's original language he termed the flow of highly charged unconscious content into the realm of thought or action as "drives." He thought of those forces which opposed or contained such drives as the similarly unconscious forces of repression. Later psychoanalysts would come to identify many ego mechanisms at work along the repression barrier and, after the study of borderline and narcissistic disorders, would divide defense constellations along a spectrum ranging from archaic or primitive defenses (i.e., splitting, projective identification, somatization, denial, dissociation, and omnipotent and paranoid thinking) through intermediate defenses (i.e., displacement, externalization, isolation, reversal, identification with the aggressor, and counterphobia) to more advanced defenses (i.e., intellectualization, sublimation, creativity, humor, and wisdom) (A. Freud, 1966; Kernberg, 1971; Kohut, 1966).

PSYCHOANALYSIS AND ALLOSTASIS

Sigmund Freud would have found it intriguing and challenging to bring the language of defense into alignment with the language of altered neurohumoral circuits or allostasis. He would understand that the energy required for splitting, disavowal, and magical thinking to defend against the incessant demands of traumatic disruption to the repression barrier would wear down the organism, leading to a new steady state, one which was, for example, numb, avoidant, and alienated. As new or recurrent trauma-related stressors strain the defensive psychological constellations trying to protect the organism, there is malfunction of neurohormonal networks. In other words, allostatic load and allostasis are both physiological and psychological phenomena. *As with Freud's model of the psyche, allostatic models are epiphenomenal representations of organismic functioning.*

Indeed, as we examine patients with chronic PTSD in analytic psychotherapy, we see not a temporary aberration from a homeostatic state but an organism chronically distressed as it uses more maladaptive (pathological) defenses trying to hold at bay the disruptive breakthrough of trauma.

FREUD'S METHODS AND THE PATHOGNOMONIC TRANSFERENCES OF PTSD

Freud, who was unable on his own to complete his ideas on the psychodynamic pathology in the traumatic neuroses (Freud, 1919/1955), would have insisted that psychoanalysts systematically collect their experiences relating to the pathognomonic transferences which arise in PTSD much as he did for hysteria. He would then want to know what intrapsychic systems became engaged in the treatment and, in particular, which ones permitted the patient to recover, to grow, or to restore former function. For example, in disorders characterized by guilt, sexual inhibition, and symbolic somatization, Freud found through transference that "cure" occurred when the patient not only understood the meaning of fantasies and symptoms but was able to replace an excessively rigid superego with a more benign, flexible superego which he or she found present in the analyst. Hysteria, Freud concluded, was structurally a disorder of the superego drive system. He would have asked (Strachey, 1934): Are there comparable processes at work in patients with PTSD, so that we can locate the site of intrapsychic damage?

We believe that strides have been made in this direction (Lindy, 1989; Lindy & Wilson, 1994) and that, on the basis of studying transference and the restoration of function in patients with PTSD, we can identify three intrapsychic systems at risk for impairment in the disorder: (1) the perceptual system, (2) the affect-regulating system, and (3) the self-esteem system. We explore each of these in the following sections, illustrating allostatic maladaptations which have replaced homeostasis, and demonstrating how these posttraumatic dysfunctional systems become engaged in the therapeutic process and how attention to the protective function that allostasis serves can assist the therapist and the patient.

THREE DYSFUNCTIONAL SYSTEMS IN PTSD: PERCEPTION, AFFECT, AND SELF-REFERENCE

In PTSD, chronic defensive operations leading to allostasis or posttraumatic character change (Titchener & Kapp, 1976) evolve primarily for three reasons: (1) to preempt perceptive distortion, (2) to numb or control affect dysregulation, and (3) to disavow self-fragmentation. Survivors with PTSD are all too aware that unless they guard themselves carefully, misperceptions will re-create the traumatic condition; that unless they block out certain emotions, they will be overwhelmed in the present precipitating affect dysregulation; and that unless they adopt a discontinuous, constricted view of themselves and the world, they are exposing themselves to disillusionment and despair. This new alloplastic equilibrium comes at a great personal cost and further distances these survivors from intimate relationships. It damages work and destroys ambition.

PERCEPTUAL DYSFUNCTION IN PTSD

In PTSD, perceptual functioning can become reequilibrated at a pathological level following trauma. The evenly hovering attention with which we normally scan our horizon enables us to pick up and respond smoothly to both expectable and unexpectable events of day-to-day living. As we drive down a street, we are alert to anything outside the routine—to the child who is about to run into the street, to the cyclist nearby who is unsteady, or to the car ahead which seems to be weaving. These are preparatory signals which alert us to a state of readiness but do not startle us into premature action. We may momentarily grip the wheel with firmness or slow down. After the momentary threat, our perception reequilibrates at its homeostatic position.

But posttraumatically disrupted patients find it impossible to maintain that evenly hovering attention. Rather, in order not to stumble inadvertently onto a replay of the traumatic situation, their perception is hyperalert, suspicious of massive trauma conditions which threaten life or bodily integrity. To preempt being overwhelmed, all modes of sensory perception are prepared to identify (or misidentify) the trauma situation and to institute emergency efforts to prevent it or survive in it once it has been identified. The perceptual apparatus is reset at an allostatic level. Startle replaces signal; action replaces thought. Dissociation replaces ego activity. Traumatic dreams replace normal ones which ordinarily protect sleep, while sleep itself is perceived as dangerous rather than as a replenisher. When asked about their symptoms, posttraumatically disturbed patients say that they are tense, anxious, unable to cooperate, sleepless, and irritable.

How do survivors with PTSD use the clinical situation and the presence of the analytic therapist to engage and then alter this disequilibrium, this perceptual and psychobiologically based allostasis? In treatment, trauma survivors defend against and then gradually experience the therapist's office as a safe place. They defend against and then gradually accepts the therapist's intention to help. They narrate external events and then reveal in the sessions their distress at PTSD-related misperceptions. Subtle verbal and nonverbal cues such as disruptive sounds or activities including those of the therapist illustrate problems with perception. As the alliance grows, not only does the survivor understand better what sets off these disruptions and misperceptions, but they also come to rely on the therapist's input to modify thier own assessment of external danger. Each patient will only alter his or her pathological hyperalertness if there is something safe to replace it. He or she will not relinquish defenses against perceived and emotionally experienced vulnerability until a genuine sense of trust and safety exist. *The therapist comes to play a role "as if" he or she is located at the site of the damaged perceptual apparatus. Now the therapist is able with the patient's help to elaborate trauma-specific meanings of such sounds and perceptions from within the trauma perspective to help the patient find words to name such phenomena and the distressing states of mind they set in motion.* As already mentioned by Wilson, Friedman, & Lindy in Chapters 1 and 2, this ego state is the configuration of trauma-specific PTSD and all of its derivatives. It is the phenomenological manifestation of PTSD for the patient.

In the following case a hyperalert allostasis was interfering with adjustment to the trauma survivor's current tasks. Residual war trauma became animated due to states of vulnerability caused by illness.

Allostasis, Ego Vulnerability, and PTSD Transformation

Frank is a 50-year-old veteran of combat in the Vietnam War whose chronic PTSD and adaptations to it made it difficult to cooperate with doctors as he later experienced the debilitating effects of a life-threatening lymphoma and chemotherapy. Asked to lead his squad on numerous long-range reconnaissance and search-and-destroy missions, Frank had responded with high energy and a no-stretch-is-too-great attitude. Asked now to rest in order to recover from his chemotherapy, Frank could only respond by the PTSD-related adaptation of heroic action, thereby worsening his condition. In the treatment Frank searched for and found in the therapist a presence which warned of danger and valued conserving energy, dosing it for current tasks. The therapist interpreted how the patient's understandable coping styles growing from his experiences in the field of combat now stood in the way of recovery from his medical condition. At the same time the therapist functioned in a protective role as a calmer, more reliable and perceptive individual. Gradually Frank's allostatic load from the current stress of illness reequilibrated. Signaling his arrival at a new allostatic state, he reported a dream in which he saw in his peripheral vision the comforting presence of a soldier on sentry duty who was looking out for him, protecting him from tasks that would involve too much fatigue. The figure in the dream seemed to represent a calmer and more reliable perceptive system which allowed him to rest when he needed it most. It also seemed to be representing the internalization of the therapist's function, integrating the treatment efforts into cognitive processing of the "flow" of memory activated by therapy.

In the next case, treatment helped a PTSD patient to restore the capacity to delay potentially self-destructive behaviors following perception of threat.

Allostasis, Perceived Threat, and Affect Modulation

Mitch had been a scout in the Vietnam War. As a "tunnel rat" he took risks to explore highly dangerous situations. In fact, that was his "job assignment" in Vietnam. He had been successful because of his caution, suspiciousness, and willingness to make preemptive (i.e., hyperalert) strikes. But now, many years later, rage attacks, set off by perceived threatening behavior by friends and family, including his wife, formed an ongoing allostatic load. The threat of outbursts led to his referral for treatment. Over time a strong trusting relationship developed with his therapist in which he disclosed the details of his many trauma experiences. His therapist explained that while the impulse toward protective preemptive action made sense in combat, it was destructive in current relationships. Gradually Mitch replaced abrupt rage attacks with the more measured thinking which his therapist demonstrated. Marking his improvement, Mitch described a curious event. A car nearly cut him off on the highway. Mitch at first reacted characteristically, feeling the impulse to retaliate by running that car off the road and bashing the driver's head against a tree. Becoming aware of these thoughts and the discomfort at them, he glanced for a moment in his rear view mirror perceiving a car on the track of the offending driver. He relaxed and slowed down, thinking to himself that the proper agent to reprimand the bad driver (a policeman) was in position to apprehend the offender, so Mitch could get on with his own business. He felt relief and noted a sharp decrease in his level of tension, with no need to retaliate even though, he later realized, the car behind turned out not to be that of a policeman.

Mitch and his therapist thought this symbolized the beginning of a restoration of control over rage attacks as they had existed before the stressful motor vehicle event. The phenomenon represents his restoring an earlier function: the judicious flow between perception, its processing, and delay of affect release in action, processes which he seemed to relearn through his work in treatment.

AFFECT DYSREGULATION IN PTSD

Affect regulation has been severely disturbed in PTSD. Ordinarily the emergence and awareness of emotional states is a useful and integral part of healthy functioning. We become aware of anger or shame, for example, and then allow these feelings to bring to mind an emotional configuration which relegates meaning to the affect and guides us in our further thoughts and plans. For example, the information is useful that we are angry when something is interfering or disrupting our plans. It leads us to remove the annoying element, provided that this creates no harm, and/or alter our behavior or expectations, assess the situation and its context, and respond adaptively. The information, for example, that we are feeling shame might usefully inform us to back up from an exhibitionistic plan. Also, we have some capacity to block off disruptive emotion when such emotion adversely affects our ability to integrate a configuration of information correctly. Thus, both awareness of affect and ability to reduce affect intensity are within the ego's adaptive capacity. But the posttraumatically disturbed person has lost this comfort with affect as a useful, informative, and controllable part of psychic functioning. *The posttraumatically injured person tries desperately to ward off a state of uncontrollable rage, anxiety, helplessness, shame, or guilt. In order to protect against setting into motion affective dyscontrol, the PTSD patient disavows the offending affect and feels numb.* On the one hand, the PTSD sufferer notes that he or she has a tendency to lash out and fears that his or her anger will get out of control; on the other hand, there is an unconscious resort to numbness in an attempt, often unsuccessful, to suppress these affect-driven impulses.

Because affect discharge is connected with extreme states and trauma-related fantasies (often unconsciously driven by prior trauma), its presence is only a sign that things are out of control. In psychodynamic terms, affect has lost its signal function (Freud, 1919/1955). Powerful affects such as disgust, rage, and shame cease to alert the mental apparatus of a situation that needs to be understood so that appropriate action can be taken. Rather, such affects overload the psychic apparatus, constituting an overwhelming and abhorrent experience in the present. Once overwhelmed, there is no observing ego nor self-soothing functions to help process and manage the state. The actual nonverbal behavior during the affect overload may in fact constitute a trauma reenactment. Stated simply, one form of allostasis is simply that of a system out of control. Numbing of affect now produces a temporary salutary effect. *It minimizes the risk of overreaction; numbing becomes the defensive (or allostatic) counterpart of reenactment.* Posttraumatically disturbed persons make great efforts to keep their emotions under control; to block out intrusive reminders of the trauma, and to reestablish an equilibrium albeit at an allostatic level which diminishes healthy optimal adaptation. For purposes of this discussion we divide the way in which allostasis, as defense against affect overload, enters the treatment situation from the way in which allostasis as numbing enters the clinical picture.

Affect Overload and Psychic Numbing: Allostatic Sides of a Coin

We begin with affect overload because in some instances this state is a major part of the presenting set of symptoms flooding the clinical picture, well before any significant clinical understanding or therapeutic alliance has been built.

In the following case displaced hyperalertness regarding her children was a thin barrier covering the patient's childhood trauma. Hyperalertness was the trauma-specific cue to traumatic memory and reenactments.

Annette, a 35-year-old mother of two preschool children, was referred by her pediatrician because she was hypervigilant in monitoring normal gastrointestinal functions of her children. In her sessions, tension was rising as she pressed herself for some memories which could explain her anxieties. Her therapist suggested that she was displacing her own anxieties onto the children and said, "The next time we will need to go deeper." During the next session, she dissociated, writhing on the floor in agony, then leaping up and turning the light on and off. Trying to help her settle down, the therapist poured her some water. But the sound of the water precipitated another round of severe dissociation. Later, clues from the dissociated behavior led Annette to recover the memory that her mother had given her frequent stimulating and painful enemas when she had a fecal blockage as a toddler. Her mother, frantic that surgery would be necessary, administered the high-powered enemas with great energy while the child screamed out of control. The enemas were themselves a form of intrusive, controlled violation of the child's body. Once words were placed on the traumatic reenactment which had occurred in the office, Annette and her therapist jointly could piece together the sources of her hypervigilance with her children and this allostatic adaptation disappeared. Her behaviors were dual levels of reenactment of her own trauma.

Allostasis and the Therapeutic Alliance

How does the therapist respond when affect overload enters the therapeutic space, especially before a solid therapeutic alliance is built? First, the therapist distinguishes between abreaction, often characterized by unworkable affect overload, and dosed dysphoric affect states, which are more limited in nature and therefore more amenable to potentially working through. Here the therapist has a dosing function. When this dosing is impossible, as is often the case in the first onslaught of traumatic material, the psychodynamic therapist functions as the "container for affect overload" (i.e., being there during the reaction, without making demands or judgments, or stimulating shame while the patient is out of control). The therapist must maintain his or her own boundaries even as the patient, under the throws of expectable traumatic regression, challenges the therapist to lose sight of those boundaries by rescuing, rejecting, nurturing, reacting counterphobically, or acting out. The therapist empathizes with the discomfort of the out-of-control feeling and then, later, when the patient has regained emotional composure, reconstructs with the patient those events which seem to link up with the overwhelmed response. Together with the patient's "observing ego," the therapist attempts to help the survivor find words to identify the landmarks and transition points of the analytic process. In all of this, the therapist has attempted to provide a temporary psychic structure to contain allostatic load. But it is precisely at this juncture that the therapist needs to know how to use trauma-specific transference interpretation to facilitate processing countertransference in him- or herself.

By carefully monitoring countertransference, the therapist will intuit spaces in the trauma sequence for which we have no firm data as yet but will be learning more, as for example, an inhibited revenge fantasy in the midst of humiliation and pain (Lindy & Wilson, 1994). The intent here is to further elaborate the "space" and psychic dimensions of the trauma itself. The analytic therapist links the onset of this episode to specifics in everyday experience and demonstrates the presence of the disturbed perception which triggered the event, thereby also demonstrating the plausibility of such affective responses given the traumatic origins on which the misperception is based. The therapist returns to early stages in the reaction and elaborates an unconscious decision tree which can potentially serve as a signal for the entire episode. The psychodynamically oriented therapist helps the patient search for words to encapsulate major configurations of the traumatic episode. The empathic attunement of the therapist then facilitates the patient's motivation to move toward cognitive processing and integration of stress and traumatic experiences.

Allostasis, Shame, and Defensive Compensation

In the next case, an allostatic adaptation, the incessant efforts to do good deeds, broke down as a protection against shame from trauma as an adult and as a child.

Tina, a woman in her mid-40s, had entered treatment with overwhelming anxiety, suicidal thoughts, and somatic dissociative reactions. At some level she was aware that her symptoms were connected with the anniversary of the death of her congenitally impaired 8-year-old child. During a brief psychodynamic treatment her therapist clarified the many emotions condensed in somatic reenactments which connected her with her dead child and helped her find words for these emotions with good results. She disliked side effects of fluoxetine (Prozac, an antidepressant) and preferred to keep the treatment free of medication rather than try other medications. Tina demonstrated an all-consuming allostatic (i.e., overdriven, hyperaroused motive) effort to help everyone in her life. She felt that she was allowed to live so long as she was the good "angel." She experienced her relationships as pervasively masochistic and was devastated when others attributed destructive intent to her actions. Because of these ongoing relationship difficulties, she decided to enter long-term psychotherapy.

In the midphase of treatment, prior to the end of each session, Tina would often cry in heaving sobs, unable to pass from the doctor's office into the hallway. Wishes to be understood in the hour had triggered wishes to be held by her father, who—under such circumstances—seduced her sexually as a child. She felt then the fused affects of longing, overstimulation, failure to achieve discharge, and intense shame (i.e., extreme allostatic dysregulation, which had become chronic). The release, in the presence of unmodulated shame, was in itself the offending agent. Undeniable shame in the present now interfered with the defensive or alloplastic solution which Tina had acquired at much personal expense over the years. Beneath the allostatic adaptation of being the angel of goodness "to all in need" was severe early childhood sexual trauma. While the content of the incest trauma could be reconstructed fairly quickly from the somatic reenactments in the office, there could not be effective work on the trauma (i.e., engagement of a healthy observing ego and dosed working through) until the intense shame at the breakthrough of affect overload recurring in the present could be understood, accepted, and contained.

Allostasis, Numbing, and Posttraumatic Decline

Numbing, as an aspect of affect dysregulation, can be seen as a defensive structure attempting to reequilibrate the mental apparatus in its allostatic form. It becomes an alternative to affect overload. But unfortunately for so many PTSD patients, the price is of the grave. Numbing constricts the experience of life in the present and its aspirations for the future, and it deprives relationships of their meaning. It leads to what Titchener and Kapp (1976) have called *posttraumatic decline*.

An analytic approach to numbing is to appreciate its value within the trauma context (i.e., protection from threatened affect overload). By patiently listening to that which the patient feels ready to share, the therapist builds a safe therapeutic space (Lindy & Wilson, 1994). The patient presenting with numbness has anything but a static "deserted" inner life. Rather, his or her dreams are rich in trauma content; the task is less to get to the bottom of all this and more to assess readiness to move deeper without causing harm. Thus, numbing calls on the therapist to appreciate and to empathize with energy involved in maintaining the numbed state. Numbing is an allostatic condition reflective of dysregulation. Blocks in communication in the present will help inform the trauma configuration, and waiting rather than plunging in will get the better results. The analytic therapist and the patient build a therapeutic alliance on what the patient can safely share and not on what the therapist in his or her zeal demands from the still unready patient.

Abraham, a veteran with PTSD, daily relived the death in his arms of a 12-year-old Vietnamese boy after he had shot the boy and his grandfather in a free-fire zone. But to the outside world Abraham only communicated a cut-off coldness interrupted by bursts of anger. It took over a year before he was ready to explain to the therapist that the Vietnamese boy (long dead) was present in the room with them and refused to go, fearing that Abraham might show affection for his own 12-year-old son. His therapist empathized with how attached he was to the boy he had killed and how much energy had been going into the preservation of his memory out of guilt for the wartime event. He explained that it took great courage and trust to share the boy's presence in the hope that he could move beyond where he had been stuck for so many years.

DISCONTINUITY IN SELF-STRUCTURE

Each day we awaken, confronted by today's challenges, and comforted to some degree by the knowledge that all our preceding life has helped us to cope with this day and to maximize its value to us. We are reassured when our values today are the same as they were yesterday, and our ambitions are continuous. We can plan and we can reflect. The future, while not necessarily as bright as we might want, is at least an extension of the past and likely to be a fully lived one. But posttraumatically disturbed persons awaken alienated from the persons they were pretraumatically. Their view of the world is of something unpredictable and malevolent, often a radically different view than they had before the trauma. A more cynical and fractured belief system and loss of self-soothing functions create a marked contrast between the pretrauma self and the posttrauma self. The deidealized functioning of self and objects within the trauma experience become generalized to most situations and therefore to most people. Expectations of self and others as part of what pretraumatically seemed a generally ethical, benevolent world are now altered in permanent ways. The future now seems dark and ominous. Posttraumatically, such persons often view themselves as indecisive and guilty, while their relationships with others are riddled with suspicion and mistrust.

Continuity and Dissociation in the Self and Clients' Mistrust of Therapists

How does discontinuity of self present itself in an allostatic form and affix itself to the treatment? PTSD sufferers bring with them to the potential treatment alliance a brittle hopefulness, one that can easily become discouraged and disillusioned. They are leery of overly optimistic promises and often reluctantly participate in the therapeutic endeavor; at some level they believe that this effort too will fail, confirming the uselessness of their wish to rebuild hope and confidence. They anticipate that the therapist will not understand why they have fallen short, as they believe they did in the trauma situation. Alternatively, they may attribute unrealistically ideal attributes to the therapist. The therapist needs to be comfortable both with idealizing and deidealizing, and anticipate that both will likely make their way into the treatment. As patients evaluate and reevaluate specific decision points within the trauma and magnify the impact of what they did or did not do, they are vulnerable to the therapist's overt or covert responses, confirming him or her in transference as a new perpetrator, false comforter, or condemning judge (Lindy & Wilson, 1994). In contrast to this, when the therapist is able to monitor and understand countertransference tendencies and to listen empathically and nonjudgmentally, he or she performs a soothing function. When the therapist is able to assist the survivor's own efforts to understand the sociocultural contributants to the trauma (e.g., the military strategy and tactics which produced the trauma circumstance, or the patriarchal structures which affected the rape and its processing by society), he is placing the traumatized self in a believable and authentic context, more readily continuous with the past.

POLITICAL OPPRESSION AND TORTURE: PSYCHODYNAMIC CASE ILLUSTRATION OF PTSD

Mihai, a former political prisoner in Eastern Europe during the Stalinist era, was forced to undergo continuous life-threatening, degrading and humiliating torture for many months (Cucliciu, in press). At one time he truly yielded internally to the power of the brainwashing and adopted the torturer's frame of reference, even participating in the beating of fellow prisoners (students) equally innocent of any crime. Subsequent guilt and shame for that betrayal of his own beliefs led to many years of self-doubt and self-recrimination, altering him from an outgoing and energetic person of lively conviction to an excessively cautious, inhibited, and frightened one. Only after the therapist was able to identify the tendency to yield to totalitarian authority in himself could he respond empathically to a phenomenon which affected two generations of people, not only Mihai but many others who suffered a similar fate.

TRAUMA AND REFORMULATION OF THE SELF

Sometimes the negative fragmented posttrauma self is hidden by unconscious efforts to replace it with another self born from defensive activity. Here the therapist may interpret the defensive function of regressing to grandiose omnipotent thinking in the face of trauma-producing circumstances as a more general and understandable human response to an enormously inhuman event in childhood. When therapists contain and accept retaliatory fantasies of sadistic counterattack, they oppose the view of the survivor as non-self. When they make plausible the context for actions and fantasies of the self and others in the trauma context while remaining morally centered in the process, they assist the process of meaning-making and sublimation of experience.

Damage to self may originate in childhood trauma, and the allostasis which has followed may contain fragmented, omnipotent, and guilt-ridden elements which appear in the treatment. These psychic forces inevitably present in treatment.

Tina (see above) was horrified in her session when she revealed her loving yearnings for her therapist which might elicit an out-of-control sexual assault on her. She called herself a "whore" and "bad, bad." She repeated, "I'm sorry, I'm so sorry." Even in fantasy she was not aware of anger at her therapist/seducer, but rather was stricken with guilt for omnipotently initiating what might become an incestuous encounter. The two selves—one, a child yearning for love; the other, the posttraumatic self of that child as a whore—stood side by side and interacted within the safe space of the therapeutic encounter. It was explained that thinking of herself as a powerful seductress was an understandable protective response to being overwhelmed by repeated incest as a child, and that turning that experience, which had been out of her control, to one that at least in fantasy was the result of her extraordinary powers was a posttraumatic adaptation, albeit one that caused her great ongoing pain.

Sometimes it is possible to discover and point out aspects of a positive pretrauma self at work even within the experience itself. By linking its presence before the trauma, during the trauma, and in the survivor's current daily life, the therapist is in a position to help reweave self-continuity. Lee, a combat veteran with severe PTSD, had seen himself as an altruistic protector of the weak before the Vietnam War, but as a dangerous destroyer of all whom he touched afterward. As Lee recounted a crucial traumatic episode, he illustrated in the session the movement of his arms and shoulders as he killed a booby-trapped child approaching from the side. As the therapist watched how these movements were occurring in his office, he noticed that they would have protected him had he been exposed to such an explosion. At that point, he understood that in this very movement which Lee dreaded recalling, he was knocking down his friend (the therapist, in the office) away from the anticipated explosion in an effort to save him even as he was shooting the endangering booby-trapped child. Lee's altruistic protective self had not died in Vietnam; it had survived under the worst of circumstances (i.e., by revivifying allostatic reenactment).

In such activities the therapist is appreciating as understandable and meaningful the patient's paradoxical efforts within the trauma and afterward to survive, to protect, and to repair the discontinuous self.

SUMMARY

Allostasis provides a useful way to describe the adaptations the patient with PTSD makes in order to deal with damaged intrapsychic structures. Chronic stable yet pathological defenses which attempt to protect defects in perception, affect regulation, and self-continuity characterize the internal state of the survivor with PTSD.

The chronic efforts which the PTSD sufferer makes to preempt intrusion, to disavow affect, and to split off self-fragments achieve a more or less steady but maladaptive state, or allostasis. These related psychological systems interact with each other, forming posttrauma character change. In treatment each element becomes engaged in the transference, and in some cases restoration of previous function seems possible.

Each component of this intrapsychic model connects to neurophysiological, neuroanatomical, and neuroendocrine components. The mind and brain reinforce this maladaptive allostatic state. Each is responsive to the other, psychology setting off biology and biology setting off psychology.

REFERENCES

Cucliciu, I. (in press). Chapter, Romania, a time of yielding. In J. D. Lindy & R. J. Lifton (Eds.), *Beyond imaginary walls: Legacy of Soviet trauma*. New York: Brunner and Routledge.

Freud, A. (1996). *The ego and the mechanisms of defense* (Rev. ed., Vol. 2). New York: International Universities Press.

Freud, S. (1966) Project for a scientific psychology. In *Standard edition*. (Vol. 1, pp. 281–397). London: Hogarth Press. (Originally published 1950 [from an 1895 draft])

Freud, S. (1986). *Draft K of The neuroses of defence* (Vol. 1, pp. 220–226). (Originally published 1896)

Freud, S. (1955). Introduction to *Psychoanalysis and the war neuroses*. In *Standard edition* (Vol. 17, pp. 205–215). London: Hogarth Press.

Kernberg, O. (1971). Prognostic considerations regarding borderline personality organization. *Journal of the American Psychoanalytic Association, 19*, 595–635.

Kohut, H. (1966). Forms and transformations of narcissism. *Journal of the American Psychoanalytic Association, 14*, 243–272.

Lindy, J. D. (1989). Transference and post-traumatic stress disorder. *Journal of the American Academy of Psychoanalysis, 17*, 397–413.

Lindy, J. D., & Wilson, J. P. (1994). *Countertransference and the treatment of PTSD*. New York: Guilford Press.

Strachey, J. (1934). The nature of the therapeutic action of psychoanalysis. *International Journal of Psychoanalysis, 15*, 126–159.

Titchener, J., & Kapp, F. (1976). Family and character change at Buffalo Creek. *American Journal of Psychiatry, 133*(3), 295–299.

6

Acute Posttraumatic Interventions

BEVERLEY RAPHAEL and MATTHEW DOBSON

To suggest the possibility of acute posttraumatic interventions, there must be a belief that they are of value, or that they may be beneficial, and that they do no harm. Current popular belief, and indeed many scientific views, would suggest that it is essential to provide acute posttraumatic interventions for every exposure; indeed, it is often suggested in both the media and some professional literature that "debriefing" or "trauma counseling" is essential for the survivors or even for the bereaved. An earlier community view held that such matters should not be talked about, that it would be better to put what happened "behind you" and to "try to forget about it." The change of culture has not only been driven by the rapid expansion of scientific understandings of trauma and its effects, particularly its adverse psychological consequences such as disabling posttraumatic stress disorder (PTSD), but also by popular "victim" movements demanding a supportive response.

In this context numerous intervention frameworks have evolved to deal with the reaction to trauma in the acute phase. They are motivated as well by a powerful and altruistic human need to assist those who have been "hurt" and to undo what has happened. They are also influenced by the view that to respond may prevent adverse psychosocial outcomes following disaster. It is now time to state that these many types of intervention, now so frequently provided, at least in developed countries, have not, with a few exceptions, been demonstrated to achieve the hoped-for benefits.

The whole field of acute posttraumatic intervention requires analysis; conceptual and theoretical development which is linked to the rapidly grow-

139

ing science of trauma effects; and systematic research with rigorous method-ologies to establish potential benefits—or otherwise. These issues will be ad-dressed below.

THE NATURE OF PSYCHOLOGICAL TRAUMA

There has been considerable diversity in the definition of the type of experi-ence that might be psychologically traumatic. Views range from those that suggest that any significant life event may come into this category to those that support criterion A of DSM-IV, with its inherent life threat. The field has been confused by the inclusion of normal bereavement as a potential traumatic stressor when there is no evidence to suggest this to be the case. The reactive processes to bereavement are those of separation distress with anger and protest and those of separation-related arousal. The bereaved is aroused with a focus on the lost attachment figure and scans the environ-ment, seeking the return of that person, searching for his or her image or fact. This gradually resolves with psychological mourning processes which in-volve reviewing the lost relationship and memories of the loved one and gradually undoing the bonds of attachment. On the other hand, the psycho-logically traumatized person is aroused with intense anxiety and fear that the threat will return and scans the environment to negate or prove this. This is not separation anxiety but anxiety related to life threat. The bereaved yearns and longs for the loved one to return; the traumatized longs for the trauma not to have happened, for his or her world to be as it was—there are some similarities in this. The preoccupations of traumatized persons are of the horror, threat, and helplessness that pervade their sleeping and waking hours. The preoccupations of bereaved individuals are with memories and images of the lost person—there is pleasure in the preoccupation, pain in the recog-nition of the absence (Raphael, 1977, 1986; Raphael & Martinek, 1997). Both these sets of reactive processes usually settle in the days and weeks fol-lowing the experience; that is, both resolve in a natural and progressive miti-gation of distress, lessening of intrusive preoccupations, and a return of feel-ings of well-being. In these circumstances they do not lead to morbidity and the justifications for intervention, apart from a normal and comforting re-sponse, must be few.

In addition, other reactive processes are likely in response to the differ-ent types of experience that have been classified as "traumatic" at some time. Some of these include general life events such as difficulties at work, upset in a relationship, or financial difficulties. These may be expected to lead to dis-tress, perhaps for a period of time, but as the individual adapts and copes, this lessens. It may be that these life events contribute to increased vulnerabil-ity for some, but the majority deal with these successfully. Other experiences are much more severe and out of the ordinary, for instance, being a victim of violence, being in an accident, hearing of or witnessing another's horrendous experience, or being threatened with death. Such experiences are more likely to be traumatic.

It is established that the co-occurrence of life event stressors may complicate the adaptive resolution of either trauma or loss, so understanding the effects of such variables is also very important.

These issues are highlighted here to emphasize that even the basis for what is determined to be an acute posttrauma period or situation for intervention is not automatically clear. This has lead to confusion in the provision of interventions to deal with any or all such experiences, and the interventions provided are frequently rather generic (e.g., debriefing), not formulated in terms of specificity of stressors or reaction or timing. Other interventions target groups who might be determined to be at higher risks of adverse outcomes, but usually not with specific focus on the stressor or timing.

In this chapter traumatized populations will be considered to be those who have been exposed to severe life threat, either to the self or to significant others; those who have been exposed to violence or the gruesome and mutilating deaths of others; or those who have experienced a "death encounter." Whether this leads to feelings of helplessness will be considered, but both dissociative reactions and intense arousal without dissociation have been shown to heighten risk of posttraumatic morbidity, specifically PTSD. Interventions for normal bereavement are unnecessary, but if the bereavement has been associated with a traumatic experience through the circumstances of the death, then the resulting traumatic bereavement will be considered as a potential context for acute posttrauma intervention. This chapter will not, however, provide substantial discussion on the management of other high-risk bereavements (see Raphael & Minkov, 1999).

WHAT IS AN ACUTE INTERVENTION?

While models such as psychological first aid and debriefing suggest an almost immediate posttrauma intervention, especially in the first 48 hours or so, the provision of trauma counseling may take place in the early days or even weeks and can still be considered acute. This is the more readily understandable when there is an awareness of the longitudinal phenomenology of PTSD. The merging of acute stress disorder (ASD) into PTSD may be quite subtle, or PTSD may only become apparent in the weeks and months after the trauma. Research shows that acute PTSD settles in these early months and that only if distress continues at a high level after 3–4 months is chronic PTSD likely (Davidson, Hughes, Blazer, & George, 1991). Thus to some degree *acute* interventions could be considered to apply at least in the early phases of this period (i.e., during the early weeks and possibly the first 1–2 months). Sadly much of the research into posttrauma interventions has not examined the time of intervention and its relevance in terms of timing to the phases of acute posttrauma response. Acute posttrauma response has usually been seen as a positive action in its own right, but this is now open to question with the recognition that the universal application of debriefing as an acute posttrauma intervention may be quite inappropriate, and possibly harmful, and that many other endeavors at this time are unproven as to their effectiveness. Some important research questions have yet to be addressed, such as who should be offered intervention, what sort of intervention, and when. Anecdotal reports often suggest that current interventions such as debriefing were "too soon" for some participants and that later would have been better for certain individuals. This is more relevant in light of recent suggestions that too early an intervention may heighten arousal, retraumatize the individual, or even help to create a "catastrophic" memory, because of interference with neuropsychophysiological adaptation mechanisms (Shalev, 2000). In addition, there is the possibility that later timing may be appropriate when two models of posttrauma intervention (Chemtob, 2000; Stallard, 2000) suggest that a "debriefing" intervention model applied many months after the incident was effective as an intervention when earlier it had not been. Thus timing may be a critical issue. This relates not only to knowledge of normal or maladaptive responses in posttrauma adaptation but also to the model of intervention that may be applied (e.g., debriefing versus trauma counseling). Another factor that is frequently highlighted in terms of the timing of debriefing interventions is that they may be provided at a time when it is not possible for those debriefed to utilize them, for instance, when still in a traumatic or dangerous situation or having to return to one.

THE PURPOSES OF ACUTE POSTTRAUMA INTERVENTIONS

The potential purposes of these interventions are many. They include the following:

- The wish to help others, to "make better"
- Interventions to educate, to prepare those affected by informing them of what to expect and what they can do
- Interventions to return the person to necessary task-related functioning
- Interventions to assist with recovery
- Interventions to prevent adverse affects
- Interventions to treat problems or disorders that are considered to be present
- Interventions to facilitate trauma resolution, whatever that may mean

MODELS OF ACUTE POSTTRAUMA INTERVENTIONS

There are a number of models of acute posttrauma intervention that are in current use. These will be reviewed below. It should be noted that while some of these share similarities with interventions for the treatment of established and even chronic PTSD, their focus is different in that they primarily aim for the fullest possible recovery, although this may not be clearly articulated. The chronicity of longer-established disorder means that the focus of interventions is usually on the maintenance of function and the diminution of symptoms.

Emergency Interventions

These interventions would be provided in the immediate aftermath of the traumatic experience. They aim to protect the person from further harm and to prevent deterioration. This could include rest and protection for the highly aroused and acutely distressed, and even the provision of short-term psychopharmacological intervention. However, in the majority of instances this type of intervention is protective and supportive. It is ensuring safety, providing comfort, and meeting basic needs. It is not intrusive and makes no attempt to help the person to actively work through the trauma.

Psychological First Aid

This term arose in the disaster context (Raphael, 1986) and is increasingly used in these and other situations of trauma. It involves a number of models including those of Foss (1994), a semistructured support process (Raphael & Meldrum, 1994), a model linking to the culture of physical first aid, and more recently a similar approach from the World Health Organization (WHO) (Mocellin, 1998). While these are intended to be generic and supportive, they have not been subjected to research and evaluation, so that the usefulness and validity of their application needs to be established. Their general supportive nature and nonactive intervention suggest that they are unlikely to do harm.

Debriefing

There is a range of debriefing models that have arisen, generally from the military psychiatry approach to deal with combat stress reactions, one pattern of acute posttrauma reaction. While Dunning (1988) has critically reviewed models and placed these in educational and psychoeducational contexts, the popularity of the "Mitchell model" (Mitchell, 1983) means that this is usually equated to debriefing. This model has been widely used across the

world, and extensive presentation and training concerning its use has occurred. Debriefing was originally suggested as an intervention for emergency
service workers such as police, rescue, fire services, and other emergency personnel. It was situated in an occupational health context with aims of diminishing adverse consequences of "critical incidents" experienced in the course
of work, such as job turnover, stress, and sick leave. As the model evolved it
became situated in a "critical incident stress management" (CISM) framework and became known as CISD (critical incident stress debriefing). It was
seen as on a continuum with other acute interventions, including defusing,
peer support, crisis intervention and possibly counseling (Mitchell & Bray,
1989).

This debriefing model has a number of stages and is intended to be carried out in the earliest days posttraumatization. It provides a structured
group process in which the incident is reviewed, knowledge shared, feelings
expressed, and education provided about symptoms that may occur. While it
is frequently perceived as helpful by those who receive it, this helpfulness does
not appear to correlate with improved outcomes. Nevertheless, Mitchell and
Everly (2000), following a range of reviews of their own and others work,
conclude there is ample evidence of its effectiveness in reducing symptoms of
stress in the posttraumatic period, of increasing workers' capacity to function, and of lessening levels of sick leave and job turnover in the emergency
professions. Thus it can be seen, if this proves to be the case, as a form of
stress management relevant to "critical incident stress." The authors carefully delineate this from traumatic stress and do not claim that it lessens risk for
or levels of PTSD, although this possibility is frequently inferred by those
who use this debriefing model. Furthermore, the extensive spread of CISD
and the social demand generated have occurred alongside a reluctance to
evaluate it, and to systematically examine any negative effects, while claiming
its undoubted benefit.

Recent studies such as those of Ørner (1995), Watts (1994), and Kenardy and Carr (1996) contest the benefits of debriefing. They have not
found it to be beneficial in their studies of disaster-affected populations or, in
Ørner's case, for those workers using a CISD model for support. This leads
to considerable debate between those supportive of the Mitchell model
specifically or debriefing generally, on one side, and those who do not find
benefit and even suggest that there is the potential for those provided with
this type of acute intervention to fare worse, on the other. Furthermore, studies using the model as an acute one-off intervention in other settings such as
acute intervention for psychological traumatization following serious burn injuries (Bisson, Jenkins, & Bannister, 1997) and following the trauma of motor
vehicle accidents (Hobbs, Mayou, Harrison, & Worlock, 1996) have found it
to be of no benefit in reported trials. A recent Cochrane review came to the
same conclusion (Wessely, Rose, & Bisson, 1998). Thus there must be a call
for caution in the broad use of the model, concern about the potential to

"make worse," perhaps through mechanisms suggested by Shalev (see above). Moreover, some of these studies have suggested that those who have had several debriefings were worse. Many research criticisms can be placed on the findings of both groups of protagonists, but there is certainly a growing body of negative findings which must challenge any universal application of debriefing as an acute posttraumatic intervention (Rose & Bisson, 1998; Raphael, Meldrum, & McFarlane, 1995; Raphael & Wilson, 2000).

Military Interventions

These interventions evolved with the recognition of combat stress and its detrimental effects on soldiers, in the immediate period of the battle, when their ability to continue fighting was critical to the achievement of military goals, and subsequently when long-term disability brought a burden of personal damage and social cost.

Two types of intervention which have been utilized in this setting sit in the acute posttraumatic framework. These are *forward psychiatry*, based on the principles of proximity, immediacy, and expectancy (PIE), and debriefing. The former intervention is a specific treatment format for soldiers who develop combat stress reactions and are unable to continue to fight effectively. They are taken from their unit but kept close to the front (proximity), treated immediately with supportive measures including rest and possibly medication (immediacy), and with an orientation to return them rapidly to their unit where they will continue to function as soldiers (expectancy). This treatment modality has been studied and validated (e.g., Solomon & Benbenishty, 1986).

It has been found to be very effective in achieving its goals, with the soldier usually reengaging with his unit and returning to combat (Solomon, Weisenberg, Schwarzwald, & Mikulincer, 1987). Thus it is effective in diminishing symptoms and supporting function. Whether or not it can prevent PTSD has not been established, however. Solomon and associates' work and longer-term follow-up of these men in the Israeli army and subsequently have shown that those with repeated combat stress reaction, even though continuing to function as soldiers at the time, were in many instances later more vulnerable to developing chronic and disabling PTSD (Solomon et al., 1987; Solomon, 1989). Whether keeping people functional but in so doing keeping them in a situation where they may be traumatized again (and again) is ultimately helpful to outcomes is a critical question for future research. Here as elsewhere findings need to be extended to better encompass the role of pretrauma factors such as the following: previous experience and mastery or vulnerability; vulnerable personal styles such as those of obsessive rumination; resilience characteristics such as those of hardiness and personal hopefulness; and background preparation and training. Posttrauma interventions cannot be really evaluated without taking these things into account.

Debriefing in military contexts has evolved somewhat differently. Marshall (1944), a U.S. military historian, undertook to interview soldiers in groups to get a full and clear picture of what had happened in combat in particular battles. All were treated as equal, every soldier's story was encouraged, and no interpretations were made. These narratives appeared to help the soldiers (as well as the interviewer) to gain a coherent or "whole" picture of what had gone on and appeared to be helpful to them psychologically, although no specific research was done to formally establish this. While debriefing has been widely used in the military since that time, it has, with the recent uptake of interest in debriefing models, usually been in the CISD format. More recent concerns about debriefing have called this into question, and this review suggests that it may be more appropriate to return to the use of the earlier type of model. Shalev (2000) describes the effectiveness of this "historical group debriefing" in decreasing arousal in soldiers and suggests that, as this is a crucial pathway to PTSD, this intervention may help to prevent it. Weisaeth (2000), again talking of the military context, suggests that debriefing is of most use when it is for those who have been briefed for an incident and that the leaders of groups of soldiers or emergency workers, for instance, should be trained and supported to provide this type of debriefing as part of their leadership roles. Weisaeth adds that other debriefing formats should only be used for incidents where stresses are so severe as to disrupt the unit's functioning (e.g., when there are deaths of several soldiers or emergency workers of a unit).

Combat is a stressor that is associated with a relatively high risk of PTSD, and those interventions that can potentially diminish this risk are very important. But what is not clear in the above is how much the debriefing provided is more a form of stress management for the "critical incidents" that are very much part of warfare, as opposed to interventions for those psychologically traumatized and at risk of PTSD.

People in the military are exposed to stressors other than combat, and these may be traumatic (Dobson & Marshall, 1997). Reports of soldiers who were involved in body recovery in the Gulf War provide important insights. This is a high-stress situation, linked to vulnerability to posttraumatic morbidity. Deahl, Gillham, Thomas, Searle, and Srinivasan (1994) reported that soldiers of one group who had been debriefed were compared with another, which, for operational reasons, had not. The debriefed group was no better at longer-term follow-up: no benefits could be demonstrated for the debriefing in groups that appeared to be equivalent in experience and vulnerability to these stressors. PTSD was not prevented by this intervention.

Peacekeepers also suffer experiences which may be psychologically traumatic—for instance, witnessing genocide, violence, bombing, or deaths from famine, without being able to intervene. Ward (1995) has demonstrated significant psychological morbidity in a group of peacekeepers, and cases of PTSD have also been reported in such groups. Yet these groups have had extensive briefing *and* debriefing in recent times. For many, however, their experiences in the developing countries where they had these peacekeeping roles were overwhelming and may well have added to their vulnerability.

Soldiers, like emergency workers and others in structured crisis response services, may have their own informal "debriefing" mechanisms in socially sanctioned modalities and in more secure settings.

Crisis Intervention

This modality developed from Caplan's (1964) original ideas of preventive intervention following stressful life events. It has been applied as a brief intervention in association with bereavement (Raphael, 1977), motor vehicle accidents (Bordow & Porritt, 1979), and acute injury and illness (Bunn & Clarke, 1979). When provided in accordance with this theoretical modality, it has been shown to be effective in high-risk populations in lessening the likelihood of morbidity. Although potentially "traumatic" stressors could have been identified in each of these studies, the traumatic stress model did not inform them. While it is now known that traumatic bereavements can be associated with PTSD, that motor vehicle accidents may lead to the development of PTSD, and that life-threatening illness and injury may be associated with vulnerability to PTSD, further research in crisis intervention is needed to test this model as an acute posttraumatic intervention. Nevertheless, it is potentially so. The recontextualizing of debriefing in the crisis intervention framework is not really helpful, as its format, intervention, timing, and hypothesized mode of action are quite different.

Trauma Counseling

This modality has become a subject of research in recent times, with studies showing that specific focused counseling can lessen the risk of PTSD after acute rape trauma (Foa, Rothbaum, Riggs, & Murdock, 1991).

"Trauma counseling" has often been provided as a nonspecific general counseling aimed at both making better the psychological hurt and preventing the development of PTSD. Unfortunately, the marketplace demand for trauma counseling and the belief in its value have far outstripped the knowledge base of what is effective and the skills of many would-be providers.

The effectiveness of focused interventions which are provided over a number of sessions in the later (2 weeks or more) acute posttrauma period appears to be established (Bryant, Harvey, Basten, Dang, & Sackville, 1998). These interventions are chiefly in cognitive behavioral formats which focus on the specific trauma and support reconfrontation and working through.

Foa, Hearst-Ikeda, and Perry (1995) carried out a pilot study of a brief preventive intervention program for female sexual assault survivors. The intervention built on what was known to be effective in the treatment of some chronic PTSD in such circumstances (e.g., Foa et al., 1991) and included exposure, relaxation training, and cognitive restructuring. The authors compared intervention and nonintervention subjects, both groups having an intervention, of four weekly 2-hour sessions which began within a month of the assault. Although numbers were small and it was not a controlled trial, those who would have met criteria for PTSD diminished significantly in the intervention group and did not in the control group. Symptoms were far less severe for the intervention group. These benefits were sustained. The authors note that intervention did not start until 2 weeks later. While they initially believed this might contribute a difficulty, they subsequently considered that those affected may have been better able to benefit from these interventions at this later time. This would fit with findings of bereavement counseling.

With these findings in mind, and the comparative effectiveness of cognitive behavioral interventions for treatment of some cases of established PTSD, there is a sound framework for using this modality of trauma-focused cognitive behavioral therapy in short-term counseling as the basis for an acute posttrauma intervention provided in the early weeks *but not* immediately posttrauma.

Structural and Integrated Interventions

Some debriefing and other acute posttraumatic interventions are provided in a structured and integrated framework which seems to have been associated with some positive results. This is exemplified in Tyrer's (1989) rotation and support for officers working after the Lockerbie plane crash in Scotland and Alexander's structural support of police body recovery workers after the North Sea oil rig disaster. In the latter case, a support system was provided by briefing workers. This consisted of pairing a younger with an older, more experienced officer and providing informal debriefing merged with support by a psychiatrist known to and trusted by these men (Alexander, 2000). The security provided by such a structured environment, where there was a need to get on with the work, which was continuing, suggests that such a model could be of value in other such circumstances. This could become a structural approach as part of an occupational health program.

System-based interventions include those in postdisaster response programs such as those of consultation with affected communities, as well as supportive interventions such as group meetings for relatives of those killed in a plane crash or other disasters where information can be provided and mutual support and reassurance can be built.

Information plays a central part in recovery processes, and emergency organizations in the posttrauma period frequently develop systematic formats to provide this. This in itself is likely to be a supportive posttrauma intervention.

Education and Learning Interventions

While there is general agreement that education about anticipated responses is helpful, and it is reported to be so when it is provided, for instance, in debriefing or support programs. There has been inadequate investigation of this intervention method and its effectiveness. It is of interest that the formal learning of debriefing in the CISD model is toward a pathology focus (e.g., symptom lists). Other learning in debriefing formats has been highlighted by Weisaeth (2000), who suggests that the learning a group may do with the use of its own processes and without the intervention of a mental health professional may be very helpful to the future functioning of its members. They may develop a sense of positive mastery. It might also be said that the cognitive behavioral interventions listed above promote a specific and focused learning to undo the fear response to the trauma that was involved.

This whole area promises to be a valuable field for further research.

Other Potential Interventions

The possibility of pharmacological interventions in the acute posttrauma period is of interest, particularly in view of the greater understanding of neurophysiological, and neuroendocrine reactive processes following trauma. Yehuda and McFarlane (1997) have suggested that there is an alteration in the acute stress process that reflects an overreactive system and that with such understandings a biological method may be able to alter vulnerability. While there are a number of clinical hypotheses, there is no clearly determined appropriate intervention in the acute posttrauma period. Rather, the decision for such interventions should have a strong clinical rationale (i.e., for those most distressed and dysfunctional, and addressing these two parameters).

Other Interventions

Several other interventions have been developed, but as of this writing their overall effectiveness has not been established. Eye movement desensitization and reprocessing (EMDR) is one such intervention—attractive to many, but not as yet with evidence of significant benefits as an acute intervention (Shapiro, 1989, 1996).

Other interventions have had a vogue but not been continued, and there is little evidence of their effective use in the acute posttrauma period; where benefits are claimed, these have not been substantiated by scientific trials.

SPECIAL ISSUES WITH CHILDREN

The nature and effectiveness of acute posttrauma interventions with children is yet to be established. Wraith (2000) has described a model of psychological first aid followed by "clinical debriefing" that she has evolved to stand in place of debriefing. Nevertheless, she stresses that this model is primarily for critical incidents. She believes that it is necessary to first assess whether the child has suffered psychological traumatization and, if this is the case, individual and focused counselling is seen as necessary because of the high risk to the child's development. Other workers in this field (e.g., Pynoos & Nader, 1989) have suggested a framework for preventive intervention with children who have suffered potentially traumatic incidents in a disaster. This also stands on good theoretical and clinical grounds, but there has been no systematic evaluation. Yule (1992), working with children and adolescents, reports some benefits of intervention, but this is not a controlled trial. For younger children, for instance, to deal with parents' needs is often critical so that a progressive desensitization and resolution of the issues can be achieved.

There have also been a number of structured programs such as that of Storm, McDermott, and Finlayson (1994) that help children to work through their experiences in a school setting with books focused on the disaster, in this case a forest fire. The degree to which this is appropriate for the earliest stages is not clear, but it may be, like trauma counseling, appropriate when there is a "readiness" a few weeks later—still within the relatively acute period.

CLINICAL PROCESSES AND INTERVENTIONS

The interventions described in the literature occur for the most part in the context of a clinical system of understanding. The knowledge of the reactive processes following trauma and how these may indicate or be linked subsequently to the spectrum of posttraumatic morbidity has evolved from clinically oriented studies. Much of the understanding has arisen with work with populations who have established PTSD—often Vietnam veterans populations. More recently, there have been studies which throw light on the acute posttrauma response, including studies of disasters and other acute traumatic situations such as rape and violent incidents.

The experience of clinicians in these settings is of enormous value, both as researchers (e.g., Weisaeth, 2000) or when they are involved in acute disaster response, or are called to provide advice and assistance, or to treat those already requiring mental health attention through heightened risk or actual disorder. These experiences have been distilled into a number of useful clinically oriented approaches.

The "Trauma Membrane"

This refers to the sealing off of traumatic experience, as an adaptive process in the initial phase and leads to a questioning of the appropriateness of any techniques which disrupt this, for instance, early demands for catharsis.

The "Dosing of Affect"

Lindy (1996), in discussing the management of disaster victims, has spoken of the degree to which people affected by trauma, especially in the acute period, may only be able to deal with the intense affect involved in small "doses." This may mean that therapeutic or other interventions should be provided in ways that are cognizant of this.

Trauma and Grief

As noted earlier, there are situations where those afflicted may be affected by both traumatic stressors and intense personal losses in the case of traumatic bereavements, for instance, homicide, mass killings, or deaths of family members in accidents or disasters. Clinicians working in this field suggest that the two sets of phenomena may need to be dealt with separately—frequently the traumatization first. This will require sensitivity and skill so that the bereaved and traumatized person is not overwhelmed or pushed to further decompensation (Lindy, 1996; Raphael, 1986).

Forgetting

Forgetting may be the best or only option. There is a widespread belief that people who "forget"—or "deny" the severity of what has occurred—may be pathological and must be made to "go through it" or "get it out." For some people, at some time, "forgetting" is the only option: they must go on   the circumstance is too terrible to encompass at this stage. People *must* be allowed to handle things in their own way, at their own pace, in their own time. Natural "forgetting" may be the most normal of adaptations, even though all is not really forgotten, but rather set aside and moved on from.

Victim Dynamics

The status of the victim role and its associated dynamics need to be well understood; otherwise there is a risk that acute interventions, focused as they are on the traumatic experience, may reinforce this as the most valued and sought after part of the individual. In addition, the helplessness so consonant with victim status may be imprinted and natural recovery and resilience inhibited by the therapeutic stance.

The Wrong Trauma

At a time of major catastrophe it is easy to believe, as the affected persons may, that this is the source of all their ills. Careful assessment is necessary of the contribution of the present catastrophe, or posttraumatic experience, of other traumas past or present, and of other life difficulties or pathologies, including those related to marriage, family, and workplace. This should inform the provision of interventions to deal with any current trauma.

Unmeetable Needs

The provision of trauma or grief counseling may seem simple, clear cut, and with achievable ends. For some people these will open into a devastating emptiness of unmet needs, early deprivations, and few psychological resources. It is critical that anyone providing acute interventions realizes this possibility—fortunately not frequent, but very serious when present. This may mean that great care should be taken in what is being opened up and how, and that ongoing support is available to assist this client to maintain his or her fragile integration.

Vicarious Trauma and Indulgence

Therapists should be aware of their own dynamics about dealing with the traumatic experiences of their clients and the risks of both vicarious indulgence in their horror as well as secondary traumatization.

A professional role and skills, as well as supervision, can assist this. Further issues that arise include the risks of boundary violations in the intense circumstances of acute trauma, where there are powerful affiliative tendencies and the wish to comfort and to undo what has happened. While human comforting is part of all natural response in such circumstances, it is clearly distinct from the crossing of therapeutic boundaries—a move likely to be harmful to both the client and the therapist.

THE PRACTICE OF ACUTE POSTTRAUMA INTERVENTIONS

As is clear from the issues reviewed above, there are a range of formats, formulas, and frameworks for acute posttrauma intervention. Most are driven by hopefulness and the wish to help. A great many of those actually provided are, however, based neither on scientific evidence of effectiveness nor on an in-depth understanding of the phenomenology of posttrauma reactions and their interaction with individual psychodynamics or psychopathology. The beginnings of a scientific base for these interventions is now present, for instance, in the work of Foa and Bryant and their colleagues, and in the growing understanding of acute phenomenology and its evolution in the work of Davidson, McFarlane, Yehuda, and many others. This means that there are a number of key issues that should inform the provision of acute posttrauma intervention.

First, Do No Harm

As there is now evidence that acute posttrauma interventions may, for some at least, disrupt normal adaptive process and potentially link to more adverse outcomes, they should not be provided indiscriminately for all, or by those not knowledgeable of and sensitive to the potential for harm.

Assessing Need

There has been a failure in many formats of acute posttrauma intervention to develop and utilize a systematic, scientifically based, and clinically appropriate framework for assessing need. While those providing interventions in research studies in the cognitive behavioral trauma focus, such as Foa, Bryant, and others have provided interventions based on assessed trauma-related symptomatology, the debriefing movement and the vast majority of trauma counselors do not do so. In a different and clinical context the concept of *therapeutic assessment* for determining the need for grief counseling has been utilized (Raphael, 1977). This model is based on a knowledge of demonstrated risk factors for adverse psychosocial outcomes following bereavement and is a clinical interview formatted to encompass these while allowing review of the experience and response to it.

There can be no justification for providing universal acute posttrauma interventions beyond information, general support, comfort and safety, and perhaps psychological first aid. Thus, there needs to be nonintrusive, reliable, and valid methods of identifying those who on the basis of current knowledge are likely to be at risk of adverse health outcomes if interventions are not provided. Such assessment must be simple, able to be widely used, and also be nonstigmatizing (i.e., with no inference that those so screened will automatically go on to adverse outcomes). Screening or therapeutic clinical assessment is only ethically valid if there is the possibility of providing appropriate interventions that may modify risk and influence outcomes positively.

Targeting Intervention

On the basis of such assessments, interventions should be targeted to alleviate distress, provide support, and facilitate processes of resolution. Intervention may be individual—such as focused and specific short-term trauma counseling (Bryant et al., 1998; Foa et al., 1995), or bereavement counseling for high-risk bereavements (Raphael & Minkov, 1999) or clinically based crisis intervention or brief therapy in recognized formats of established effectiveness. Naturally any such approaches, whether based on clinical guidelines, manuals, or knowledge of effective practice, may need to be tailored to individual requirements while monitoring fidelity to original effective elements.

Family interventions have not been systematically addressed but may need to be provided in ways guided by the above principles as well as knowledge and skills relevant to family dynamics and family reactions to trauma (poorly studied) and effective family-based interventions (also requiring much further research).

Group interventions have often been seen as the norm, particularly if following the debriefing modality. While they may be generally supportive for those similarly effected, they may have the potential to provide a milieu in which further traumatization may occur. Thus any group-based intervention should chiefly be informative and supportive, and not geared to therapeutic interventions in this acute period.

A further clinical issue with regard to targeted interventions for those at higher risk is the follow-on that may be required. There is nothing to support "endless" posttrauma counseling, and much to suggest it may be ill informed and in some instances potentially damaging to the affected person's capacity to move on realistically from the experience. A flexible short-term contractual arrangement for acute and brief posttrauma interventions should be the goal. Any long-term intervention should be linked to detailed further assessment and identification of its specific purposes, which should then be negotiated with the client—probably through more routine systems of care, for instance, public or private mental health service providers, also operating in an evidence-based framework.

Who Provides Acute Posttrauma Interventions?

As debriefing is inappropriate and not claimed to be effective as an acute posttrauma intervention, trained or accessible providers of this modality do not have a role in systematic evidence-based provision of acute posttrauma interventions. Skilled and knowledgeable mental health professionals with specific training in the area of trauma-related phenomenology and intervention would be appropriate. Such training should focus on a strong knowledge base, be cognizant of its rapid evolution and of the scientific criteria for appraising effectiveness, and emphasize the need to monitor outcomes in the short and long term.

It is fair to say that there is much to be done in increasing skills in this sphere, in putting in place requirements for appropriate knowledge and attitudes, demonstrated competencies, and recognition of the need first of all not to harm. Linked to this must be public and workplace education to protect people from the convergence of "trauma counselors" who do not possess the necessary skills, even if behaving as if they do, and even if wishing to do well.

Further there is need to educate and inform those affected by potentially traumatic events as to the issues of resilience and risk and what they can do to help themselves, what may be effective self-care for the process of recovery for them. Such education must move from the current negative view of outcomes of all being traumatized, to a more realistic appraisal of human strengths and adaptation, while skills are built for providing for those in need. These aspects are in need of much further research.

Evaluation and the Research Cycle

Acute posttrauma interventions have evolved in an appropriate recognition of the adverse and long-term effects that may result from psychological traumatization and in an effort to lessen human distress and suffering. Because of the needs of survivors ("victims") and the often highly charged environments that follow traumatic events, there has been a reluctance to evaluate the interventions applied and at times suggestions that to even think of doing so is wrong because everything provided with such goodwill for those so badly affected must be of benefit. This is further emphasized by public demand and the perceived helpfulness of much that is provided. It is only now—with a growing body of evidence that much may not be of benefit, may be costly for no good reason, and may even for some possibly produce harm—that requirements for evaluation can really gain acceptance.

It should be clear that any interventions must be accountable and that their outcomes must be systematically evaluated in the shorter and longer term. Thus the requirement should be in place and a culture developed to evaluate all acute posttrauma interventions and their effectiveness or otherwise. Such evaluation should be developed in ways that allow core data to be gathered and comparison of interventions in different settings. The findings can then be utilized to improve practice, develop or relinquish programs to achieve better results, and indicate areas for further research.

Evaluation as a cycle should link back to the interventions provided and their aims, and both should be linked to the research cycle of growing knowledge that should inform practice and be informed by it. It is only by such processes that an ultimate impact can be made on posttraumatic morbidity.

REFERENCES

Alexander, D. (2000). Debriefing and body recovery: Police in a civilian disaster. In B. Raphael & J. P. Wilson (Eds.), *Stress debriefing: Theory, practice and challenge* (pp. 118–130). London: Cambridge University Press.

Bisson, J. I., Jenkins, J. A., & Bannister, C. (1997). Randomised controlled trial of psychological debriefing for victims of acute burn trauma. *British Journal of Psychiatry, 171,* 78–81.

Bordow, S., & Porritt, D. (1979). An experimental evaluation of crisis intervention. *Social Science and Medicine, 13,* 251–256.

Bryant, R., Harvey, A., Basten, C., Dang, S., & Sackville, T. (1998). Treatment of acute stress disorder: A comparison of cognitive-behavioural therapy and supportive counselling. *Journal of Consulting and Clinical Psychology, 66,* 862–866.

Bunn, T., & Clarke, A. (1979). Crisis intervention: An experimental study of the effects of a brief period of counselling on the anxiety of relatives of seriously injured or ill hospital patients. *British Journal of Medical Psychology, 52,* 191–195.

Caplan, G. (1964). *Principles of preventive psychiatry.* New York: Basic Books.

Chemtob, C. (2000). Delayed debriefing: After a disaster. In B. Raphael & J. P. Wilson (Eds.), *Stress debriefing: Theory, practice and challenge* (pp. 227–240). London: Cambridge University Press.

Davidson, J., Hughes, D., Blazer, D., & George, L. (1991). Post-traumatic stress disorder in the community: An epidemiological study. *Psychological Medicine, 21*(3), 713–721.

Deahl, M., Gillham, A., Thomas, J., Searle, M., & Srinivasan, M. (1994). Psychological sequelae following the Gulf War: Factors associated with subsequent morbidity and the effectiveness of psychological debriefing. *British Journal of Psychiatry, 265,* 60–65.

Dobson, M., & Marshall, R. (1997). Surviving the war zone experience: Preventing psychiatric casualties. *Military Medicine, 162*(4), 283–287.

Dunning, C. (1988). Intervention strategies for emergency workers. In M. Lystad (Ed.), *Mental health response to mass emergencies* (pp. 284–307). New York: Brunner/Mazel.

Foa, E. B., Rothbaum, B., Riggs, D., & Murdock, T. (1991). Treatment of posttraumatic stress disorder in rape victims: A comparison between cognitive-behavioural procedures and counseling. *Journal of Consulting and Clinical Psychology, 59,* 715–723.

Foa, E. B., Hearst-Ikeda, D., & Perry, K. J. (1995). Evaluation of a brief cognitive-behavioural program for the prevention of chronic PTSD in recent assault victims. *Journal of Consulting and Clinical Psychology, 63,* 948–955.

Foss, O. T. (1994). Mental first aid. *Social Science and Medicine, 38,* 479–482.

Hobbs, M., Mayou, R., Harrison, B., & Worlock, P. (1996). A randomised control trial of psychological debriefing for victims of road traffic accidents. *British Medical Journal, 313,* 1438–1439.

Kenardy, J. & Carr, V. (1996). Imbalance in the debriefing debate: What we don't know far outweighs what we do. *Bulletin of the Australian Psychological Society, 18,* 4–6.

Lindy, J. (1996). Psychoanalytic psychotherapy of posttraumatic stress disorder: The nature of the therapeutic relationship. In B. van der Kolk, A. McFarlane, & L. Weisaeth (Eds.), *Traumatic stress: The effects of overwhelming experience on mind, body and society* (pp. 525–536). New York: Guilford Press.

Marshall, S. (1944). *Island victory.* New York: Penguin Books.

Mitchell, J. (1983). When disaster strikes: The critical incident stress debriefing process. *Journal of Emergency Medical Services, 8,* 36–39.

Mitchell, J., & Bray, G. (1989). *Emergency services stress.* Englewood Cliffs, NJ: Prentice Hall.

Mitchell, J., & Everly, G. (2000). Critical incident stress debriefing: Evolutions, effects and outcomes. In B. Raphael & J. P. Wilson (Eds.), *Stress debriefing: Theory, practice and challenge* (pp. 71–90). London: Cambridge University Press.

Mocellin, J. (1998). *Psychosocial division of disaster: Reference manual* (2nd draft). Geneva: World Health Organization.

Ørner, R. (1995). Intervention strategies for emergency response groups: A new conceptual framework. In S. Hobfoll, M. deVries, et al. (Eds.), *Extreme stress and communities: Impact and intervention* (pp. 499–521). Dordrecht, Netherlands: Kluwer Academic Publishers.

Pynoos, R., & Nader, K. (1989). Children's memory and proximity to violence. *Journal of the American Academy of Child and Adolescent Psychiatry, 28,* 236–241.

Raphael, B. (1977). Preventive intervention with the recently bereaved. *Archives of General Psychiatry, 34,* 1450–1454.

Raphael, B. (1986). *When disaster strikes: How individuals and communities cope with catastrophe.* New York: Basic Books.

Raphael, B., & Martinek, N. (1997). Assessing traumatic bereavements and PTSD. In J. P. Wilson & T. Keane (Eds.), *Assessing psychological trauma and PTSD* (pp. 373–395). New York: Guilford Press.

Raphael, B., & Meldrum, L. (1994). Helping people cope with trauma. In R. Watts & D. Horne (Eds.), *Coping with trauma: The victim and the helper.* Melbourne: Australian Academic Press.

Raphael, B., Meldrum, L., & McFarlane, A. (1995). Does debriefing after psychological trauma work? *British Medical Journal, 310,* 1479–1480.

Raphael, B., & Minkov, C. (1999). Abnormal grief. *Current Opinion in Psychiatry, 12,* 99–102.

Raphael, B., & Wilson, J. P. (Eds.). (2000). *Stress debriefing: Theory, practice and challenge.* London: Cambridge University Press.

Robinson, R. (2000). Debriefing with emergency services: Critical incident stress management. In B. Raphael & J. P. Wilson (Eds.), *Stress debriefing: Theory, practice and challenge* (pp. 91–107). London: Cambridge University Press.

Rose, S., & Bisson, J. (1998). Brief early psychological interventions following trauma: A systematic review of the literature. *Journal of Traumatic Stress, 11,* 697–710.

Shalev, A. (2000). Historical concepts and present patterns: Stress management and debriefing. In B. Raphael & J. P. Wilson (Eds.), *Stress debriefing: Theory, practice and challenge* (pp. 17–31). London: Cambridge University Press.

Shapiro, F. (1989). Eye movement desensitization. A new treatment for post-traumatic stress disorder. *Journal of Behaviour Therapy and Experimental Psychiatry, 20*(3), 211–217.

Shapiro, F. (1996). Eye movement desensitization and reprocessing (EMDR): Evaluation of controlled PTSD research. *Journal of Behaviour Therapy and Experimental Psychiatry, 27*(3), 209–218.

Solomon, Z. (1989). Psychological sequelae of war: A 3-year prospective study of Israeli combat stress reaction casualties. *Journal of Nervous and Mental Disease, 177*(6), 342–346.

Solomon Z., & Benbenishty, R. (1986). The role of proximity, immediacy, and expectancy in frontline treatment of combat stress reaction among Israelis in the Lebanon war. *American Journal of Psychiatry, 143*(5), 613–617.

Solomon, Z., Weisenberg, M., Schwarzwald, J., & Mikulincer, M. (1987). Posttraumatic stress disorder among frontline soldiers with combat stress reaction: The 1982 Israeli experience. *American Journal of Psychiatry, 144*(4), 448–454.

Stallard, P. (2000). Debriefing adolescents after critical life events. In B. Raphael & J. P. Wilson (Eds.), *Stress debriefing: Theory, practice and challenge* (pp. 213–224). London: Cambridge University Press.

Storm, V., McDermott, B., & Finlayson, D. (1994). *The bushfire and me*. Sydney, Australia: VBD Publications.

Tyrer, M. (1989). The Lockerbie air disaster. *Journal of the Royal Army Medical Corps, 135*, 93–94.

Ward, W. (1995). *Psychological adjustment in Australian veterans of the United Nations peacekeeping force in Somalia*. Dissertation, University of Queensland, Brisbane, Australia.

Watts, R. (1994). The efficacy of critical incident stress debriefing for personnel. *Bulletin of the Australian Psychological Society, 16*, 6–7.

Weisaeth, L. (2000). Briefing and debriefing: Psychological interventions in acute stressor situations. In B. Raphael & J. P. Wilson (Eds.), *Stress debriefing: Theory, practice and challenge* (pp. 43–57). London: Cambridge University Press.

Wessely, S., Rose, S., & Bisson, J. (1998). A systematic review of brief psychological interventions (debriefing) for the treatment of immediate trauma-related symptoms and the prevention of post-traumatic stress disorder [Cochrane Ceutoe: review]. In *The Cochrane Library, Issue 3*. Oxford, UK: Update Software.

Wraith, R. (2000). Children and debriefing: Theory, interventions and outcomes. In B. Raphael & J. P. Wilson (Eds.), *Stress debriefing: Theory, practice and challenge*. London: Cambridge University Press.

Yehuda, R., & McFarlane, A. (1997). *Psychobiology of posttraumatic stress disorder*. New York: New York Academy of Sciences.

Yule, W. (1992). Post-traumatic stress disorder in child survivors of shipping disasters: The sinking of the *Jupiter. Psychotherapy and Psychosomatics, 57*, 200–205.

7

Cognitive-Behavioral Approaches to PTSD

LORI A. ZOELLNER, LEE A. FITZGIBBONS, and EDNA B. FOA

THE AFTERMATH OF TRAUMA

After a traumatic experience such as combat or assault, individuals differ in their rate and extent of recovery. Many develop symptoms of posttraumatic stress disorder (PTSD), which include reexperiencing of the trauma memory, avoidance of thoughts and feelings associated with the trauma, and hyperarousal symptoms. From reports of retrospective studies, approximately 15% of theater veterans of the Vietnam War (Kulka, Schlenger, Fairbank, & Hough, 1990), 17.8% of female victims of aggravated assault, 12.4% of rape victims, and 3.4% of female victims of a noncrime assault (Resnick, Kilpatrick, Dausky, Saunders, & Best, 1993) exhibit chronic posttraumatic stress disorder (PTSD). From reports of prospective studies, higher rates of chronic PTSD have emerged. For example, Rothbaum, Foa, Murdock, Riggs, and Walsh (1992) found that within 3 weeks following an assault almost all rape victims (94%) showed emotional disturbance severe enough to meet symptom criteria for PTSD. Over time, the percentage of rape victims with PTSD declined gradually; however, 3 months after the assault, 47% of rape victims remained disturbed enough to meet diagnostic criteria for PTSD, and 6 months after the assault, 38% of rape victims still had PTSD (Foa, 1995). Thus, while the number of victims that naturally recover increases substantially within the first 3 months after the assault, most victims with PTSD at 3 months postassault tend to still have chronic symptoms. This finding that many but not all victims recover from their trauma underscores the importance of identifying factors that promote or hinder recovery. Indeed, this knowledge is vital in order to inform us about the psychopathology and treatment of chronic PTSD.

In this chapter, we first summarize the research treatment efficacy. Next, mechanisms underlying natural recovery and response to treatment are discussed. Finally, we describe how prolonged exposure treatment for chronic PTSD is conducted and we illustrate this treatment with two case examples.

COGNITIVE-BEHAVIORAL TREATMENT

The introduction of the PTSD into the DSM-III (American Psychiatric Association, 1980), gave impetus for the development of cognitive behavioral programs for this disorder. In the initial treatment literature for chronic PTSD, the cognitive-behavioral program utilized was often determined based on the type of traumatic event experienced: exposure therapy was used for war veterans (e.g., Keane & Kaloupek, 1982; Fairbank, Gross, & Keane, 1983) and stress inoculation training was used for rape victims (e.g., Kilpatrick, Veronen, & Resick, 1982). Several reports of treatment of Vietnam veterans with PTSD demonstrated that variants of exposure therapy produced positive, although sometimes modest, improvement in chronic PTSD (e.g., Keane, Fairbank, Caddell, & Zimering, 1989). However, the effects of stress inoculation training for rape victims were not systematically studied until more recent years.

Exposure Therapies: Prolonged Imaginal and *In Vivo* Exposure

Exposure programs usually involve the confrontation of feared stimuli either through imagination or in person. In the treatment of chronic PTSD, exposure therapy usually involves repeated confrontation both with the memories of the trauma (i.e., imaginal exposure) and with trauma-related situations that give rise to unrealistic fears (i.e., *in vivo* exposure).

Systematic desensitization (SD) was one of the earliest exposure techniques used to treat posttrauma reactions (Wolpe, 1958). In this treatment, after a physiological state inhibiting anxiety has been induced in the patient using muscle relaxation, the patient imagines a weak anxiety-arousing stimulus for a few seconds. As the exposure is repeated, the stimulus progressively loses its ability to evoke anxiety. Successively stronger stimuli are then treated. Uncontrolled studies and case reports (e.g., Frank & Stewart, 1983, 1984) indicated that SD was partially effective in reducing trauma-related symptoms.

In succeeding years, prolonged exposure with or without relaxation gradually replaced SD. For war veterans, several controlled studies using imaginal exposure have been conducted (Cooper & Clum, 1989; Keane et al., 1989; Boudewyns & Hyer, 1990; Boudewyns, Hyer, Woods, Harrison, & McCranie, 1990). In the first controlled study of exposure therapy for PTSD, Cooper and Clum (1989) found that the addition of imaginal exposure to individual and group counseling yielded a greater decrease in PTSD symptoms in comparison to individual and group counseling alone. However, there was no additive effect of imaginal exposure for depression or trait anxiety; and by 6-month follow-up, some posttreatment differences disappeared. Keane et al. (1989) found that imaginal exposure preceded by relaxation had a greater reduction in reexperiencing symptoms, anxiety, and depression than a no-treatment wait-list condition; however, there were no differences between groups in numbing or social avoidance. Treatment gains were maintained through the 6-month follow-up. Finally, Boudewyns and colleagues published two reports (Boudewyns & Hyer, 1990; Boudewyns et al., 1990) examining group treatment supplemented with either traditional weekly psychotherapy or weekly imaginal exposure. The group who received imaginal exposure evidenced more improvement on self-reported psychological functioning than did the control group; however, no group differences in physiological responding were found. For a subset of the original sample, at 3-month posttreatment follow-up, the exposure group exhibited better adjustment and fewer PTSD symptoms than did the control group.

For female assault victims, two controlled studies have examined the efficacy of exposure treatment for chronic PTSD in comparison to other cognitive behavioral treatments and to wait-list controls. Foa, Rothbaum, Riggs, and Murdock (1991) compared prolonged exposure (PE) treatment, stress inoculation training (SIT, to be described below), supportive counseling (SC), and a wait-list control. At posttreatment, SIT and PE conditions showed improvement on all three PTSD symptom clusters, whereas the SC and wait-list conditions only showed improvement on PTSD arousal symptoms. By 3-month follow-up, PE appeared superior to the other groups on all measures of psychopathology: 55% of the PE group, 50% of the SIT group, and 45% of the SC group no longer met diagnostic criteria for PTSD.

A second study conducted by Foa and colleagues compared PE alone, SIT alone, the combination of SIT and PE, and a wait-list control (Foa, Dancu, et al., 1998). At posttreatment, all active treatments showed improvement on PTSD symptoms, state anxiety, and depression; the wait-list group did not show improvement on these measures. Some 57% of the patients in the PE group, 42% of the patients in the SIT group, 36% of the patients in the SIT/PE group, and 0% of the wait-list reached good end-state functioning (as defined by low scores on measures of PTSD, depression, and anxiety). At 12-month follow-up, 52% of the PE, 42% of the SIT group, and 36% of the SIT/PE group had good end-state functioning. At present, several studies with female assault victims are in progress. For example, Foa and her colleagues are comparing PE alone with PE plus cognitive restructuring

(PE/CR), and Resick and her colleagues are comparing PE with cognitive processing therapy (CPT, which is described in more detail later).

With mixed forms of trauma, one controlled study and several quasi-experimental studies provide additional evidence for the efficacy of exposure-based techniques. Marks, Lovell, Noshirvani, Livanou, and Thrasher (1998) randomly assigned trauma victims with chronic PTSD to either PE alone, CR alone, PE/CR, or relaxation (R) alone. Using good end-state functioning measures at posttreatment, 53% of the PE group, 32% of the CR group, 32% of the PE/CR group, and only 15% of the R group achieved these criteria. At 6-month follow-up, overall treatment gains appeared to be maintained. In a cross-over design, Richards, Lovell, and Marks (1994), compared the results of four sessions of imaginal exposure followed by four sessions of *in vivo* exposure with those of four sessions of *in vivo* exposure followed by four sessions of imaginal exposure. In both groups, reduction in PTSD ranged from 65% to 80% on different measures. Overall, *in vivo* exposure was more effective for social avoidance than imaginal exposure, regardless of the order of treatment. Thompson, Charlton, Kerry, Lee, and Turner (1995) conducted an open trial of eight weekly sessions using imaginal and *in vivo* exposure. Patients improved significantly on a number of posttreatment measures such as PTSD symptomatology, general health, and general symptoms.

Anxiety Management Programs Including Stress Inoculation Training

A number of variants of anxiety management programs have been utilized for the treatment of chronic PTSD. The primary goal of these procedures is to provide a means to manage distressing anxiety, employing a variety of strategies such as biofeedback, relaxation, social skills techniques, and distraction. One of the most studied anxiety management programs for PTSD is stress inoculation training (SIT; Kilpatrick et al., 1982). SIT incorporates a number of components such as education, relaxation, breathing control, cognitive restructuring, covert modeling, and thought stopping. Several uncontrolled studies have supported the efficacy of SIT (e.g., Veronen & Kilpatrick, 1982).

In a controlled study, Resick, Jordan, Girelli, Hutter, and Marhoefer-Dvorak (1988) compared SIT, assertion training, or supportive psychotherapy plus information to a naturally occurring wait-list control. The SIT condition was slightly modified from the earlier version in that cognitive restructuring, assertiveness training, and role playing were excluded and some *in vivo* exposure was added. In comparison to the wait-list control, all three treatments were effective in reducing PTSD symptoms and gains were maintained at 6-month follow-up. However, improvements on depression, self-esteem, or social fears were not maintained.

As described earlier, two other controlled studies by Foa and colleagues have examined the efficacy of SIT (Foa et al., 1991; Foa et al., 1999). In both studies, SIT was found to be an effective treatment for PTSD albeit somewhat less effective than PE.

Cognitive Processing Therapy

Resick and Schnicke (1992) compared cognitive processing therapy (CPT) to a wait-list control. CPT contains three components: education about PTSD symptoms and information processing theory, exposure, and cognitive therapy. Rather than using imagery, the exposure component involves writing a detailed account of the rape and reading it in sessions. Therapy was conducted weekly in a group format. Patients receiving CPT improved on symptoms of both PTSD and depression and maintained their gains at 6-month follow-up. The wait-list control did not show evidence of any changes from pre- to posttreatment. A follow-up study (also reported by Resick & Schnicke, 1992) examined a larger sample of women, including the 19 from the previous study. This report continued to support the usage of CPT. Although other comparison groups were not used and dismantling procedures regarding the components of CPT have not been examined, CPT appears to be a relatively effective treatment for rape-related PTSD.

As mentioned above, Resick and colleagues are comparing the efficacy of a 12-sessions CPT to a 9-sessions PE program. At the present time, both treatments appear highly effective in reducing PTSD compared to a wait-list control condition, but no differences between treatments have emerged at any assessment point (P. A. Resick, personal communication, 1998).

Eye Movement Desensitization and Reprocessing

Eye movement desensitization and reprocessing (EMDR; Shapiro, 1989, 1995) has recently gained considerable notoriety. EMDR may be considered a special application of imaginal exposure, because it utilizes the repeated guided visual imagery of the traumatic memory; however, it has been considered unique because it involves the elicitation of rapid, saccadic eye movements during the imaginal exposure session and these movements are considered to be an important treatment element. Most of the studies that examined the efficacy of EMDR suffer from methodological problems which render their results inconclusive (see Foa & Meadows, 1997, for a more complete review); however, several studies warrant discussion. In a well-controlled study, Rothbaum (1997) compared the efficacy of four weekly sessions of EMDR to a wait-list control in female rape victims. On PTSD symptoms, EMDR produced more improvement than the control condition, with gains maintaining at 3-month follow-up. This study suggests that a brief course of

EMDR can effectively reduce symptoms of PTSD; however, since the author conducted all of the treatment, general treatment effects cannot be removed from therapist effects. Several other studies also support the efficacy of EMDR (e.g., Vaughan et al., 1994; Wilson, Becker, & Tinker, 1995; Carlson, Chemtob, Rusnak, Hedlund, & Muraoka, 1998; Scheck, Schaeffer, & Gillette, 1998).

In a well-controlled dismantling study of Pitman and colleagues (1996), male veterans with PTSD were assigned to up to six sessions of EMDR either with saccadic eye movements or with eyes in a fixed position. Neither treatment produced clinically significant improvement. On average, EMDR produced 11% reduction and the fixed-position condition produced 16% reduction. Based on these findings, Pitman et al. concluded that eye movement per se was not the active ingredient in EMDR. A similar dismantling study (Renfrey & Spates, 1994) also suggests that EMDR was not more beneficial than standard exposure treatment for PTSD. In conclusion, the advantage of EMDR for chronic PTSD, beyond that of other exposure techniques, remains questionable (see Tolin, Montgomery, Kleinknecht, & Lohr, 1996).

Combined Treatment Programs

With the advent of effective treatments, studies have examined whether treatment efficacy can be enhanced by combining individually effective treatment components. As described earlier, two studies explored this possibility: Foa et al. (1999) compared PE alone, SIT alone, the combination of PE and SIT, and a wait-list control; and Marks et al. (1998) compared PE alone, CR alone, the combination of PE and CR, and relaxation only (R). Contrary to clinical expectations, the results of both studies did not support the use of combination treatments over individual treatment components.

Overview of Cognitive-Behavioral Treatment Efficacy

At present, both SIT and PE alone appear to perform well, but their combination does not seem to enhance the efficacy of either alone. PE seems to have some advantage over SIT and SIT/PE. CPT has also shown promising results but is not more effective than PE alone. However, the techniques involved in CPT may require more training than those of PE, and PE was conducted over a shorter time frame than CPT. The efficacy of a program that includes PE and one component of SIT, cognitive restructuring, is currently being studied with female assault victims (Foa, 1997). However, Marks and associates' (1998) results do not show an advantage in the addition of cognitive therapy to PE over PE alone. EMDR awaits further empirical verification, and at present its efficacy beyond that of exposure techniques has been questioned.

PSYCHOLOGICAL PROCESSES UNDERLIE NATURAL AND THERAPEUTIC RECOVERY

We propose that the processes involved in successful treatment for PTSD can be best understood if we construe treatment as encouraging the same processes that are involved in natural recovery from a trauma. Data relevant to mechanisms underlying natural recovery and successful therapy are considered next.

Emotional Engagement and Habituation of Traumatic Memories

As early as the 19th century (Janet, 1889), and later (Freud, 1933/1973), trauma theorists have postulated that emotional engagement with traumatic memories is essential for successful processing of the traumatic event and the consequent recovery. Many contemporary theorists also hold this same assumption (Horowitz, 1986; Foa & Jaycox, 1999). A parallel assumption is that the lack of emotional engagement with the traumatic memories such as deliberate avoidance of trauma reminders, emotional withdrawal, and dissociation may hinder recovery. Support for the emotional engagement hypothesis derives from several empirical investigations.

Retrospective reports of dissociative symptoms during or immediately after the trauma have been found to be related to the severity of later PTSD (Bremner et al., 1992; Marmar et al., 1994; Tichenor, Marmar, Weiss, Metzler, & Ronfeldt, 1996). In two prospective studies, dissociative symptoms immediately after natural disasters have been associated with greater long-term PTSD symptoms (Cardeña & Spiegel, 1993; Koopman, Classen, & Spiegel, 1994).

If early engagement promotes recovery, then victims who exhibit high PTSD severity shortly after the trauma should evidence faster recovery than victims with delayed peak symptom severity. To examine this hypothesis, Gilboa and Foa (1998) examined the magnitude and the delay of the peak reaction in a prospective study of trauma reactions. As predicted, 14 weeks after the trauma, victims whose peak reaction occurred within the first 2 weeks exhibited less severe PTSD and depression than victims whose peak reaction occurred later. Thus, initial emotional engagement appears to facilitate natural recovery.

In therapeutic recovery, two studies have found that fear activation, or emotional engagement, during treatment is associated with successful therapeutic outcome. Foa, Riggs, Massie, and Yarczower (1995) found that patients who displayed more intense facial fear expressions during the first exposure session benefited more from treatment than those who displayed less intense fear. Interestingly, patients who reported more anger prior to treatment displayed less fear during reliving of the trauma and benefited less from treatment than patients who were less angry. These data are corroborated by another study of recent assault victims that found that anger impeded natural recovery (Riggs, Dancu, Gershuny, Greenberg, & Foa, 1992). Thus, the relationship between anger immediately after the trauma and later psychopathology may be mediated by the failure of angry victims to engage emotionally with trauma-related fear. While anger may be protective in the short run, in the long run it may interfere with emotional processing of the traumatic event.

Further support for the role of emotional engagement in promoting treatment outcome comes from a study examining the patterns of subjective distress reported by patients during their recounting of the traumatic event in the context of exposure therapy (Jaycox, Foa, & Morral, 1998). Average distress levels during each of the imaginal exposure sessions were submitted to a cluster analysis. Three distinct clusters of patients emerged, differing with regard to their patterns of distress: (1) those with high distress in the first session and gradual decline in distress over the remaining sessions; (2) those with high distress during the first session and no habituation over the course of treatment; and (3) those with moderate distress during the first sessions and no change in distress over time. As would be predicted by the engagement hypothesis, patients from group 1 improved more after treatment than did patients belonging to the groups 2 and 3. Overall, there is converging evidence from two types of studies—one examining natural recovery in recently assaulted victims and the other examining patients with chronic PTSD during treatment—that emotional engagement and habituation promote recovery.

Organization and Elaboration of Traumatic Memories

Many trauma theorists believe that traumatic memories are qualitatively distinct from other types of memories and that recovery involves special processing. In understanding the nature of trauma memories, the research of trauma experts such as Koss (e.g., see Tromp, Koss, Figueredo, & Tharan, 1995) and Pennebaker (e.g., see Harber & Pennebaker, 1992) suggests that study of trauma narratives is promising. Indeed, clinical observations of trauma narratives recounted by patients with chronic PTSD appear to be characterized by an abundance of speech fillers, repetitions, and incomplete sentences. On this basis, Foa and Riggs (1993) hypothesized that the natural process of recovery involves the organizing and streamlining of the traumatic memory and that individuals who fail to organize the memory would exhibit more trauma-related pathology.

In a study of narrative organization, Amir, Stafford, Freshman, and Foa (1998) examined the level of articulation in rape narratives. The degree of articulation was operationalized as the reading level and reading ease of the narratives recounted by victims approximately 2 weeks after the assault. Awir et al. found that a low level of articulation of the trauma narrative, both in grade level and reading ease, was related to later PTSD. Interestingly, the correlations between the level of articulation and both severity of depression and anxiety were not significant, suggesting a more specific relationship between the level of processing the traumatic memory and PTSD.

Likewise, successful treatment should result in more organized and less fragmented trauma memories. Foa, Molnar, and Cashman (1995) hypothesized that the repeated reliving of the traumatic event during exposure therapy would produce changes in the trauma narrative and that these changes would be related to improvement after treatment. To test these hypotheses, they examined rape narratives from the first and last sessions of exposure therapy. They found that the last narratives contained less actions and dialogues and more thoughts and feelings, and were more organized than the first narratives. Also, as hypothesized, the reduction in narrative fragmentation and increase in organization was highly correlated with reduction in trauma-related psychopathology. These findings are consistent with Amir and colleagues' (1998) findings that victims whose trauma narratives were articulated well exhibited less PTSD. Thus, the two studies that investigated trauma narratives—one utilizing narratives of recent victims who had not been treated and the other examining narratives of chronically disturbed victims during therapy—converged to suggest that narrative organization is implicated in recovery from trauma.

Changes in Core Beliefs

Many trauma theorists also argue that successful processing of a trauma requires adjustments of core schemas, that is, changes in beliefs about the world and about oneself (e.g., Epstein, 1991; Horowitz, 1986; Janoff-Bulman, 1992; McCann & Pearlman, 1990). Janoff-Bulman (1992) suggested that traumatic experiences violate the belief that the world is a good place and that the self is invulnerable. Accordingly, victims who previously viewed themselves as invulnerable and perceived their world as extremely safe would be more likely to show trauma-related disturbances than victims who had not held these beliefs. However, victims who had previously experienced multiple traumas have a greater likelihood of developing PTSD (e.g., Burgess & Holstrom, 1978; Resick, 1993). Presumably, these individuals would not perceive the world as extremely safe or themselves as extremely competent. Rather, they would be more likely to perceive the world as extremely dangerous and themselves as extremely incompetent.

In trying to understand this discrepancy, Foa and her colleagues (Foa & Jaycox, 1999; Foa & Riggs, 1993) have suggested that holding an extremely rigid view, either in the positive or negative direction, renders an individual less able to process traumatic events. Therefore, when the trauma either severely violates existing knowledge or when the trauma primes existing knowledge, natural recovery will be less likely to take place. Those trauma victims whose life experiences have allowed them to make refined discriminations of degrees of "dangerousness" and "competence" would be better able than others to process the trauma as a unique and unusual event. Therefore, the trauma would not substantially change their evaluations of themselves and of the world, and natural recovery would be more likely to take place.

Data supporting the hypothesis that rigid beliefs concerning individual competence and the safety of the world are implicated in PTSD have been reported by Foa (1995). In a prospective study, beginning about 2 weeks after the assault, self-esteem and perception of the world were assessed monthly by means of the World Assumption Scale (WAS; Janoff-Bulman, 1989, 1992) and the Personal Beliefs and Reactions Scale (PBRS; Mechanic & Resick, 1999). As expected, individuals who had PTSD 3 months after the trauma exhibited a less positive view about the world and about themselves immediately after the trauma than did victims who recovered. Similarly, using the Post-traumatic Thoughts Inventory (PTTI), Foa, Ehlers, Clark, and Tolin (1999) found that core schemas following an assault were related to PTSD severity. Specifically, three factors discriminated trauma victims with PTSD from those without PTSD: negative thoughts about self, negative thoughts about others, and self-blame. Furthermore, the hypothesis that chronic PTSD is marked by negative cognitions about the self and world has been examined using content analysis of trauma narratives (Ehlers et al., 1998). Ehlers and colleagues found that permanent changes in one's self or life and a sense of alienation impeded recovery from trauma.

Indeed, changes in core schemas have also been implicated in therapeutic recovery. Results from a study reported by Foa and Jaycox (in press) lend support to the hypothesis that cognitive-behavioral therapy induces change in world and self schemas. Female victims of assault who manifested chronic PTSD completed the WAS and the PBRS before and after therapy. In each of these assessments, they were asked to indicate how positively they viewed the world and themselves, both before the assault and at the time of the pretreatment interview. Specifically, at the pretreatment assessment, victims indicated that their current perception of the world and of themselves was less positive than their perception before the trauma. At the posttreatment, these perceptions were more positive than before treatment. Although these data suffer from self-report biases, the investigation of natural recovery from a trauma and the study of treatment outcome both suggest that negative evaluations of the world and of oneself are associated with PTSD and that modification of these evaluations are related to recovery.

Summary of Mechanisms for Recovery

Thus, there is good preliminary evidence to suggest that the degree to which the trauma victim engages trauma memory, organizes and articulates it, and maintains a balanced view about the world and self determine whether natural recovery or therapeutic recovery will take place.

PROLONGED EXPOSURE TREATMENT OVERVIEW

Having examined the mechanisms underlying recovery from a trauma, we now describe a treatment program designed to target a number of these mechanisms. As noted above, the PE program is one of most studied cognitive-behavioral programs and in some studies shows superiority over other treatments. In this section, we describe the PE program that has been developed at the Center for the Treatment and Study of Anxiety in Philadelphia and present two cases: one illustrating a successful treatment outcome; the other, a treatment failure. For a detailed description of the program, see Foa and Rothbaum (1997).

The PE treatment program contains four main components: education about PTSD symptoms, breathing retraining, imaginal exposure, and *in vivo* exposure. The goal of the program is to help the patient resume preassault functioning and be able to remember the trauma without undue anxiety and distress. Patients are seen for 9–12 weeks, for approximately an hour and a half each session. After 9 weeks, treatment progress is reviewed; if the patient has not improved markedly (at least 70% reduction of PTSD symptom severity), an additional three sessions are offered. At the end of each session, homework is assigned to be completed during the subsequent week.

Education

Treatment begins with education about common reactions to a traumatic event. This presentation takes the form of a dialogue allowing the therapist to tailor the presentation to match the patient's symptom presentation. The definition of PTSD, the role of fear and anxiety, and a description of common PTSD symptoms are all discussed. Furthermore, other common trauma-related disturbances such as depression, guilt, loss of sexual interest (particularly with rape victims), and disruptions in social support are discussed. Careful attention is paid to suicidal ideation, and appropriate risk assessment is conducted. These factors are all discussed in detail, and their relationship to the traumatic experience is emphasized. Following this discussion, the patient is provided with a handout that summarizes common reactions to trauma. The patient is encouraged to reread the handout and to share this information with important people in his or her life.

Breathing Retraining

Breathing retraining is taught to help the patients manage anxiety and distress. The therapist briefly explains the relationship between the physical symptoms of anxiety and hyperventilation. The therapist first models the diaphragmatic breathing, taking a breath and exhaling very slowly, quietly uttering the word "calm." After a brief pause, another breath is taken. This sequence is repeated approximately 10–15 times. After that, the therapist and patient conduct the exercise together. Finally, the therapist watches the patient breathing, monitoring problems and making appropriate recommendations. The therapist highlights the role of practice in developing this skill for managing anxiety. As homework, the skill is practiced three times daily.

In Vivo Exposure

Before *in vivo* exposure is started, the rationale and procedures are explained in detail. The therapist explains that fears associated with the trauma are often unrealistic or excessive. Prolonged and repeated confrontation (i.e., *in vivo* exposure) with situations that are anxiety provoking but not objectively dangerous results in reduction of anxiety. The beliefs that particular situations are unsafe and that escape is necessary for anxiety reduction are disconfirmed. Furthermore, *in vivo* exposure helps increase both self-esteem and self-efficacy.

In PTSD sufferers, avoidance behavior is often trauma specific. Typical situations can be highly specific ones, such as reading about a similar event in the paper or seeing a person who resembles the assailant. More general fear-evoking cues are being touched, being alone, or going into a crowded store. The therapist and patient carefully discuss the patient's daily functioning, focusing on changes since the assault. Avoided situations are rated for degree of fear, using the Subjective Units of Discomfort scale (SUDs), which ranges from 0 to 100. Next, a hierarchy is constructed from lowest to highest fear-producing situations or objects. The objective safety of the situation must be assessed. Confrontation with realistically dangerous situations should not be introduced into the hierarchy. The therapist and patient choose situations that evoke moderate levels of anxiety (e.g., SUDs = 50) for the first exposure homework. The patient is instructed to stay in each situation for 30 to 45 minutes, or until his or her anxiety drops considerably (at least 50%). Eventually, more anxiety-producing items on the hierarchy are assigned for practice until the patient can comfortably confront most of them. Toward the end of therapy, SUDs scores are obtained again for each situation in order to evaluate progress and assess areas for future intervention.

Imaginal Exposure

During imaginal exposure, the patient recalls the memory as vividly as possible, imagining the trauma as if it is happening at that moment. First, the patient is given a detailed rationale for imaginal exposure. The therapist explains that the goal of the reliving is to help process and organize the traumatic memory. During this repeated reliving, the patient learns that traumatic memories are not dangerous and gains confidence in his or her ability to manage distress. See Foa and Rothbaum (1997) for a detailed description of the rationale for imaginal exposure.

During imaginal exposure, the patient is encouraged to describe the trauma in the present tense and recount as many details as possible, including specific thoughts and specific feelings. The therapist monitors the SUDs level during the reliving approximately every 5 minutes and asks the patient for vividness ratings on a scale from 0 to 100 as to how real the image feels.

Imaginal exposure continues for approximately 45–60 minutes, repeating the story several times if necessary. The therapist helps the patient obtain a vivid image of the memory during the exposure. Although details are helpful in enhancing vividness, the goal is not to recall as many details as possible or recover "lost" memories. Following the reliving, time is allotted for discussion of the patient's reaction to the reliving experiences as well as to the content of the exposure. The patient is instructed to listen to the audiotape of the imaginal exposure daily and to record pre, post, and peak SUDs levels.

As therapy proceeds, the imaginal exposure focuses on the most difficult parts of the trauma, or "hot spots," to promote anxiety reduction. The therapist must help to titrate distress by either encouraging more detail and affect if the patient is not sufficiently emotionally engaged or by diminishing detail and affect if the patient becomes overwhelmed.

CASE DESCRIPTIONS

To illustrate the process of delivering exposure therapy, we have selected two cases of patients who exhibited some reluctance to comply with treatment requirements and difficulty in treatment implementation. We also selected one person, Alice, to illustrate the efficacy of exposure and a second person, Rebecca, to illustrate its limitations.

Case Illustration 1

The patient, Alice, was a 58-year-old divorced African American woman, a mother of two adult children and living alone. At the time she presented for treatment she was working part-time as a real estate agent. A year prior to treatment, Alice was out walking her dog in the early morning when a man with a gun approached her on the street. The assailant forced her into an alleyway, where he robbed her and raped her both vaginally and anally. At intake, Alice reported symptoms that were clearly related to the assault, including recurrent thoughts about the assault, nightmares, and intense emotional and physical reactions when reminded of the assault. She avoided all possible contacts with strangers, did not leave her home after dark, and did not ride public transportation. She also reported difficulty falling asleep (taking an average of 3 hours to fall asleep), continuous irritability, and hypervigilance.

Initial Assessment

Alice was assessed extensively as part of our ongoing treatment research project. This included a full diagnostic interview (SCID: Structured Clinical Interview for DSM-IV Axis I Disorders; First, Spitzer, Gibbon, & Williams, 1995), a structured interview for PTSD (PTSD Symptom Scale—Interview, PSS-I; Foa, Riggs, Dancu, & Rothbaum, 1993) conducted by an independent evaluator, and several self-report measures including the Posttraumatic Diagnostic Scale (PDS; Foa, Cashman, Jaycox, & Perry, 1997), the Beck Depression Inventory (BDI; Beck, Ward, Mendelsohn, Mock & Erbaugh, 1961), and the Beck Anxiety Inventory (BAI; Beck, Epstein, Brown, & Steer, 1988). Alice was diagnosed with PTSD in the moderate-to-severe range, subthreshold prior major depression, and prior alcohol dependence. She also reported current depressive symptoms in the moderate range (BDI = 21) but did not meet diagnostic criteria for a current depressive disorder. Her major trauma prior to the index rape and robbery was domestic violence (including rape) from her former husband, approximately 10 years earlier. During the first treatment session, additional information was gathered by the therapist.

Alice's beliefs about herself, others, and the world were also assessed. She held the view that the world was a dangerous place, noting that "because I was assaulted in a situation I thought was safe, I never feel safe anymore." Alice also strongly endorsed feelings of low self-esteem and incompetence.

Alice's treatment focused on the reduction of symptoms of PTSD via imaginal exposure and *in vivo* exposure. Special attention was paid to her severe avoidance and hyperarousal symptoms. Because she evidenced moderate depression, depressive symptoms were closely monitored. Her sobriety, on the other hand, did not appear to be an issue, as she had remained abstinent for the entire year since the assault and prior to that was abstinent for 10 years.

Course of Treatment

The initial treatment session focused on explaining the rationale for treatment and its procedures. Alice easily grasped the rationale for treatment but expressed some concern about the exposure practices because of her advanced age and the unsafe areas in her neighborhood. She was convinced that some of her avoidance was reasonable. Alice was reassured that each exposure practice would be carefully assessed for realistic risk. Finally, the rationale for breathing retraining was explained and the therapist modeled the procedure before Alice attempted it. Alice mastered the exercise easily and reported that she felt calmer at its completion.

During the second session, common reactions to trauma were described. Alice actively participated in the discussion, noting that she felt less alarmed for having these reactions. Alice and her therapist identified patterns of avoidance and together created a hierarchy for *in vivo* exposure practices. The hierarchy ranged from going to dinner with a girlfriend (SUDs = 5) to going back to the place of the assault (SUDs = 100). Her first *in vivo* homework assignment involved walking slowly to the grocery store (SUDs = 40), smoking outside at work (SUDs = 55), and waiting at the train station (SUDs = 70). All of these exposures represented activities that Alice had routinely done without fear prior to the assault.

In the third session, Alice reported that she found the *in vivo* exercises to be extremely helpful. She had practiced each situation at least twice during the week and was pleased with the anxiety reduction she experienced (i.e., the highest post SUDs score was 15). The main objective of the third session was the introduction of imaginal reliving. While Alice expressed initial hesitation, she was convinced by the rationale for the treatment and cooperated with the therapist. The exercise progressed well. Alice recounted her trauma in a quiet voice and maintained the present tense with little prompting. She was able to generate vivid imagery (vividness = 100) and evidenced high emotional engagement (peak SUDs = 100). Her narrative began with her leaving the apartment and ended with her boyfriend's reaction of shock and support. Her initial SUDs score was 60, increasing to 100 within the first 5 minutes. The second repetition of the narrative caused an initial SUDs score of 50, increasing again to 100. Her anxiety peaked when she described the rape itself and her fear of HIV afterward. After the reliving, Alice voiced skepticism about the usefulness of the reliving but agreed to take the tape home and listen to it daily. Alice expressed amazement that she was able to tell the story, noting that she had believed she would not be able to do so.

As treatment progressed, Alice continued to experience success with her *in vivo* exposure, gradually moving up her hierarchy. She continued by visiting banks, going to the back of bookstores, and walking with a friend to the place of the assault. With each of these exercises Alice reported initial moderate-to-high anxiety, which subsequently decreased. She was pleased with her progress, and this success bolstered her self-esteem. However, she found imaginal exposure to be much more difficult. Alice listened to the imaginal tape five times during the first week, with limited reduction in anxiety. Consequently, in the next session, Alice expressed reluctance to continue the reliving homework assignments. The therapist reassured her that if she continued with the process her anxiety would decrease, linking this process with that of *in vivo* exposure where Alice experienced habituation of anxiety. Alice agreed to continue, despite the persistence of anxiety during the reliving in the first four sessions.

With the help of the therapist, Alice was able to identify her emotional reactions during the imaginal exposure. In addition to the high level of anxiety, the reliving elicited intense anger toward the assailant. Alice was encouraged to focus on the fear rather than on the anger when recounting her trauma. This modification, as well as her persistence with the imaginal homework, resulted in a substantial anxiety reduction to the trauma memories during the fifth imaginal exposure session. As her anxiety decreased, her PTSD symptoms began to abate. Because of her substantial progress, Alice and her therapist decided to terminate treatment after the ninth session.

Outcome

At the end of treatment Alice was again assessed by an independent evaluator. This evaluation corroborated Alice's self-report of vast reduction in PTSD symptoms. Indeed she no longer met diagnostic criteria for PTSD, although she still reported occasional feelings of irritability (PSS-I = 3). Notably, her depressive symptoms had dissipated (BDI = 2), as did symptoms of general anxiety (BAI = 2). By the 6-month follow-up, Alice reported no symptoms of reexperiencing, avoidance, or arousal. After treatment, she moved with her boyfriend to another state, adjusting well to her new environment and reporting no trauma-related daily dysfunction.

Case Illustration 2

The patient, Rebecca, was a 34-year-old single Caucasian woman receiving disability from her job as a restaurant manager. During the year prior to her treatment, Rebecca had been stalked by one of the male patrons of the restaurant, who used to wait for her in the parking lot of the restaurant and had occasionally followed her home after hours. Six months prior to seeking treatment, Rebecca was shot by the stalker in the restaurant parking lot. The stalker had been caught and was in custody awaiting trial. Rebecca sustained considerable physical injuries, but at the time of intake was only experiencing some pain and limited movement in her left leg. Her psychological symptoms included recurrent thoughts about the assault, disturbing nightmares, and intense emotional and physical responses when reminded of it. She invested much effort in avoiding thoughts and feelings about the assault and situations or places that might remind her of it. She was unable to go back to work or to even drive by the restaurant and had great difficulty falling asleep.

Initial Assessment

Rebecca was initially diagnosed with PTSD (lifetime and current), recurrent major depression (current), and subthreshold panic disorder. Her PTSD and depression were of moderate intensity (PDS = 26 and BDI = 16). She reported panic attacks, but all were all related to the assault. Her only prior traumatic event was a brutal rape when she was 17, from which she had PTSD symptoms that diminished over time.

Course of Treatment

Rebecca's treatment program was similar to Alice's, focusing on the reduction of symptoms of PTSD via imaginal exposure and *in vivo* exposure. Again, in the initial treatment session the therapist presented the rationale for treatment and described the treatment process. In discussing the assault circumstance, Rebecca expressed extreme anger and resentment that she had to permanently suffer from the criminal behavior of another person. As was the case with Alice, Rebecca also comprehended the rationale for treatment but expressed reluctance to engage in the exposure exercises, communicating trepidation about deliberately confronting trauma reminders and believing that she would be unable to execute such practices. Rebecca was reassured that the exposure would be done gradually with easier items confronted first and more difficult ones introduced after those had been mastered. Finally, the rationale for breathing retraining was explained and the therapist modeled the procedure before Rebecca attempted it herself. Rebecca mastered the exercise easily and reported that she felt much calmer at its completion.

The second session began with a discussion on common reactions to trauma. Rebecca actively participated in the discussion, at one point breaking down in tears, noting that she should have been over it by now. In this session, Rebecca and her therapist developed an *in vivo* hierarchy. Although she objectively knew that the stalker was in jail, Rebecca reported intense fear of any reminders of the assault and of social situations in general. These situations ranged from going to a mall alone (SUDs = 50), sleeping with the lights and television turned off (SUDs = 100+), and going back to the place of the assault (SUDs = 100+). Her first *in vivo* homework assignment involved sitting or standing in parking lots, going to the gym, and walking along a popular street. Prior to the assault Rebecca had routinely engaged in these activities without any fear, but she avoided them after the assault.

In the third session, Rebecca reported that she found the common reactions handout extremely helpful and the *in vivo* exercises only somewhat helpful. She had attempted each exercise at least once and experienced only mild anxiety reduction. On further inquiry, it became clear that Rebecca had terminated her *in vivo* exposures too soon for habituation to have occurred. Rebecca's therapist reminded her that she needed to "stay in situation until her anxiety was at least 50% lower than its peak level or until one hour had passed." The main objective of the third session was to introduce the imaginal reliving. While Rebecca expressed some reluctance, she understood the rationale and complied willingly. However, she was quite agitated prior to start of the reliving, with her SUDs at 90 before she started. Rebecca was able to generate quite vivid imagery (vividness = 85) but evidenced low emotional engagement (i.e., during the narrative her peak SUDs only reached 50 while she was imagining being in the parking lot). She had a hard time keeping the narrative in the present tense and told the story in a distant manner.

She repeated the story twice during the hour of reliving. Like Alice, Rebecca was reluctant to take the tape home. Her next *in vivo* assignments focused on confronting routine activities alone, such as food and clothing shopping and sitting in her car alone, incorporating the assignments from the last session.

In the fifth treatment session, Rebecca reported using the breathing exercises frequently and finding them very helpful. She noted "hatred" for imaginal reliving but said that she listened to the tape three times during the week with only slight anxiety reduction. She reported success with the low *in vivo* exposure exercises and felt much more able to do routine activities. However, she failed to approach moderately difficult assignments, noting that any reminder of the assault itself still seemed impossible to confront. Her therapist proposed to facilitate exposure to these situations by accompanying her. Rebecca was visibly fearful and upset by this suggestion. Tearfully, she voiced deep resentment that she had to suffer unjustly and that she needed to go through therapy because of it. She also expressed anger at her employers for not taking her concerns regarding the stalker seriously, and she expressed rage at the stalker for being "crazy." Sobbingly, she accused the therapist of not understanding the extent of her distress. After considerable effort to calm Rebecca using the breathing exercise, the therapist discussed Rebecca's anger and resentment about being saddled with PTSD. Rebecca acknowledged being extremely angry and felt comforted by her therapist's understanding of the unfairness of her circumstances. The therapist then explained to Rebecca that as much as it was justified, her anger was unhelpful because it kept her from taking positive steps toward recovery, including completing exposure practices. This discourse was completed with the therapist reviewing the rationale for treatment.

To help Rebecca experience a success in trauma-related exposure practice, she (accompanied by the therapist) entered a dark closet in order to confront her fear of the dark. During this exercise, Rebecca's initial anxiety level was an 80, but within 20 minutes it decreased to a 40. Rebecca appeared far more confident and hopeful at the end of this exercise but began the imaginal exposure with some reluctance. During the imaginal exposure, Rebecca evidenced avoidance by rushing through the story, repeating it six times within 30 minutes and glossing over many important details. As usual, her anticipatory anxiety was higher than her anxiety during the reliving. For *in vivo* homework, she was assigned practices of sitting in her car alone and sitting in the dark (first with someone and then alone).

Prior to the sixth session, Rebecca left a message with the secretary that she was recommended to another therapist by her psychiatrist and would not be continuing with the treatment program.

Outcome

Rebecca refused to come in for a termination session or to participate in a phone evaluation. Her self-report data at the fourth session indicated that her

PTSD symptoms remained at the initial level (PDS = 23). Notably, her depressive symptoms had increased (BDI = 20) and her general anxiety had nearly doubled. At Rebecca's request, a detailed summary of the treatment was sent to her new therapist.

Summary of the Case Illustrations

The cases presented clearly demonstrate divergent outcomes for the same treatment program for chronic PTSD. Alice definitely demonstrates the value of a brief exposure treatment that targets symptoms of PTSD, whereas Rebecca demonstrates the limitation of this therapy. The divergent course of response to treatment is puzzling because of the apparent similarity between the two cases. Both Alice and Rebecca expressed concern as to their ability to follow exposure procedures, and both women experienced considerable anger associated with the traumatic event and its sequelae. However, Alice complied with treatment, emotionally engaging with the traumatic memory during reliving, and diligently persevered with homework assignments despite the distress they caused her. Rebecca, on the other hand, remained focused on the "unfairness" of her circumstances and on her anger about being condemned to suffering for no fault of her own. This perspective, together with her low tolerance of distress, interfered with her ability to comply with treatment guidelines; she refused to engage emotionally with the traumatic images and failed to conduct homework assignments in the prescribed manner. Exposure treatment was effective in presenting Alice with information that disconfirmed her erroneous cognitions (e.g., "anxiety stays forever"), resulting in symptom reduction. In contrast, Rebecca's inadequate exposures served to confirm her dysfunctional beliefs, intensifying her sense of being incompetent, and thus perpetuating her PTSD symptoms and even amplifying her depression.

CONCLUSION

In this chapter, we have argued that several cognitive-behavioral treatments are effective in reducing PTSD and related symptoms and that prolonged exposure may have some advantage over other programs. In an attempt to explain natural recovery and treatment efficacy, we have focused on three psychological factors that are involved in the successful processing of a traumatic event: emotional engagement with the trauma memory, organization and articulation of the trauma narrative, and modification of basic core beliefs about the world and about oneself. To illustrate the process of exposure therapy and the mechanisms involved in its success, we have presented two case examples, one describing recovery and the other failure to benefit from treatment. These cases also demonstrate the complexity and intricacy inherent in delivering this seemingly straightforward treatment program.

ACKNOWLEDGMENTS

We would like to thank Rosemary Gruber for her help in the manuscript preparation. The preparation of this chapter was supported in part by two grants from the National Institute of Mental Health (Nos. MH-52272 and MH-42178) awarded to Edna B. Foa.

REFERENCES

American Psychiatric Association. (1980). *Diagnostic and statistical manual of mental disorders* (3rd ed.). Washington, DC: Author.

Amir, N., Stafford, J., Freshman, M. S., & Foa, E. B. (1998). Relationship between trauma narratives and trauma pathology. *Journal of Traumatic Stress, 11*(2), 385–392.

Beck, A. T., Epstein, N., Brown, G., & Steer, R. A. (1988). An inventory for measuring clinical anxiety: The Beck Anxiety Inventory. *Journal of Consulting and Clinical Psychology, 56*, 893–897.

Beck, A. T., Ward, C. H., Mendelsohn, M., Mock, J., & Erbaugh, J. (1961). An inventory for measuring depression. *Archives of General Psychiatry, 4*, 561–571.

Boudewyns, P. A., & Hyer, L. (1990). Physiological response to combat memories and preliminary treatment outcome in Vietnam veteran PTSD patients treated with direct therapeutic exposure. *Behavior Therapy, 21*(1), 63–87.

Boudewyns, P. A., Hyer, L., Woods, M. G., Harrison, W. R., & McCranie, E. (1990). PTSD among Vietnam veterans: An early look at treatment outcome using direct therapeutic exposure. *Journal of Traumatic Stress, 3*(3), 359–368.

Bremner, J. D., Southwick, S., Brett, E., Fontana, A., Rosenheck, R., & Charney, D. S. (1992). Dissociation and posttraumatic stress disorder in Vietnam combat veterans. *American Journal of Psychiatry, 149*(3), 328–332.

Burgess, A. W., & Holmstrom, L. L. (1978). Recovery from rape and prior life stress. *Research in Nursing and Health, 1*, 165–174.

Cardeña, E., & Spiegel, D. (1993). Dissociative reactions to the San Francisco Bay Area earthquake of 1989. *American Journal of Psychiatry, 150*(3), 474–478.

Carlson, J. G., Chemtob, C. M., Rusnak, K., Hedlund, N. L., & Muraoka, M. Y. (1998). Eye movement desensitization and reprocessing (EMDR) treatment for combat-related posttraumatic stress disorder. *Journal of Traumatic Stress, 11*(1), 3–25.

Cooper, N. A., & Clum, G. A. (1989). Imaginal flooding as a supplementary treatment for PTSD in combat veterans: A controlled study. *Behavior Therapy, 20*(3), 381–391.

Ehlers, A., Clark, D. M., Winton, E., Jaycox, L. H., Meadows, E., & Foa, E. B. (1998). Predicting response to exposure treatment in PTSD: The role of mental defeat and alienation. *Journal of Traumatic Stress, 11*(3), 457–471.

Epstein, S. (1991). The self-concept, the traumatic neurosis, and the structure of personality. In D. Ozer, J. M. Healy, & A. J. Stewart (Eds.), *Perspectives in personality* (Vol. 3, Pt. A, pp. 63–98). London: Kingsley.

Fairbank, J. A., Gross, R. T., & Keane, T. M. (1983). Treatment of posttraumatic stress disorder: Evaluation of outcome with a behavioral code. *Behavior Modification, 7,* 557–568.

First, M. B., Spitzer, R. L., Gibbon, M., & Williams, J. B. W. (1995). *Structured Clinical Interview for DSM-IV Axis I Disorders—Patient Edition* (SCID-I/P, Version 2.0). New York: Biometrics Research Department.

Foa, E. B. (1995, March). *Cognitive behavioral treatment of post-traumatic stress disorder in female assault victims.* Paper presented at the Symposium on Sexual and Physical Abuse and Its Clinical Impact, at the 53rd annual scientific meeting of the American Psychosomatic Society, New Orleans, LA.

Foa, E. B. (1997, September). *Psychopathology of PTSD and its treatment: New findings.* Keynote lecture presented at the Conference of the European Association for Cognitive and Behavioral Therapies, Venice, Italy.

Foa, E. B., Cashman, L., Jaycox, L., & Perry, K. (1997). The validation of a self-report measure of PTSD: The Posttraumatic Diagnostic Scale™ (PDS™). *Psychological Assessment, 9*(4), 445–451.

Foa, E. B., Dancu, C. V., Hembree, E., Jaycox, L. H., Meadows, E. A., & Street, G. P. (1999). The efficacy of exposure therapy, stress inoculation training, and their combination in ameliorating PTSD for female victims of assault. *Journal of Consulting and Clinical Psychology, 67*(2), 194–200.

Foa, E. B., Ehlers, A., Clark, D. M., & Tolin, D. F. (1999). The Post-traumatic Thoughts Inventory (PTTI): Development and validation. *Psychological Assessment, 11*(3), 303–314.

Foa, E. B., & Jaycox, L. H. (1999). Cognitive-behavioral treatment of posttraumatic stress disorder. In D. Spiegel (Ed.), *Psychotherapeutic frontiers: New principles and practices* (pp. 23–61). Washington, DC: American Psychiatric Press.

Foa, E. B., & Meadows, E. A. (1997). Psychosocial treatments for posttraumatic stress disorder: A critical review. In J. Spence, J. M. Darley, & D. J. Foss (Eds.), *Annual Review of Psychology* (Vol. 48, pp. 449–480). Palo Alto, CA: Annual Reviews.

Foa, E. B., Molnar, C., & Cashman, L. (1995). Change in rape narratives during exposure therapy for PTSD. *Journal of Traumatic Stress, 8*(4), 675–690.

Foa, E. B., & Riggs, D. S. (1993). Post-traumatic stress disorder in rape victims. In J. Oldham, M. B. Riba, & A. Tasman (Eds.), *American Psychiatric Press review of psychiatry* (Vol. 12, pp. 273–303). Washington, DC: American Psychiatric Press.

Foa, E. B., Riggs, D. S., Dancu, C. V., & Rothbaum, B. O. (1993). Reliability and validity of a brief instrument for assessing posttraumatic stress disorder. *Journal of Traumatic Stress, 6*(4), 459–473.

Foa, E. B., Riggs, D. S., Massie, E. D., & Yarczower, M. (1995). The impact of fear activation and anger on the efficacy of exposure treatment for PTSD. *Behavior Therapy, 26,* 487–499.

Foa, E. B., & Rothbaum, B. O. (1997). *Treating the trauma of rape.* New York: Guilford Press.

Foa, E. B., Rothbaum, B. O., Riggs, D. S., & Murdock, T. B. (1991). Treatment of posttraumatic stress disorder in rape victims: A comparison between cognitive-behavioral procedures and counseling. *Journal of Consulting and Clinical Psychology, 59*(5), 715–723.

Frank, E., & Stewart, B. D. (1983). Physical aggression: Treating the victims. In E. A. Bleckman (Ed.), *Behavior modification with women* (pp. 245–272). New York: Guilford Press.

Frank, E., & Stewart, B. D. (1984). Depressive symptoms in rape victims. *Journal of Affective Disorders, 1,* 269–277.

Freud, S. (1973). *The new introductory lectures in psychoanalysis.* New York: Penguin Books. (Original work published 1933)

Gilboa, E., & Foa, E. B. (1998). *Patterns of recovery after trauma: Individual differences and trauma characteristics.* Manuscript submitted for publication.

Harber, K. D., & Pennebaker, J. W. (1992). Overcoming traumatic memories. In S. Christianson (Ed.), *The handbook of emotion and memory: Research and theory* (pp. 359–387). Hillsdale, NJ: Erlbaum.

Horowitz, M. J. (1986). *Stress response syndromes* (2nd ed.). Northvale, NJ: Aronson.

Janet, P. (1889). *L'automatisme psychologique.* Paris: Alcan.

Janoff-Bulman, R. (1989). Assumptive worlds and the stress of traumatic events: Applications of the schema construct. *Social Cognition, 7*(2), 113–136.

Janoff-Bulman, R. (1992). *Shattered assumptions: Towards a new psychology of trauma.* New York: Free Press.

Jaycox, L. H., Foa, E. B., & Morral, A. (1998). The influence of emotional engagement and habituation on exposure therapy for PTSD. *Journal of Consulting and Clinical Psychology, 66*(1), 185–192.

Keane, T. M., Fairbank, J. A., Caddell, J. M., & Zimering, R. T. (1989). Implosive (flooding) therapy reduces symptoms of PTSD in Vietnam combat veterans. *Behavior Therapy, 20,* 245–260.

Keane, T. M., & Kaloupek, D. G. (1982). Imaginal flooding in the treatment of posttraumatic stress disorder in Vietnam veterans. *The Behavior Therapist, 8,* 9–12.

Kilpatrick, D. G., Veronen, L. J., & Resick, P. A. (1982). Psychological sequelae to rape: Assessment and treatment strategies. In D. M. Doleys, R. L. Meredith, & A. R. Ciminero (Eds.), *Behavioral medicine: Assessment and treatment strategies* (pp. 473–497). New York: Plenum Press.

Koopman, C., Classen, C., & Spiegel, D. A. (1994). Predictors of posttraumatic stress symptoms among survivors of the Oakland/Berkeley, Calif., firestorm. *American Journal of Psychiatry, 151*(6), 888–894.

Kulka, R. A., Schlenger, W. E., Fairbank, J. A., & Hough, R. (1990). *Trauma and the Vietnam War generation: Report of findings for the National Vietnam Veterans Readjustment Study.* New York: Brunner/Mazel.

Marks, I., Lovell, K., Noshirvani, H., Livanou, M., & Thrasher, S. (1998). Treatment of posttraumatic stress disorder by exposure and/or cognitive restructuring: A controlled study. *Archives of General Psychiatry, 55,* 317–325.

Marmar, C. R., Weiss, D. S., Schlenger, W. E., Fairbank, J. A., Jordan, B. K., Kulka, R. A., & Hough, R. L. (1994). Peritraumatic dissociation and posttraumatic stress in male Vietnam theater veterans. *American Journal of Psychiatry, 151*(6), 902–907.

McCann, I. L., & Pearlman, L. A. (1990). *Psychological trauma and the adult survivor: Theory, therapy, and transformation.* New York: Brunner/Mazel.

Mechanic, M. B., & Resick, P. A. (1993). *The Personal Beliefs and Reactions Scale: Assessing rape-related cognitive schema.* Paper presented at the annual meeting of the International Society for Traumatic Stress Studies, San Antonio, TX.

Pitman, R. K., Orr, S. P., Altman, B., Longpre, R. E., Poire, R. E., & Macklin, M. L. (1996). Emotional processing during eye-movement desensitization and reprocessing therapy of Vietnam veterans with chronic post-traumatic stress disorder. *Comprehensive Psychiatry, 37*(6), 419–429.

Renfrey, G., & Spates, C. R. (1994). Eye movement desensitization: A partial dismantling study. *Journal of Behavior Therapy and Experimental Psychiatry, 25,* 231–239.

Resick, P. A. (1993). The psychological impact of rape. [Special Section: Rape.] *Journal of Interpersonal Violence, 8*(2), 223–255.

Resick, P. A., Jordan, C. G., Girelli, S. A., Hutter, C. K., & Marhoefer-Dvorak, S. (1988). A comparative outcome study of group behavioral therapy for sexual assault victims. *Behavior Therapy, 19,* 385–401.

Resick, P. A., & Schnicke, M. K. (1992). Cognitive processing therapy for sexual assault victims. *Journal of Consulting and Clinical Psychology, 60*(5), 748–756.

Resnick, H. S., Kilpatrick, D. G., Dansky, B. S., Saunders, B. E., & Best, C. L. (1993). Prevalence of civilian trauma and posttraumatic stress disorder in a representative national sample of women. *Journal of Consulting and Clinical Psychology, 61,* 984–991.

Richards, D. A., Lovell, K., & Marks, I. M. (1994). Post-traumatic stress disorder: Evaluation of a behavioral treatment program. *Journal of Traumatic Stress, 7*(4), 669–680.

Riggs, D. S., Dancu, C. V., Gershuny, B. S., Greenberg, D., & Foa, E. B. (1992). Anger and post-traumatic stress disorder in female crime victims. *Journal of Traumatic Stress, 5*(4), 613–625.

Rothbaum, B. O. (1997). A controlled study of eye movement desensitization and reprocessing in the treatment of post-traumatic stress disordered sexual assault victims. *Bulletin of the Menninger Clinic, 61*(3), 317–334.

Rothbaum, B. O., Foa, E. B., Murdock, T., Riggs, D. S., & Walsh, W. (1992). A prospective examination of posttraumatic stress disorder in rape victims. *Journal of Traumatic Stress, 5*(3), 455–475.

Scheck, M. M., Schaeffer, J. A., & Gillette, C. (1998). Brief psychological intervention with traumatized young women: The efficacy of eye movement desensitization and reprocessing. *Journal of Traumatic Stress, 11*(1), 25–44.

Shapiro, F. (1989). Efficacy of eye movement desensitization procedure in the treatment of traumatic memories. *Journal of Traumatic Stress, 2*(2), 199–223.

Shapiro, F. (1995). *Eye movement desensitization and reprocessing: Basic principles, protocols, and procedures.* New York: Guilford Press.

Thompson, J. A., Charlton, P. F. C., Kerry, R., Lee, D., & Turner, S. W. (1995). An open trial of exposure therapy based on deconditioning for posttraumatic stress disorder. *British Journal of Clinical Psychiatry, 34,* 407–416.

Tichenor, V., Marmar, C. R., Weiss, D. S., Metzler, T. J., & Ronfeldt, H. M. (1996). The relationship of peritraumatic dissociation and posttraumatic stress: Findings in female Vietnam theater veterans. *Journal of Consulting and Clinical Psychology, 64*(5), 1054–1059.

Tolin, D. F., Montgomery, R. W., Kleinknecht, R. A., & Lohr, J. M. (1996). An evaluation of eye movement desensitization and reprocessing (EMDR). In L. Vander-Creek, S. Knapp, et al. (Eds.), *Innovations in clinical practice* (Vol. 14, pp. 423–437). Sarasota, FL: Professional Resources Press.

Tromp, S., Koss, M. P., Figueredo, A. J., & Tharan, M. (1995). Are rape memories different?: A comparison of rape, other unpleasant, and pleasant memories among employed women. *Journal of Traumatic Stress, 8*(4), 607–627.

Vaughan, K., Armstrong, M. S., Gold, R., O'Connor N., Jenneke, W., et al. (1994) A trial of eye movement desensitization compared to image habituation training and applied muscle relaxation in posttraumatic stress disorder. *Journal of Behavior Therapy and Experimental Psychiatry, 25,* 283–291.

Veronen, L. J., & Kilpatrick, D. G. (1982, November). *Stress inoculation training for victims of rape: Efficacy and differential findings.* Paper resented in the Symposium on Sexual Violence and Harassment, conducted at the 16th Annual Convention of the Association for the Advancement of Behavior Therapy, Los Angeles, CA.

Wilson, S. A., Becker, L. A., & Tinker, R. H. (1995). Eye movement desensitization and reprocessing (EMDR) treatment for psychologically traumatized individuals. *Journal of Consulting and Clinical Psychology, 63,* 928–937.

Wolpe, J. (1958). *Psychotherapy by reciprocal inhibition.* Stanford, CA: Stanford University Press.

8

Group Psychotherapy for PTSD

DAVID W. FOY, PAULA P. SCHNURR, DANIEL S. WEISS, MELISSA S. WATTENBERG, SHIRLEY M. GLYNN, CHARLES R. MARMAR, and FRED D. GUSMAN

In this chapter we present an overview of three types of group therapy supportive, psychodynamic, and cognitive-behavioral—currently used in the treatment of posttraumatic stress disorder (PTSD). Preliminarily, the historical development of group treatment for PTSD is briefly reviewed, including several advantages offered by group therapy, followed by an overview of evidence providing empirical support for group treatment. Next, for each type of group therapy the treatment rationale and description of procedures are presented, along with a case example. Considerations for offering group therapy as a primary mode of therapy are enumerated. Finally, we discuss matching criteria for use in selecting the type of group intervention that best fits a particular client, and areas of necessary further investigation are identified.

HISTORICAL DEVELOPMENT OF GROUP TREATMENT FOR PTSD

Chronic PTSD typically involves a disruption of trust in others (Janoff-Bulman & Frieze, 1983; McCann & Pearlman, 1990). By their very nature, many traumatic experiences involve interpersonal violence (e.g., rape, physical assault, domestic violence, torture, or combat) and incorporate at their core information about how humans are capable of harming other humans. Other traumas, especially those resulting from natural disasters or accidents, may not involve interpersonal violence per se but often include responses of fear, helplessness, or horror. These emotions may cause survivors to question whether others are really available to assist and support them in times of extreme need, and result in a subsequent disruption of trust. The disruption in trust seen in trauma survivors is reflected in the DSM-IV PTSD avoidance symptom, "feeling of detachment or estrangement from others."

Given the prominence of disturbances in trust in the responses of trauma survivors, it is not surprising that *group* treatment of traumatic responses has been a common form of intervention. The appeal of group interventions for PTSD rests, to a large extent, on the clear relevance of joining with others in therapeutic work when coping with a disorder marked by isolation, alienation, and diminished feelings (Allen & Bloom, 1994). A group intervention seems even more suitable for populations such as Vietnam veterans or sexual assault survivors, who often feel ostracized from the larger society, or even judged and blamed for their predicament. Bonding with similar others in a supportive environment can be a critical to regaining trust. Beyond its obvious cost advantage, group therapy may be particularly useful for those individuals who fail to meet common assumptions (e.g., psychological mindedness and responsibility for life choices and outcomes) thought necessary for individual psychotherapy (Klein & Schermer, 2000).

Inherent in the earliest forms of group intervention for PTSD was the notion that survivors must rely on other survivors, often without benefit of professional assistance (Brende, 1981). Veterans' groups and women's groups were often left to address trauma issues with little professional input or guidance. In part, this emphasis on self-help reflected the lack of clear PTSD diagnostic criteria offered by professional organizations such as the American Psychiatric Association or the American Psychological Association during the 1960s and 1970s. In addition, it probably also reflects many survivors' general distrust of other people, especially those who have never been traumatized. It is not at all surprising that, among these individuals who felt alienated from and distrust of the greater community, group interventions originally tended to adopt a "survivor helping survivor" or "band of sisters/brothers" model in which the group facilitator(s), in fact, shared the same traumatic exposure history as those seeking counseling (Lifton, 1973; Shatan, 1973). These interventions emphasized communality and mutual commitment—in short, the engendering of trust. The genesis of veterans' "rap groups" and the creation of the VA (Veterans Administration) Readjustment Counseling Service, in which Vietnam veterans were hired to assist other veterans outside of the traditional hospital setting, epitomizes this type of approach.

While groups of survivors assisting and witnessing for each other have often offered participants comfort and support, there have been no controlled trials to establish an empirical basis for their efficacy in promoting recovery from traumatic events. In contrast, mental health professionals from several theoretical orientations have refined and tested a number of more systematic group interventions for PTSD since its inclusion in the psychiatric nomenclature in 1980. In contrast to rap groups, these interventions hold to clearly delineated lines between the therapist and clients, and are intended for group members who share a specific, well-diagnosed, acknowledged psychiatric disorder. Some have argued that they are especially appropriate for more chronic forms of PTSD (Walker & Nash, 1981).

In surveying the scientific literature on types of group therapy for PTSD, distinctions can be drawn between "covering" and "uncovering" methods utilized to address the traumatic experiences of members. *Supportive groups* represent a "covering" approach in which the emphasis is placed on addressing current life issues, whereas *psychodynamic* and *cognitive-behavioral* approaches are designed to address members' specific traumatic experiences and memories directly (i.e., "uncover" the trauma). In fact, current group treatments from either psychodynamic or cognitive-behavioral perspectives are often described as "trauma focus" groups wherein members' recounting of their traumatic experiences is a primary feature. Trauma focus groups of either type are more likely to be conducted as "closed" (or cohort) groups, while supportive groups are amenable to an "open" format in which members can be added after the group begins. Some clinicians have posited that a combination of approaches, tailored to the individual's specific phase of the disorder and clinical status, may be most appropriate (e.g., Herman, 1992).

The theoretical contributions of Yalom's (1995) principles of group process to the conduct of each of the three types of trauma group treatment have often been acknowledged (e.g., the importance of the instillation of hope). Nevertheless, it is imperative to note that none of these approaches is "process oriented" strictly defined. That is, the critical therapeutic ingredient is *not* thought to be the corrective recapitulation of the primary family group nor expression of intense affect between members about their relationship. While they may differ in their underlying formulations of symptom etiology and maintenance, these three approaches share some basic features: (1) homogeneous membership in the group by survivors of the same type of trauma (e.g., combat veterans or sexual assault survivors); (2) acknowledgment and validation of the traumatic exposure; (3) normalization of traumatic responses; (4) utilization of the presence of other individuals with a similar traumatic history to dispel the notion that the therapist cannot be helpful to the survivors because he or she has not shared the experience; and (5) adoption of a nonjudgmental stance toward behavior required for survival at the time of the trauma. Incorporating these principles facilitates the development of a psychologically safe, respectful therapeutic environment which permits members to address issues of trust.

EVIDENCE SUPPORTING GROUP THERAPY

Recently, we have reviewed in detail the published reports of clinical trials of group psychotherapy for adult trauma survivors (Foy et al., 2000). We found that group therapy was typically conducted over 10–15 weekly sessions (range = 6 weeks to 1 year), and session length was usually set at 1½ or 2 hours. Most studies were conducted with female survivors of childhood or adulthood sexual abuse; very few published reports have included male participants.

Overall, the current literature provides consistent evidence that group psychotherapy, regardless of the type, is associated with favorable outcomes across a number of symptoms. PTSD and depression are the most commonly targeted, but efficacy has been demonstrated for a range of other symptoms as well, including global distress, dissociation, self-esteem, and fear. Elsewhere we have delineated a number of significant methodological issues—including random assignment of participants, ensuring adequate statistical power, and use of standardized treatment manuals—that currently constrain the causal inferences that can be drawn about the efficacy of group treatment (Foy et al., 2000). These limitations are particularly important for informing future research in this area. In the next sections we offer a treatment rationale and description of procedures in some detail for each of the three types of group treatment. Further, to illustrate the application of these group treatments, case illustrations are offered for the three treatments.

SUPPORTIVE GROUP PSYCHOTHERAPY

Rationale

The supportive tradition stems largely from the humanistic and experiential movements in psychotherapy. These movements suggest a natural healing process that occurs through actively experiencing interpersonal contact in the present, in an atmosphere of acceptance and emotional safety. In group therapy, "the whole is greater than the sum of its parts," taking on a life of its own beyond that of the individual members within it. Participation in this powerful environment can enhance and accelerate progress toward emotional health. Schema theory (McCann & Pearlman, 1990; Neisser, 1976), often applied to understanding the alteration of cognitions in PTSD, similarly suggests that healthy cognitive schemas automatically incorporate new information, flexibly recalibrating and reorienting toward optimal adjustment in the current environment. For individuals with PTSD, trauma-based intrusions, affects, and attitudes interfere with this automatic process of digesting and assessing new information (Zlotnick et al., 1997). Therapy which provides consistent access and attention to the current environment will allow members' trauma-influenced worldviews to gradually readjust, resulting in healthier functioning. From this perspective, supportive group therapy may offer a corrective context in which to modify the effects of trauma.

As in any therapy, clients with PTSD may be reluctant to give up patterns learned in the interest of survival under traumatic conditions of threat and danger. A pseudomutual, premature cohesion (Parson, 1985) can develop in groups, one in which group members validate each others trauma-based attitudes while dismissing the value of change. The symptoms and features of PTSD can also present challenges to group treatment (e.g., difficulty verbalizing feelings, distrust of authority, control issues, hyperarousal, and distracting intrusions). Supportive group therapy for PTSD addresses these issues in a number of ways. The active therapist style and moderate structure assists in diffusing a countertherapeutic stance. Groups often include segments of psychoeducational discussion on PTSD which validate the potentially interfering symptoms while asserting that these issues are grist for the (therapeutic) mill. And the therapeutic factors offered by supportive group therapy (e.g., universality, interpersonal learning, development of social skills, cohesion, and containment) can offer particular advantages for PTSD treatment.

Description

Supportive group therapy for PTSD is problem oriented, providing members with additional social support in the group to improve current coping. Groups may differ in their theoretical underpinnings, but they do share some characteristic features. Supportive groups typically avoid actual details of members' traumatic experiences, although personal consequences of trauma are acknowledged and validated. Groups are managed so that there is some emotional engagement of members' middle-range affects (e.g., frustration, sadness, happiness, or hurt), while rage and terror are diffused. Supportive groups infrequently use structured materials, and expectations for members' participation rarely involve homework or testing for mastery of material. Unlike Tavistock-style experiential groups, supportive groups attempt to maintain a sense of interpersonal comfort and to keep transference at a low-to-moderate level. Other features of supportive groups include an active, facilitative leadership style, emphasis on members' strengths, process-encouraging interventions, combination of pragmatic and "here-and-now" focus, low-to-moderate structure, and view of change as gradual and incremental. Level of confrontation is generally low to moderate.

Chronic PTSD often interferes with responses to current circumstances and may lead to gradual deterioration in functioning. Intrinsic therapeutic factors found in group psychotherapy (Yalom, 1995) help mobilize the personal resources of group members, thereby helping to control interference from symptoms and trauma-based attitudes, as reflected in social, emotional, occupational, and recreational functioning. Supportive groups are used in a variety of settings to promote a sense of community among "fellow strugglers" dealing with isolating chronic conditions and circumstances. These include crisis intervention (e.g., for divorce, job loss, recent rape or other victimization), adjustment to life transition (e.g., retirement), and stabilization of an acute or exacerbated condition (e.g., following psychiatric hospitalization). In PTSD programs, supportive groups may serve as a primary therapy modality, or they may provide support and preparation for other therapies. In many programs for PTSD, supportive groups help members positively participate in their overall treatment, providing cohesion and comfort for coping with more demanding therapies.

Case Example

The group, facilitated by two cotherapists, offered supportive, present-focused psychotherapy for a homogeneous, closed cohort of six Vietnam combat veterans with PTSD. Running for 30 weekly sessions and 5 monthly follow-up sessions, it featured orientation, psychoeducation, and goal-setting in the first four sessions, and open current-day discussion in the remaining sessions. The client, Sam, a 50-year-old, service-connected Army veteran with combat-related PTSD secondary to two tours in Vietnam, had just returned to live with his wife and 15-year-old daughter, after a series of separations. His presenting problems included intrusive recollections, sleep loss, nightmares, irritability, depression, occasional flashbacks, emotional numbing, alexithymia, panic disorder, mild agoraphobia, isolation, depression, poor concentration, intermittent self-medication with alcohol, and family problems.

Case History

Sam described a "happy" early family, school, and social adjustment. Drafted in 1966, he "did well" in the military prior to going to Vietnam. He completed two tours in Vietnam, spending most of 18 months "in the bush." Traumatic events included being ambushed twice on patrols, seeing a buddy killed in front of him, engaging in "body counts," and witnessing deaths of civilians during two incursions into villages. He recalls experiencing his first PTSD symptoms toward the end of his second tour, exacerbated on return to the United States by unreceptive "homecoming" experiences. Drinking heavily, experiencing flashbacks and sleep disturbance, and oscillating between suicidal and homicidal urges, he was hospitalized for psychiatric treatment within a couple months after discharge, receiving a diagnosis at that time of "schizophrenia, paranoid type" (prior to recognition of PTSD diagnosis). He left treatment upon release, coping through avoidance, numbing, and alcohol use. He walked away in anger from a variety of jobs and now has not worked for 20 years.

Case Formulation

Reexperiencing, hyperarousal, and avoidance of intimacy had limited Sam's postcombat functioning. His Vietnam experiences contributed to his difficulty in maintaining a consistent family life. His distressing homecoming from Vietnam, aversive early treatment experiences, and subsequent avoidance of treatment all suggested a need for supportive therapy.

Course of Treatment

Beginning Phase of Group: *Group Forming/Setting Norms (Sessions 1–7).* Sam initially responded more to the male facilitator (a Vietnam veteran) than to the female facilitator. He often appeared distracted in group and reported, "I'm having more nightmares, not sleeping—my wife wonders if this is right for me—is this supposed to happen?" Facilitators helped the group understand that the group itself could be a "trigger" initially and that comfort was likely to increase as members got to know each other. Sam occasionally made abrupt, disconnected trauma references; facilitators helped him identify these as resulting from intrusive recollections and encouraged refocusing on the present. In early discussion of family issues, Sam joined with members about how family members "push their buttons." During the fifth group, Sam departed from the group norms by leaving early, without explanation. After missing the sixth session, he returned and explained, "I had an argument with my daughter. She was writing a report on Laos for her history class—well, I was in Laos, so I tried to help her. She wouldn't listen—she kept saying, 'Never mind, Dad, never mind!' Then she wanted me to check her spelling, and I blew up! My wife took her side. I didn't sleep all night, and when I came to group, somebody else was talking; and I didn't want to interrupt . . . I know I shouldn't have left . . . I started drinking on my way home . . . I was embarrassed to come to group last week." Facilitators helped the group consider the impact of intrusive memories and hyperarousal (triggered by the topic of Laos) on Sam's reaction to his family. Group members shared similar experiences, suggested coping strategies, and recommended Alcoholics Anonymous (AA). Sam was receptive but made "no guarantees."

Middle Phase of Group: *Cohesion (Sessions 8–16).* Sam discussed the fear, anger, and shame he experienced in his early contact with the VA, which he initially associated with the group and with the female facilitator. He identified more with other members ("We're all in the same boat") and directed comments toward them rather than toward the facilitators. He began to confront members if they missed a group (as members started to "own" group norms) but uniformly supported his peers in their interactions with people outside the group.

Later Phase of Group: *Awareness and Changes (Sessions 17–24).* Sam and other members began to actively confront each others' contributions to problems in personal and family relationships ("Sounds like it's 'your way or the highway'!"). By week 19, Sam announced that he hadn't had a drink in 2 months. His occasional trauma references were connected to current issues (e.g., "It's hard for me to get close to people now, because of the way I lost my buddy"). At the group's urging, Sam explained his actions and needs more clearly to his family, in place of yelling, intimidating, or projecting a stony silence. Group members encouraged Sam to accompany his family on a vacation—an activity he had avoided in previous years. The group helped him problem-solve how to manage his hyperarousal during the trip, and he returned reporting success.

Ending Phase of Group: *Consolidation (Sessions 25–30, and Monthly Follow-Up Sessions 1–5).* As the group neared the end of its weekly sessions, members revealed more personal issues. Sam described the drinking and outbursts of temper that led to years of alienation from his family. On the group's advice, he talked with his daughter about how his PTSD had affected him through the years and reassured her that it wasn't her fault. As the group terminated, he articulated a relationship between leave-taking in group and in Vietnam: "Back then, we said, 'It don't mean nothing,' and moved on. But now, I can carry the spirit of the group with me."

Outcome

Sam's initial increase in symptoms abated within 8 weeks, at which point he also appeared significantly less depressed. He spoke less about symptoms and more about positive efforts in his life. As group continued, he was able to join his family on vacations for the first time in years. He and his wife remained together throughout the period of the group and beyond—a longer period than they had experienced over the past 3 years. He was able to assert himself in group and with family members. Sam and other members moved from blaming their wives and other family members to acknowledging their own contributions to family problems. Sam himself expressed surprise at "how fast I've been making these changes," and he attributed this ability to the group.

Conclusions

Sam needed to address the confusing and shaming experiences from his early treatment in order to establish comfort with current treatment. His motivation to address this difficult issue developed from his wish to connect with other group members. As the group offered normalization and demystification of symptoms, problem solving, and practice attending to present-day environment and current feelings, Sam partially modified the worldview and automatic responses derived from his combat experiences in Vietnam. Changes were at first more evident within in the group than outside the group but eventually generalized to important family relationships. By the end of the weekly sessions, Sam reported, "My symptoms are still there, but they don't get in the way as much."

PSYCHODYNAMIC GROUP THERAPY

Rationale

The primary goal of psychodynamic group therapy for PTSD is to help members achieve new understanding of their traumatic experiences, their own reactions at the time, and continuing related psychological issues. The group seeks to help each member clarify his or her working model of self and other(s) involved in reactions to his or her traumatic events. Among these clarifications are cognitive appraisals of internal dialogues about the meaning of the event, "lessons learned," or personal meaning attributed to an event or some aspect of the event. Group process includes exploring members' conscious and unconscious self-concepts related to self-representations evoked by their traumas. These trauma-related self-representations are then related to current conflicted views of the self, and to self-representations from early development. In addition, clarification of common implicit assumptions about predictability and culpability involved in the meaning of the trauma is made in the safe context provided by the group.

Psychodynamic group therapy promotes integration of accurate recounting of events, including pre- and posttrauma issues that are important parts of each member's story. These important aspects include responses by family members and others in the trauma social milieu. Members' affective involvement is dosed to allow group work to be done without overwhelming members by precipitating dissociative reactions or flashbacks. Members' affective patterns typically involve initial anxiety prior to recounting the incident, anxiety and/or tears during the telling, and a kind of calm after the storm, when consolidation is desired. In a psychodynamic approach these painful affects are tied back to views, frequently irrational, of self and others. These irrational views may involve need for omnipotent control, the assumption that betrayal is inevitable, the belief that trauma happens only for good or understandable reason, and that avoidance of strong feelings is a necessary protective strategy.

When members are retelling their stories, recognition of the context in which the event took place (i.e., stranger vs. known assailant, use of drugs or alcohol, or ignoring of warning signs or signals) is important. During the recounting of stories, the leaders must be attuned to subtle but significant omissions or incongruities in members' narrations. When positive group process has developed, other members may also perform this function. Noticing and commenting upon the speaker's comments about her or his own dialogue as it unfolds is an especially important aspect of this attunement. Capitalizing upon these comments at the time and following up on their associative meanings is crucial. It is the importance attributed to these associative meanings that distinguishes the dynamic approach.

Description

Group Structure

The group should comprise five to seven members. There can be some variability among group members in basic demographics (e.g., time elapsed since trauma, age, ethnicity, or socioeconomic status). On the other hand, it will be helpful if they are homogeneous, as far as possible, regarding level of ego functioning, interpersonal skills, and ability to confront defenses and integrate warded off material.

Attempts to verify the veracity of events should tactfully be undertaken prior to a person's joining the group (e.g., law enforcement reports, medical records, and collateral information). Unfortunately, from time to time, there are individuals whose psychopathology leads them to want to become members of a specialized group, such as those being described here, when in reality they have not had the kind of experience that would qualify them. Such "as if" or "wanna-be" individuals are sometimes difficult to identify, but their inclusion in a group can be an extremely disruptive influence regarding safety and trust. Consequently, to the degree possible, the integrity of an individual's presentation should be examined carefully. Two group leaders are preferable, and one model (Weiss, Tichenor, Schadler, Marmar, & Koller, 1997) is designed to last for 24 weeks, with each session lasting an hour and a half. Various types of group can be formed (e.g., Koller, Marmar, & Kanas, 1992; Goodman & Weiss, 1998).

Overview

Sessions 1–7 are relatively structured by group leaders and initially include didactic presentation of psychoeducational material, preparation for group participation, and introduction by leaders of themes to be addressed in each session. Leaders will actively model frank discussion about disagreements or differences in viewpoints about how to proceed, appropriate supportive-probing questioning, and explicitly attend to within-group process (interpreting parallels to trauma-related issues). This structure will gradually be reduced as group members learn to take on this role. The content of sessions

8–22 will be dictated primarily by group members, but the main agenda will be repeated exposure to the traumatic event by the telling and retelling of each participant's story. Group leaders will actively direct the process as necessary and ensure that relevant themes are raised for consideration at some point during this middle trauma-focused phase. The leaders will help explicitly structure the focus of repeated tellings of the event for the individual participants, asking for concentration on affect, details, reactions, or other aspects as indicated by the participants' difficulties and what has occurred during previous tellings of the story. Sessions 23 and 24 explicitly focus on termination issues, with some increase in the activity and structuring by the leaders, as termination and treatment follow-up issues are addressed.

Group Leadership

Leaders must titrate the amount of structure and activity to simultaneously create an atmosphere of "safety" and sense of trust in their competence without unduly letting the group as a whole make important decisions and deal with issues that arise in the process. Leaders also need to allow for transference and working through of issues with authority figures if these exist. More active leadership is often necessary early in group development, though whenever it seems appropriate the leaders should solicit input and commentary from the group members themselves about the current theme, topic, story, or issue. Attention must always be paid to defensive within-group dynamics and behaviors. These defenses can be tied to avoidance and the need to regulate painful affective experiences using the language in the educational sessions of the group. These will also likely come up with respect to the safety of the group and if members can trust each other or the leaders. Countertransference issues regarding being too nice or too mean can both interfere here. In these circumstances, the other group leader must be assertive enough to comment on and redirect the discussion if the process has gone awry.

Case Example

Mr. B, was a 50-year-old Caucasian, a Vietnam veteran, with a childhood history of abandonment, violence, humiliation, and intimidation. Mr. B never met his real father and was removed from his biological mother's custody at age 4 when it was discovered that the mother's boyfriend was beating Mr. B and his two brothers. A newspaper article and photograph that Mr. B discovered as an adult documented the abuse. Mr. B's adoptive home was also abusive; his alcoholic adoptive father held a gun to Mr. B's head and threatened to shoot him, and his adoptive mother, whom he nevertheless loved, locked him in closets and hit him with lumber. During his service in Vietnam he participated in firefights and sustained shrapnel wounds. His post-Vietnam life included a stint of adequate functioning but also included depression, volatile anger, avoidance, numb feelings, and alcoholism. He sought treatment because of his concern about his ability to father his 7-year-old son by his third wife.

Mr. B described himself as scarred by his childhood. He had a fear of crying and inability to do so, difficulty asking for help, a tendency to sabotage relationships before they caused any pain, a questioning of his identity, and homicidal revenge fantasies toward his adoptive stepfather. Any experience of affect was equated with loss of control.

Mr. B joined a group focused on the connection between childhood and traumatic events in Vietnam. He was ambivalent about committing to the group, missing half of the first 12 sessions. When present, he sat with his head down and his chair pushed back, signaling through his body language. His initial contributions to the group focused on his lethality toward others, using as examples his killings in Vietnam and his destruction of two marriages. He highlighted his self-loathing and could not imagine anyone finding him worthwhile. He believed his only peace might be death, as suggested by a story of witnessing a dying but tranquil soldier. He took the stance that distance from his wife and son was best, as he would then be sure not to hurt them. This stance was replicated in the group, and the view of himself as a potential perpetrator of violence having to be held under check by withdrawal was prominent.

Over time, Mr. B gradually revealed more of himself, prompted by the occurrence of the holidays and the memories this evoked. As his feeling of safety increased, he related incidents from both his childhood and Vietnam in which feelings of powerlessness, "being in a jungle," not knowing who was an enemy, playing survival games, and "being lied to" prevailed. During this growing attachment to the group, Mr. B developed a positive but tenuous transference to the male cotherapist. A pattern ensued that any perceived criticism or lack of attention by the "father" of the group was experienced as "being destroyed," corroding his sense of connection and self-worth. Minor slights were experienced as "slaps in the face" and triggered flashbacks of beatings and other torture. Mr. B's capacity to continue to attend the group was strained, and he considered dropping out many times. Support and feedback from other group members enabled him to recognized his distortions and appreciate how this sequence also occurred with his wife. Equally important, the ability to negotiate and be heard by the paternal figure and perceived aggressor led to replacing anger with new ways of coping after hurt feelings.

Gradually, the meaning of his childhood experiences were connected with the painful affects associated with assumptions of being loathsome as the only explanation for being victimized. During a particularly strong and painful anniversary period, Mr. B became disorganized and began to hallucinate the voice of his mother telling him to join her in death. This allowed him, however, to acknowledge his confusion about the depth of his conflicting feelings for his mother. His anger at his wife for being unavailable for his son was helpfully interpreted as an overidentification with his son and his longing for his mother to have been available for him.

The termination of the group was difficult, since it was a loss of the group and a loss of the female cotherapist who was relocating out of state. Nonetheless, he spoke to the important changes he noted in himself and about an increased awareness of his effects on others.

COGNITIVE-BEHAVIORAL GROUP THERAPY

Rationale

Cognitive-behavioral group therapy seeks to reduce ongoing PTSD symptoms, and to enhance members' control of their symptoms when they recur. Thus, the goal of improving members' self-control and quality of life is as important as immediate symptom reduction. Recognizing that chronic PTSD frequently involves lifelong risk for symptom recurrence, cognitive-behavioral group therapy challenges members to adopt realistic goals of living fuller lives while managing risks of periodic symptom exacerbation.

Trauma processing for group members involves prolonged exposure and cognitive restructuring applied to each member's trauma story, as well as relapse prevention training to provide coping skills and resources for maintaining control over specific PTSD and related symptoms (Foy, Ruzek, Glynn, Riney, & Gusman, 1997). Repeated exposure to traumatic memories reduces trauma-related fears and desensitizes related cues. In the group, members retell their selected traumatic stories and prolonged exposure helps correct faulty perceptions of danger derived from traumatic experiences.

Some cognitive-behavioral groups are designed to help members set their traumas in a developmental perspective, taking into account the entire lifespan over pretrauma, trauma, and posttrauma time frames (e.g., Gusman et al., 1996). In these groups there is an autobiographical emphasis upon individual member's narrative construction as well as the group dynamic of having others bear witness to members' public recounting of their significant life experiences. Vicarious trauma processing may also occur through repeated exposures to the traumatic narratives of other group members. Relapse prevention planning can also be a core component of cognitive-behavioral trauma focus groups for chronic PTSD. These coping skills are useful for dealing with high-risk situations that occur during the course of group therapy, as well as after group therapy is completed.

Description

Cognitive-behavioral group treatment procedures address the need for repeated exposures to traumatic memories by devoting multiple sessions to individualized focus work on members' traumatic experiences. This extensive exposure element, along with its related cognitive restructuring (guided rethinking about the cause and meaning of the trauma), is the core treatment component. Thus, it necessarily occupies the largest percentage of the total group treatment time. It is followed by sessions teaching specific coping skills for dealing with high-risk situations that could precipitate relapse.

Table 8.1 is an example of session design and sequence of cognitive-behavioral group therapy for chronic combat-related PTSD. There are six group members and two group facilitators in each cognitive behavioral war trauma focus group. Each session is organized to include five core elements: check-in, review of homework, specific topics, assignment of homework, and check-out. There is one group meeting each week. Prolonged exposure (war-zone focus) sessions last 2 hours; other meetings last 90 minutes. As outlined here, the group meets for 30 sessions, or about 7 months, followed by 5 monthly booster sessions in the clinic and 5 telephone follow-up calls.

Case Example

Mark was a 48-year-old divorced male, service-connected Vietnam veteran, referred by his VA case manager for cognitive-behavioral assessment and treatment of his chronic combat-related PTSD symptoms. His premilitary

TABLE 8.1. Cognitive-Behavioral Group Therapy: Session Topics

Introductory sessions	
Session 1	Introductions, structure, and group rules
Session 2	PTSD education
Session 3	Coping resources
Session 4	Negative and positive coping
Session 5	PTSD symptoms and self-control
Sessions 6 and 7	Premilitary autobiographies
Session 8	Prewarzone military autobiographies
Warzone focus sessions	
Sessions 9 and 10	Warzone trauma scene identification/coping review
Sessions 11–22	Warzone trauma focus
Relapse prevention and termination	
Session 23	Developmental perspective—putting the trauma in a life history
Session 24	Improving social support
Sessions 25 and 26	Anger management
Sessions 27 and 28	Risk situations and coping strategies
Session 29	PTSD rehabilitation contracting
Session 30	Summary and transition

social history was unremarkable in that there was no reported abuse, no indications of severe family dysfunction, and indications of positive school adjustment through his timely completion of high school. He served in the Marines, with training as a rifleman and supply clerk. His tour of Vietnam duty included several instances in which his unit was exposed to heavy combat and suffered casualties, although Mark himself was not wounded.

After Mark's discharge from military service, he was employed as a stock clerk in a succession of entry-level jobs, several of which he eventually walked away from after disputes with supervisors. He had had two earlier marriages, each of which produced one child with whom he had intermittent contacts, and he was there in a cohabitation relationship which began about 2 years prior to his entering group therapy. Mark had a history of three brief psychiatric hospitalizations, and he had had two extensive attempts at individual psychotherapy on an outpatient basis. He also had a history of previous alcohol abuse, but he had been sober for approximately 2 years and attended AA meetings on a monthly basis. Mark had been maintained on antidepressant medication from which there had been modest improvement in mood but no change in his PTSD symptoms. At the time of his referral he had just left his job of 8 months as a warehouseman after a disagreement with his supervisor and was reporting increased discomfort at being around other people, combat-related nightmares, and unresolved strife with his cohabitating partner.

Case Formulation

Despite Mark's positive premilitary history his postcombat adjustment had been marginal, suggesting that profound life experiences and changes in his coping capabilities occurred during his period of military service. Although his specific traumatic experiences in combat had not yet been identified, it appeared that his primary PTSD features included both reexperiencing and avoidant symptoms in the form of recurring nightmares and disrupted interpersonal relationships indicative of social isolation and mistrust. In view of his history of insignificant gains following his two previous attempts at individual therapy and his specific interpersonal difficulties, trauma-focused group therapy (TFGT) was recommended to Mark as a new form of combat-related PTSD therapy that could possibly help him achieve improvements.

Course of Treatment

Over the course of 7 months Mark participated as a member of a VA-sponsored TFGT that included five other combat veterans and two professional cofacilitators. His group met weekly for those first 7 months and then moved to once a month for booster sessions and transitioning out of the group. For each session one of the cofacilitators made an outline of the topics to be covered on a flipchart in the group therapy room so that members could refer to the session agenda as the group sessions unfolded. Although it made him somewhat uncomfortable at first, Mark and the other members soon became accustomed to the videotaping of each session. He agreed to the taping on the condition of confidentiality and that the tapes would be used for teaching purposes and to provide feedback to the facilitators for their performances in managing each group session.

It had been many years since Mark and the other members had been assigned school homework. However, he found that doing the weekly assignments prescribed in his own member's workbook made it easier for him to prepare for and follow along with weekly session topics. He also noticed that the cofacilitators had a similar requirement to follow the session guides contained in their own leaders' manuals.

Mark's response to treatment thus far was positive. He attended sessions as scheduled and completed homework assignments on all except one occasion. Since he had been prone to social isolation, it was especially noteworthy that he related well to other members of the group and appeared well motivated to begin his warzone trauma work.

The 13th session was devoted to supporting Mark as he reviewed his specific combat-related trauma in detail (i.e., "exposure") for approximately 45 minutes and then reconsidered his assumptions and beliefs about the event for accuracy (i.e., "cognitive restructuring"), utilizing feedback and observations from both other group members and the facilitators over about an hour. For his exposure work, Mark chose to work on an explosion which occurred when he and three of his buddies were cleaning a bunker. There were two key aspects of the cognitive restructuring in the session: (1) clarifying the exact sequence of events during the trauma; and (2) ascertaining whether the events were predictable or controllable. While Mark clearly believed himself culpable for the injuries of his companions, the data did not necessarily support his assumption of guilt, according to other experienced members' observations. Thus, tension between his evaluations and those of respected others prompted him to begin reconsidering his self-appraisal of responsibility. This "cognitive shift" was accompanied by a drop in his rated anxiety level. This therapeutic work continued in Mark's second round of trauma focus 6 weeks later.

Outcome and Prognosis

Mark attended every session except one and completed almost all of his homework assignments. After years of avoidance (shutting out thoughts about the trauma), he did find listening to the taped narrative of his trauma very stressful (experiencing anxiety levels of 9 or 10 during each exercise), and reported a significant increase in sleep difficulties and nightmares inter-mittently during the 8 weeks he did his focused trauma work. As the trauma focus component of the treatment was drawing to a close, he spontaneously played the tape for his girlfriend so that "she could understand what I might have done wrong and why I was so screwed up." She was very supportive about the experience, and this greatly relieved his tension. At that point, Mark decided to go back to his boss, inform him that he had been working on some personal issues, and ask for his job back. The supervisor agreed to rehire him on a probationary status. At the conclusion of the treatment, Mark opted to transition to an anger management class at the Vet Center, in order to "get more control of my wicked temper." While he still met diagnostic criteria for PTSD, his symptom severity had declined approximately 25%. He reported that he had found the TFGT content "somewhat helpful" but was especially appreciative of the feedback from his peers and for the opportunity to bond with other veterans.

INDICATIONS FOR GROUP THERAPY FOR PTSD

Elsewhere we have detailed a number of individual characteristics that have emerged in the literature regarding the appropriateness of choosing group therapy as a primary therapy for PTSD (Foy et al., 2000). Among these factors are the following:

Has ability to establish interpersonal trust with other group members and leaders

Has prior group experience, including 12-step groups

Has completed a preparatory course of individual therapy

Is not actively suicidal or homicidal

Shares similar traumatic experiences with other group members

Has compatible gender, ethnicity and sexual orientation with other members

Is willing to abide by rules of group confidentiality

Is not severely paranoid or sociopathic

Has stable living arrangements

TREATMENT–CLIENT MATCHING CONSIDERATIONS

Since individuals recovering from traumatic experiences often show great emotional volatility and mistrust, a gradual approach has been recommended that involves three phases: (1) education and support, (2) trauma processing, (3) and longer-term reintegration (Klein & Schermer, 2000). It is striking that these phases correspond closely with the different primary aims of the three types of group treatment in this chapter. We have also enumerated factors related to matching individuals to the three types of evidence-based group therapy (Foy et al., 2000). Developing a comprehensive, effective treatment plan well suited for the individual is of paramount importance. In addition to group treatment, many individuals with severe chronic PTSD and serious comorbid conditions will need ongoing case management services.

Active psychoses, severe cognitive deficits, and pending compensation-seeking litigations may be contraindications for assignment to group therapy (Foy et al., 2000). Since these selection factors are primarily rationally derived, they do not constitute hard-and-fast criteria so much as they represent useful guidelines for informing the matching process. Relative to individual forms of therapy for PTSD, group therapies tend to be more structured and place more rigid requirements upon the individual for participation. There is less flexibility for accommodating individual needs that may arise over the course of therapy in the group format. For some individuals, extreme social interaction anxiety may block beneficial participation in group therapy activities.

When we compare possible selection factors for trauma focus groups to those for supportive groups, there are more stringent requirements for assignment to the "uncovering" modality. Generally, individuals need to be psychologically stable and be willing to undergo reexperiencing of their traumas. Supportive group therapy may be a better match for less stable individuals or for those who do not accept the rationale for personal trauma processing. Assignment considerations for the two types of trauma focus group therapy appear to be very similar. Clear factors for differentiating between assignment to psychodynamic or cognitive-behavioral focus group therapies have not been identified.

SUMMARY

Group therapy has emerged as a widely used treatment for PTSD despite the preliminary nature of the evidence from research evaluating group techniques. Despite methodological limitations that constrain the scientific conclusions that can be drawn, positive treatment outcomes have been reported in most studies, lending general empirical support for the use of group therapy with trauma survivors. While three distinct types or combinations of group therapies are represented in the literature, treatment outcome findings do not presently favor a particular type. Indeed, it may well be that the three types are best used in sequence across recognizable phases of treatment for trauma survivors. At the present time, it is clear that much more research is warranted to identify those techniques and procedures that produce superior outcomes.

ACKNOWLEDGMENTS

The authors acknowledge substantial overlap in authorship and text in portions of this chapter and some sections of a similar chapter (Foy et al., 2000) produced as a group treatment guidelines position paper for the International Society for Traumatic Stress Studies.

REFERENCES

Allen, S. N., & Bloom, S. L. (1994). Group and family treatment of posttraumatic stress disorder. *Psychiatric Clinics of North America, 17*, 425–437.

Brende, J. O. (1981). Combined individual and group therapy for Vietnam veterans. *International Journal of Group Psychotherapy, 31*, 367–377.

Foy, D. W., Glynn, S. M., Schnurr, P. P., Jankowski, M. K., Wattenberg, M. S., Weiss, D. S., Marmar, C. R., & Gusman, F. D. (2000). Group psychotherapy for posttraumatic stress disorder. In E. B. Foa, T. M. Keane, & M. J. Friedman (Eds.), *Effective Treatments for PTSD* (pp. 155–175). New York: Guilford Press.

Foy, D. W., Ruzek, J. I., Glynn, S. M., Riney, S. A., & Gusman, F. D. (1997). Trauma focus group therapy for combat-related PTSD. *In Session: Psychotherapy in Practice, 3*, 59–73.

Goodman, M., & Weiss, D. S. (1998). Double trauma: A group therapy approach for Vietnam veterans suffering from war and childhood trauma. *International Journal of Group Psychotherapy, 48*, 39–54.

Gusman, F. D., Stewart, J., Young, B. H., Riney, S. J., Abueg, F. R., & Blake, D. D. (1996). *Ethnocultural aspects of posttraumatic stress disorder: Issues, research, and clinical applications.* Washington, DC: American Psychological Association.

Herman, J. L. (1992). *Trauma and recovery.* New York: Basic Books.

Janoff-Bulman, R., & Frieze, I. H. (1983). A theoretical perspective for understanding reactions to victimization. *Journal of Social Issues, 37*, 105–122.

Klein, R. H., & Schermer, V. L. (2000). Introduction and overview: Creating a healing matrix. In R. H. Klein & V. L. Schermer (Eds.), *Group psychotherapy for psychological trauma* (pp. 3–4). New York: Guilford Press.

Koller, P., Marmar, C. R., & Kanas, N. (1992). Psychodynamic group treatment of posttraumatic stress disorder in Vietnam veterans. *International Journal of Group Psychotherapy, 42*, 225–246.

Lifton, R. J. (1973). *Home from the war.* New York: Simon & Schuster.

McCann, I. L., & Pearlman, L. A. (1990). *Psychological trauma and the adult survivor: Theory therapy, and transformation.* New York: Brunner/Mazel.

Neisser, U. (1976). *Cognition and reality: Principles and implications of cognitive psychology.* Freeman.

Parson, E. R. (1985). Post-traumatic accelerated cohesion: Its recognition and management in group treatment of Vietnam veterans. *Group, 9*(4), 10–23.

Shatan, C. F. (1973). The grief of soldiers: Vietnam combat veterans' self-help movement. *American Journal of Orthopsychiatry, 43*, 640–653.

Walker, J. J., & Nash, J. D. (1981). Group therapy in the treatment of Vietnam combat veterans. *International Journal of Group Psychotherapy, 31*, 379–389.

Weiss, D. S., Tichenor, V., Schadler, M., Marmar, C. R., & Koller, P. (1997). *Treatment manual for time-limited trauma-focused group psychotherapy of PTSD: Female sexual victimization version.* Unpublished manuscript, Department of Psychiatry, University of California, San Francisco.

Yalom, I. D. (1995). *The theory and practice of group psychotherapy.* New York: Basic Books.

Zlotnick, C., Shea, M. T., Rosen, K. H., Simpson, E., Mulrenin, K., Begin, A., & Pearlstein, T. (1997). An affect-management group for women with posttraumatic stress disorder and histories of childhood sexual abuse. *Journal of Traumatic Stress, 10,* 425–436.

III

CLINICAL TREATMENT APPROACHES FOR SPECIAL TRAUMA POPULATIONS

9

Treatment of Persons with Complex PTSD and Other Trauma-Related Disruptions of the Self

LAURIE ANNE PEARLMAN

At the end of the 19th century, Pierre Janet described some of the difficulties we now include in the rubric "posttraumatic stress disorder" (PTSD) (see van der Kolk et al., 1996; van der Kolk & van der Hart, 1991). These difficulties were described half a century later by Grinker and J. Spiegel (1945) and Kardiner and H. Spiegel (1947). Yet only lately, another half-century later, have empirically validated treatments for this disorder been emerging (Foa & Meadows, 1997; Foa, Keane, & Friedman, 2000; Solomon, 1997). So it is not surprising that now, at the start of the 21st century, we do not yet have empirically validated treatments for the trauma-related disorders of the self that go beyond PTSD. These sequelae of early childhood abuse and neglect are now commonly referred to as complex PTSD (Herman, 1992a), or disorders of extreme stress not otherwise specified (DESNOS; see Pelcovitz et al., 1997, for a discussion of this construct and terminology). It is only in the 1990s that clinicians have begun to agree on what to call the collection of difficulties that so many survivors of early or extreme stress, neglect, abuse, and other violence experience. In addition to the symptoms of PTSD (intrusive experiences, avoidance, and arousal), "complex PTSD" or complex trauma includes dissociation, relationship difficulties, revictimization, somatization (bodily expressions of psychological processes), affect dysregulation, and disruptions in identity (Herman, 1992a).

Of course, it was not so recently that these and other trauma-related difficulties were first observed or described. One of the things Janet described in the late 19th century was *dissociation,* which is notably absent from our contemporary definition of PTSD. Contemporary observers returned to an awareness of dissociation in the early 1980s (Gelinas, 1983). A few years earlier, Courtois (1979) described the *relationship difficulties* and *changes in identity* experienced by adult survivors of childhood trauma. Other researchers described *revictimization* of childhood abuse survivors in the form of rape (Miller et al., 1978), domestic violence (Briere, 1984; Walker, 1985), child prostitution (James & Meyerding, 1977), other crimes or accidents (Sedney & Brooks, 1984), self-injury (Green, 1978), and aggresson against others (Curran, DeCou, Dusek-Gomez, Haven & Rodriguez, 2000). *Somatization* has also been documented in this population for more than two decades (Hilberman & Munson, 1977/1978). van der Kolk and van der Hart (1989) have pointed out that Janet noted affect dysregulation as part of the aftermath of traumatic life experiences in the 1880s. (van der Kolk et al., 1996, have provided a concise historical description of this and other aspects of complex PTSD, from Janet to the early contemporary research.) Nakashima and Zakus (1977) described depression in incest survivors. Gelinas (1983) described *affect dysregulation* in incest survivors as well. These difficulties are well documented in adults who have experienced sexual and other physical abuse in a review (Polusny & Follette, 1995) and a meta-analysis (Neumann, Houskamp, Pollock, & Briere, 1996) of the relevant empirical literature. They have also been supported in more recent research studies (Dancu, Riggs, Hearst-Ikeda, Shoyer, & Foa, 1996; Roth, Newman, Pelcovitz, van der Kolk, & Mandel, 1997; Zlotnick et al., 1996).

But the time frame required for clinical observation to translate into theory and then into treatment research is long, as evidenced by the evolution of treatments for PTSD (Foa et al., 2000). So it is appropriate that we are just now at the point of moving from theoretical conceptualizations to the development of potentially effective clinical approaches (Turner, DeRosa, Roth, Batson, & Davidson, 1996). Testing the effectiveness of these interventions may require different assessment paradigms, yet to be developed (Richters, 1997; Kuhn, 1970). One measure of the symptoms of DESNOS, the Structured Interview for Disorders of Extreme Stress (SIDES), has been developed (Pelcovitz et al., 1997; van der Kolk & Pelcovitz, 1999) and used satisfactorily by some researchers (Ford, 1999; Jongedijk, Carlier, Schreuder, & Gersons, 1996).

In this chapter, I provide a theoretical framework for understanding the clinical observations that have been collectively termed "complex PTSD." Out of this theory, constructivist self development theory, an approach to treatment has grown which I will describe as it applies to these adaptations. I then apply that approach to case examples of three survivors of childhood trauma. In the process, I delineate some hypothetical mechanisms of change in psychotherapies with survivors of severe and early trauma. My hope is that this chapter will provide a clinical and theoretical basis for future research into these mechanisms and treatment approaches.

BACKGROUND

The lives of survivors of traumatic events or conditions often are fraught with pain as they try to live with or in spite of their distress, sometimes agonizing daily about the value of continuing life itself. Many struggle to overcome loneliness that is rooted in fear, shame, or both. Others battle to forge relationships in the face of deep-seated mistrust of others. Still others fight terror at every turn. Many must—or cannot—harness rage that seems to erupt like a volcano with any—or no—provocation. Debilitating depression thwarts efforts to work, parent, study, or survive. Who are these anguished individuals? They are the many who have been beaten, abused, neglected, and/or molested as small children. They are the people who have encountered humanity at its most gruesome—in war, in concentration camps, in their own families. They are the multitudes who have grown up without enough food, clothing, attention, or protection, often in homes that appear to be middle class and "normal." To understand their experiences, we must look beyond the symptoms of PTSD. Of course, many do show those symptoms. And many have difficulties in their inner lives that translate into serious interpersonal problems as well.

When we understand symptoms in a theoretical context, treatment options multiply. A theory is a map that provides a framework for locating our clinical observations. A symptom is like a street address; without a map, it is a meaningless piece of information. A theory that links our observations allows us to create hypotheses and investigate them. Our theories and our research are our true professional licenses; they give us authority to claim that we can help and to charge for our services. When people come to us for help and become our clients or patients, we are ethically bound to work from some theoretical base. Without a theory, clinicians are not much more useful than any other interested, kindly individual.

The theoretical basis I describe below for understanding the impact of traumatic life experiences is constructivist self development theory (CSDT). CSDT is a general personality theory developed to aid in our understanding and treatment of trauma survivors. The observations that are encompassed by complex PTSD can be understood within this framework, which then provides guidelines for treatment.

CONSTRUCTIVIST SELF DEVELOPMENT THEORY

CSDT was first described by McCann and Pearlman (1990). It has subsequently evolved on the basis of clinical experience and research and is further described by Pearlman and Saakvitne (1995) and Saakvitne, Gamble, Pearlman, and Tabor Lev (2000). Briefly, the theory is interactive; it regards psychological trauma (the effect on the person) as arising from an interaction between who that person is and the traumatic situation (the events and their context). The theory integrates cognitive theories (constructivism: Mahoney, 1981; Mahoney & Lyddon, 1988; social learning theory: Rotter, 1954; cognitive developmental theory: Piaget, 1971) with psychoanalytic theory (object relations: Mahler, Pine, & Bergman, 1975; White & Weiner, 1986; interpersonal psychiatry: Fromm-Reichmann, 1960; Sullivan, 1953); and self psychology: Kohut, 1971, 1977; Stolorow, Brandchaft, & Atwood, 1987).

Assumptions

Some of the important assumptions underlying CSDT are as follows. The theory is constructivist, meaning that individuals construct and construe their own psychologically meaningful environments. Thus, the individual defines traumatic experiences as such. This view is consistent with that of the DSM-IV (American Psychiatric Association, 1994), which identifies as a criterion A event for PTSD an event that the individual *experiences* as a threat to life; the individual defines the criterion. While external reality is important, in attempting to understand and treat survivor clients we must enter into their frameworks and meaning systems. Clients are often acutely aware of the areas that are most difficult for them (e.g., trusting others) and want to tell rather than be told. This is crucial both to our ability to understand and assist our clients and to convey to them our availability to help. Many survivors have encountered therapists who knew what they needed and told them so, re-creating the invisibility they experienced in childhood.

A natural implication of constructivism is that individual differences exist and are significant. What harms or helps one person will not necessarily harm or help another. We must learn from all of our clients about how they experience their pasts and their present lives, what was worst for them, what their experience means to them, what they need, what is helpful to each individual.

The theory is developmental. Thus the age and life stage at which the individual encounters traumatizing events suggest psychosocial developmental tasks that may be incomplete. For children who grow up in abusive, chaotic, or neglectful homes, many core tasks, like learning to trust others, may be unfinished. These tasks will need to be addressed in treatment. We cannot assume that adults who grew up in such homes will be able to trust, to take appropriate risks, to know what they feel, to assert their needs.

CSDT views symptoms as adaptations. Attempting to understand how problematic behaviors evolved, how they may have served the individual at one time, what their current functions are, and what letting go of them might mean now is part of the therapy. This exploration allows the individual far greater freedom and choices.

Therapy within a CSDT framework is relational. Interpersonal trauma must be healed in an interpersonal context (Herman, 1992b; Saakvitne et al.,

2000). The process of change in psychotherapy, as in all human development, takes place in relation to other persons. Relationships are an integral and essential part of the treatment, as discussed below.

Finally, traumatic life experiences and healing take place in a social and cultural context. That includes the family and its values, the community and its norms, society and its mores. Today's context for trauma therapy is one that questions the reality of childhood sexual abuse, of the suffering people that endure for years after active abuse has ended, of people's struggles to know and to remember. The context is also that of a society that doesn't want to pay for psychotherapy, especially for psychotherapy for trauma survivors or for the longer-term treatment that is often required for the resolution of the difficulties experienced by so many adults who have endured severe or early trauma. Our context in the United States is also one of misogyny, patriarchy, racism, and homophobia. There is still a widespread belief that people cause their own misery, that people should put their problems behind them and get on with their lives, get over it, get a life. If only it were that simple. Yet these are the beliefs that survivors encounter daily, sometimes subtly woven into the media, the so-called entertainment industry, the Sunday sermon. Sometimes these beliefs are not so subtle, coming forth as epithets, limited opportunities, and victim blaming. These are very real, integral aspects of each of our lives, of the context in which our clients were traumatized, and of our psychotherapies with survivors.

Definition of Trauma

CSDT defines psychological trauma as the experience of affect that overwhelms one's ability to respond and the experience of threat to life or bodily integrity. Note that I am using the term "trauma" to designate the response, not the stressor. For most people, experiences of childhood sexual molestation or unwanted sexual contact will be traumatizing. For most, physical abuse, emotional abuse, and neglect are traumatic. Severe stressors like those experienced by prisoners of war or people living in chronic poverty or chronic physical danger are traumatic for most. But we cannot assume that we know which aspects of events will be most traumatizing for each individual. Learning about what was most difficult is part of the therapeutic process with each client. Indeed, it is an essential part of constructing a narrative, part of the healing process of creating meaning for each victim on his or her way to becoming a survivor (Newman, Riggs, & Roth, 1997; Pearlman & Saakvitne, 1995).

Impact of Traumatic Life Experiences on the Self

CSDT delineates various aspects of the self that are impacted by traumatizing experiences. Disruptions in each of these aspects are characterized by certain "symptoms." I describe below some of these aspects of the self, related difficulties and behaviors, and therapeutic work in each area. I do not address here approaches specific to the amelioration of PTSD symptoms, as these are addressed elsewhere in this volume. The approaches I describe, however, are also helpful in addressing focal PTSD symptoms. I am focusing here specifically on healing the disruptions of the self and relationships that may be characterized as complex PTSD.

Getting Started

The tone for the therapy is set in the first contact between the therapist and the client. The therapist's job is to respond to the client's needs and concerns, help to establish realistic goals and expectations of the therapy and the therapist, and endeavor to set a frame for the treatment that will allow both parties to do the necessary work. The early part of the treatment involves establishing a mutually respectful relationship in which decisions about the frame of the therapy (such as meeting time, length and frequency of sessions, fees, and forms of address) are made jointly. Clients are invited to notice and name feelings about what happens in the therapy and to express their concerns about safety and confidentiality. This process conveys an important message to clients about the value of their input, the balance of power, and the process of negotiation. As the therapist and client address issues such as length of sessions, forms of address of both client and therapist, and telephone availability, they are developing a collaborative work style that forms the basis for healing. Clients begin to learn that their needs matter and that they can express them and expect to be heard (Pearlman & Saakvitne, 1995; Saakvitne et al., 2000)

Although it is elusive for many survivors, safety must be the first consideration in every treatment, a view that is consistent with a phase-oriented approach (Courtois, 1999; Herman, 1992; McCann & Pearlman, 1990; Steele, van der Hart, & Nijenhuis, in press). The most effective approach to safety is to embark on a collaborative process of negotiating the frame for the work (Saakvitne et al., 2000). Safety may require attention to living arrangements for people in battering relationships, hospitalization for those who need protection from self-injurious or other aggressive behaviors, medication for those whose depression, anxiety, or sleep difficulties are debilitating. Safety for clients always requires honesty on the part of the therapist and a commitment to listen to them and respect their needs. In the long term, safety is established by sharing power and naming interpersonal processes.

Psychoeducation, which can provide frameworks for understanding the survivor's responses and struggles and for understanding the therapy process itself, is essential in the early part of treatment and continues to have a role over time. Self-help resources such as reading materials and Twelve-Step Programs are useful for many survivors. Psychopharmacology has much to offer those to whom medication is acceptable. Expressive therapies allow communication through alternative channels and may provide the most effective means of addressing that which cannot be named (such as traumatic preverbal experiences). Group therapy normalizes people's responses to traumatic events and breaks the overwhelming isolation many survivors experience. Each client's treatment program is individualized and is developed by the therapist and client according to the client's evolving needs, preferences, priorities, and resources.

Taking a trauma history is a process that unfolds over the course of treatment (Pearlman & McCann, 1994). Clients must control the pace of revealing what happened to them in the past. The therapist provides assistance by encouraging clients to talk about painful events if they are reluctant to do so yet are struggling with avoidance-related problems such as depression, emotional numbing, and somatization. Alternatively, the therapist will encourage clients to slow down if they are revealing so much so quickly that they become overwhelmed and experience increased symptoms such as intrusive imagery, flashbacks, and dissociation or attempts to cope with strong feelings through self-destructive behaviors.

Self Capacities

As the frame and the therapeutic relationship are being established, the therapist begins to focus on the development of self capacities. Self capacities are inner abilities that allow individuals to manage their intrapersonal world. Collectively, they allow us to maintain a coherent and cohesive sense of self. CSDT includes three self capacities: the ability to maintain an inner sense of positive connection with others (connection—conceptualized by others as object constancy); the ability to maintain a sense of self as viable, benign, and positive (self-worth); and the ability to experience, tolerate, and integrate feelings (affect tolerance). We have written in detail elsewhere about the development of self capacities, manifestations of disruptions, and therapeutic work to restore or develop self capacities (Pearlman, 1998; Saakvitne et al., 2000). A brief summary of these issues follows:

Self capacities develop through early interactions with responsive caregivers. By naming the child's apparent psychobiological states ("You look sleepy"; "You're upset, aren't you?") and naming and responding to his or her needs ("Are you hungry? I'll feed you"), the caregiver helps the child develop an awareness of the connection among his or her biological states, affective states, and the means of satisfying needs. This validates and connects the experiences of feeling and needing. By responding to the child's needs, the caregiver demonstrates that the child is worthy of attention and that his or her needs are reasonable and can be met. Through the inevitable imperfect attunement to another's needs, the caregiver also teaches the child that we all make mistakes and that the child can tolerate frustration.

When any aspect of this process breaks down, children suffer. If the breakdowns are severe or chronic, children may not learn essential lessons that form the basis of internal stability and self-care in adulthood. As adults, they may not feel worthy of love and affection, or even of life. They may not be able to feel anything or may feel everything intensely, without modulation. They may not have internalized images of loving others to draw upon in difficult times.

How, then, do such adults deal with the inevitable disappointments, losses, and injuries of daily life? Some do so with the help of alcohol or other drugs. Others dissociate when a feeling such as fear, anxiety, or shame is on the internal horizon. Still others inflict harm upon their bodies for a variety of reasons (Connors, 2000; Deiter, Nicholls, & Pearlman, 2000). Respondents in our own research reported that their primary reasons for self-injury were to distract themselves from painful feelings (or difficulty with affect tolerance) and to punish or express anger at themselves (or problems with self-worth) (Nicholls, Deiter, & Pearlman, 2001). Others, who do not have words for their internal experiences, may find their bodies speaking for them (Rothschild, 2000; van der Kolk, 1994). Others have sexual difficulties (Briere & Elliott, 1994; Maltz, 1991; Miller, 1994). Some who experience emotional abuse may binge and purge as a way of managing their otherwise intolerable inner world (de Groot & Rodin, 1999; Kent & Waller, 2000).

The extent of development of self capacities can be assessed in various ways. When dissociation, self-harming or aggressive behaviors, substance abuse, affective lability, or numbing is significant, affect tolerance is probably not well developed. Self-denigrating statements, lack of self-care, substance abuse, and isolation may indicate undeveloped self-worth. Difficulty with self-soothing, expressions of profound isolation, the experience of self as oddly different, and habits of hiding the self from others suggest difficulty with connection with internalized loving others. We are developing a short paper-and-pencil self-report measure of self capacities, the Inner Experience Questionnaire. Preliminary data from partial hospital and outpatient psychotherapy clients indicate adequate reliabilities and promising validity (Brock, Pearlman, & Deiter, 2001).

Therapeutic Approaches to Self Capacity Deficits[1]

Where self capacities are underdeveloped, they can be developed through the therapeutic relationship. The goal of developing self capacities is to help clients move toward a fuller experience of self. This means developing an awareness of what they feel and acceptance of a full range of feelings (affect tolerance), a sense of themselves as viable beings who deserve to be alive and to be loved (self-worth), and a sense that they are cared about by others (connection). This is long-term work, requiring the authentic participation of the therapist. Authenticity on the part of the therapist means that our behavior is trustworthy, reliable, and genuine.

Therapeutic work on self capacities takes two avenues, both in the context of the therapeutic relationship: one is exploratory; the other, cognitive-behavioral. In the former, the goal is to help clients identify how their current state evolved, what the meanings of strong affect are for them, what it would mean to feel more solidly connected to life, and who are the people who inhabit their inner world. Cognitive-behavioral strategies are used to provide clients with new skills that will serve as alternatives to their current less adaptive and less satisfying responses. Over time, this work translates into clients learning to understand, accept, and regulate their feelings. In the therapy, clients learn about the connection between bodily states (such as upset stomach, neck pain, tightness in the chest, headache) and names of feelings. They learn that feelings pass with time, dissolving into something different. As affect tolerance increases, clients are a step closer to being able to put their feelings into words. Some survivors need help elaborating a lexicon for the language of feelings. This allows for symbolic expression of emotions as an alternative to expressing feelings and needs through bodily states (physical discomfort, illnesses) and actions.

Survivors then have alternatives to fleeing their feelings through illnesses, substance abuse, dissociation, numbing, tissue self-injury, bingeing and purging, driving recklessly, or striking out at others. The alternatives, activities such as writing in a journal, talking with someone, producing art, listening to music, expressing feelings through dance, engaging in soothing self-talk, connecting with nature, and helping others, can be practiced over time with the therapist serving as empathic coach.

In working with survivor clients, the therapist honors conflict and ambivalence rather than suppressing them. Gradually, the clients will begin to develop a sense that someone whom they are growing to respect and value respects and values them, that someone they are learning to trust trusts them. This process eventually results in an internalized sense of self-worth and an internalized connection with a caring other. This is one of the most delicate and important aspects of the therapy. The way things happen in these sessions—the process—is as important as the content. The therapist's attunement to clients' shifts in mood or state (which can happen swiftly and frequently) helps the client learn to notice and develop confidence in naming intra- and interpersonal processes. This development contributes to self-worth, affect tolerance, and internalization of a caring other.

But what is the content? Life difficulties, trauma-related problems (e.g., flashbacks, nightmares, relationship problems the client experiences between and sometimes during sessions), and whatever else the client chooses to discuss will be the "content" focus of the sessions. In addition, the therapist remains aware of and comments on that which is being avoided. While the pacing of the therapy must be under the client's control, the therapist must name what is missing. This can be done gently and must be done with respect for the client's defenses. The therapist might say, "I'm aware that you haven't said much about what's bothering you," or "At some point, I think it will be important for you to tell me more about what happened to you." Premature exploration of traumatic memories, before the client has developed the self capacities essential to managing the possible fear, rage, grief, and self-loathing that may accompany those memories, can be retraumatizing. Yet avoidance of memories can maintain symptoms. Balancing the need to approach the trauma material with the client's need to protect him- or herself from pain is a delicate matter (Roth & Cohen, 1986). Some research suggests that avoidance may be an adaptive coping strategy for children who are being abused (DiPalma, 1994). Yet it is the confrontation of painful memories and imagery that often brings relief from the current distress that results from a traumatic past (Foa & Meadows, 1997; Steele et al., in press). The clinician and the client must work together to move toward resolution of traumatic memories in a way that acknowledges the complexity and difficulty of this process.

Cognitive Schemas

A second area of the self that is impacted by psychological trauma is the cognitive schemas, or beliefs about self and others. CSDT identifies five central need areas—safety, trust, esteem, intimacy, and control—that are impacted by traumatic life experiences. When life experiences impinge upon these needs, which are often unconscious, beliefs are shaped to reflect that impact (see, e.g., Janoff-Bulman, 1992). Research on schemas has found a relationship between schematic or thematic disruption and trauma-related symptoms (Dutton, Burghardt, Perrin, Chrestman, & Halle, 1994; Mas, 1992; Newman et al., 1997; Pearlman & Mac Ian, 1995; Schauben & Frazier, 1995).

For each person, some need areas are more central or salient than are others. Central salient need areas are generally those which were not met or gratified adequately in childhood and which remain sensitive throughout the person's lifetime. In this way, traumatic life experiences will affect individuals differently. For example, one person who was abused in childhood may find himself experiencing others primarily through the lens of intimacy, as evidenced by beliefs such as "I can't get close to people." Another may find herself sensitive to esteem: "Other people are just no good." These beliefs in turn shape future experience. If an individual believes people are no good, it is likely that he or she will avoid relationships and find confirming evidence for that belief in interactions with others.

These beliefs are reflected and can be assessed in a variety of ways. The central disrupted need areas will be represented in the individual's reports of interpersonal relationships ("My wife is so controlling"), symbolic material (e.g., dreams, nightmares), trauma-specific experiences (trauma imagery, flashbacks, and narratives of past events), and the transference relationship with the therapist. At our Traumatic Stress Institute (TSI) we have developed a pencil-and-paper self-report measure, the TSI Belief Scale (Pearlman, in press), which assesses areas of schematic disruption (Pearlman, 1996). This nonpathologizing measure has proven useful in differentiating those with and without a trauma history, as well as pointing to potential areas of sensitivity and conflict for clients.

Therapeutic Approaches to Disrupted Schemas[2]

Like the work on self capacities (and all other realms within CSDT), the therapy takes two paths: an exploratory approach and a cognitive/behavioral approach. In general, therapeutic work on cognitive schemas requires (1) identifying areas of disruption, (2) exploring the sources of disruption, (3) exploring the meanings of the disrupted schemas and of their alternatives, (4) exploring the self-protective value of the "disrupted" schemas, (5) gently challenging the disrupted schemas, and (6) arranging small life experiments that will challenge and may expand or alter the schemas. The challenges to schemas are sometimes direct ("I understand how you see it; I see it a little differently") and often indirect (e.g., the belief that the client is not worthy of respect is challenged every time the therapist honors his or her needs or feelings). Small life experiments are conducted by supporting the client in doing something differently. For example, one childhood sexual abuse survivor client with precarious self-esteem was convinced that a particular coworker would never go to lunch with her. After she and the therapist explored the client's experiences with this coworker and possible outcomes, the client invited the coworker to lunch one day. The coworker agreed to go, and the client was invited to imagine that her self-image as loathsome and detestable might not be entirely accurate.

Research on cognitive schemas in trauma survivors has produced some findings with interesting clinical applications. Black and Deiter (1995) looked at beliefs about self and others in childhood trauma survivors and their relation to revictimization. Based on their findings, in the context of attachment theory, these authors hypothesized that early victimization may damage boundaries between self and others, making it difficult for adult survivors to differentiate their needs from those of others. This then sets the stage for revictimization; a would-be perpetrator may approach a survivor in a way that suggests he wants something that the survivor also wants. An example would be the "friend" who tries to persuade or coerce the survivor into a sexual relationship. The adult survivor may find it difficult to say no, in part because she isn't clear whether that's what she wants or not.

Black and Pearlman (1997) found a causal path among disrupted schemas as measured by the TSI Belief Scale. We found that self-esteem mediates the relationship between self-trust and self-intimacy, on the one hand, and other-trust and other-intimacy, on the other. In other words, the connection between beliefs about self and beliefs about others (in the areas of trust and intimacy) is self-esteem. This finding has important clinical implications. The areas of greatest sensitivity are often so painful that working directly on change is quite difficult: one client said, "I just don't trust people. Period." End of conversation. But moving one step away, in this example, to self-esteem, may allow for therapeutic movement. This client found it easier to work on feeling better about herself than on trusting others. The exploratory work focused on trying to understand the sources of the client's low self-esteem and their connection to her childhood and adult traumatic experiences. The cognitive-behavioral work included identifying the self-talk that maintained her bad feelings about herself, developing more positive self-statements, creating opportunities to do things that she was good at, noticing her strengths and talents, and developing new interests. Over time, this client found it possible to enter into relationships with new people and begin slowly to learn whom she could trust and with what, developing that trust through a mutual process of self-revelation and stating and responding to needs.

The cognitive-behavioral strategies will not be successful unless potential obstacles to their implementation are addressed. This requires exploratory work that must include an understanding of how the "disrupted" schema serves the person. While a belief that one is worthless (low self-esteem) may be painful, it may be more acceptable to the client than an alternative such as believing that the parent–perpetrator was bad and abusive. While a belief that one must control absolutely everything in relationships (other-control) makes relationships impossible or intolerable, it may protect the person from being injured (or so the person may believe). This exploration of the self-protective role of disrupted schemas must be done gently, to avoid accusing or blaming the client. All of us have defenses that have developed for very good reasons. Indeed, it is never our job to dismantle defenses, but rather to help survivor clients to develop alternatives.

Working on the connection between disrupted schemas and traumatic memories helps with intrusive or preoccupying trauma material. When clients relate their memory fragments or the particular aspect of a memory that is most painful, the therapist listens for the five need/schema themes. The need areas that are salient to each person (as identified by the TSI Belief Scale, the person's relationship difficulties, and the transference) will emerge in the traumatic memories. Once they are identified, the therapist and the client can work with these themes. One childhood sexual abuse survivor reported an intrusive scene in which her father was molesting her in a car in the huge parking lot of a tall apartment building. At some point she was able to recall seeing someone at a window, high above the car. She felt a moment of hope that help would be forthcoming; it was not. The theme in this image, which tormented the client for years, was betrayal and abandonment. These experiences relate to other-trust, which was this client's central disrupted need. As an adult she lived a highly counterdependent (and hence rather lonely) life, making sure she asked no one for anything. Once the other-trust theme was identified, she was able to work on that painful memory and integrate it into her life experience. The work on other-trust issues continued, and the memory ceased to have its potency.

Ego Resources

The ego resources are inner abilities that allow individuals to navigate the interpersonal world, to meet their needs, and to manage relationships. They include such things as an awareness of one's psychological needs; the ability to foresee consequences, to make self-protective judgments, to establish mature, mutual relationships with others, and to establish boundaries; perspective (which includes empathy, wisdom, and humor); willpower and initiative; and intelligence. Deficits in some of these ego resources may lead to revictimization.

To entertain the possibility of knowing one's needs requires a certain level of healthy entitlement that many survivors of childhood abuse and neglect do not have. One survivor client who grew up in circumstances of great deprivation, when asked, "What do you need?," replied, "What can I have?" The therapeutic relationship serves as a laboratory for the development of ego resources. The therapist names feelings and processes, invites the client to notice what happens between the two of them, acknowledges her own mistakes, offers perspective. Boundaries are honored in a variety of ways. The therapist adheres to appointment times, not missing appointments, starting late, rescheduling without good reason, or running sessions over time. The therapist treats the client's time with the same respect as his or her own. The therapist observes both the letter and the spirit of the client's confidentiality and privacy. Psychotherapy takes place in the office, and the therapist and the client do not have additional (social or business) relationships. The therapist is genuine, open with what he or she is experiencing in the session when doing so furthers the goals of the therapy. The therapist does not use the client's time to talk about his or her own difficulties and concerns. All of these behaviors are of course basic to any good psychotherapy. But people who grew up in chaotic or abusive homes do not take predictability and respect for granted. When the therapist behaves in this way, the client learns to expect more for—and perhaps of—him- or herself. Of course the therapist also calls attention to related behaviors as the client reports them in other relationships. When the therapist learns of someone treating the client disrespectfully, the therapist comments on it. A comment as simple as "That's distressing" can alert the client to the possibility that there is an alternative way for someone to interact with him or her.

The ability to know and ask for what one needs can also help short-circuit somatization. One childhood trauma survivor who was interviewing for a therapy group told us that she was glad the group wouldn't be starting for a while because she felt a crisis coming on. Our inquiry about this was met with the following explanation: The only way she knew to get attention was by having a crisis, usually one related to her physical health. It her way of being cared for and receiving safe (nonsexual) touch. Her sense of need was growing, so a crisis was in the offing.

Frame of Reference: Identity

van der Kolk et al. (1996) noted a variety of identity-related difficulties that may be part of the aftermath of severe or early victimization. These include "disturbances of body image [and] a view of oneself as helpless, damaged, and ineffective" (p. 86). I would add to this list an experience of self as toxic, a loser, a slut, a victim, a loner, painfully different from everyone else, or someone who has experienced devastating losses. In addition, one's identity includes characteristic affect states such as depression, loneliness, numbness; that is, one's experience of oneself as someone who feels blue, feels lonely, or doesn't feel. Finally, sexual orientation and sexuality are a central part of identity and may be affected by sexual trauma (Elliott, 1991; Gonzalez, 1993), an area about which there is suprisingly little in the literature.

Therapeutic work on identity disturbances begins with helping the client to make these issues conscious by verbalizing them. Then they are explored: Where, when, and how did they originate? What functions do they serve? What is their basis in fact? How are they limiting and how are they protective? The therapist invites the client to try to see him- or herself through the therapist's eyes. One childhood sexual abuse survivor client's experience of herself was of worthlessness and shame. After we had worked together for a year or so, I asked her to imagine how I saw her. She could barely tolerate the question. The question raised the complex issue of being seen; many survivors (like most people) long to be seen as special and yet they also dread being seen because of its association with past abuse. We processed this over many sessions, which included recalling her abusive grandfather's voice saying, "Who do you think you are?" Eventually, with encouragement, the client was able to speculate that I seemed to enjoy her and even find her likable, and she was able to hold that view without feeling frightened.

The therapist may also invite clients to "take the therapist along." "Can you imagine what I might say [or think]?" is a question I will raise with clients from time to time. This question addresses several levels simultaneously: it helps develop an inner sense of connection (self capacity); it invites perspective (ego resource); and it provides an alternative to the client's sense of identity. Developmentally, the next identity-related task is to invite clients to see themselves through their own eyes (rather than those of a harsh or abusive parent or even a benevolent other). Of course, the benefits of these interventions cross areas of the self. While this work affects identity, it also helps clients build an inner sense of connection with someone they value, the therapist, and addresses self-worth, another self capacity.

Group therapy is extremely useful to survivor clients in their identity struggles (see Klein & Schermer, 2000, for an excellent compendium of group treatments for trauma survivors, many of which pertain to work with clients with complex PTSD). Several other observers are in the room, and they are generally less harsh critics than each client is of him- or herself. Their caring can't be discounted as easily as that of the therapist ("You only like me because I'm paying you"). For example, as a survivor of childhood sexual abuse engages with the others' struggles with their own self-loathing, shame, and guilt about what they did and didn't do in response to such abuse, she learns valuable lessons. She learns that small children (even her younger self) can't stop big adults from hurting them. She learns that people who think they're awful aren't really so bad after all. She learns that she isn't the only one struggling with the painful aftermath of abuse. Of course, all of the other interpersonal benefits of group therapy (Yalom, 1975) may accrue to the trauma survivor as well, including opportunities to develop or refine interpersonal skills which are often lacking for those who grew up in abusive or neglectful homes.

One immutable aspect of being a trauma survivor is that terrible things happened and they had a negative effect. Nothing can make those facts go away. One client said she wished for a big eraser. Nothing can erase what happened. But another survivor said she views herself as an alchemist, who is "turning the lead of my suffering into the gold of wisdom and compassion."

Frame of Reference: Spirituality

Above all, sexual and physical abuse and other severe early abuse and neglect damage the victim's spirituality. We define spirituality broadly as an awareness of ephemeral aspects of life. (Neumann & Pearlman, 1994; Pearlman & Saakvitne, 1995). This definition includes the devastating impact abuse and neglect can have on meaning and hope, transcendence, openness to all aspects of life, and one's relation to nonmaterial aspects of life. This damage may be reflected in cynicism or despair; a narrow focus on self or victimhood; irreverence for nature, humanity, or life; materialism; and inability to experience love, joy, awe, wonder, gratitude, passion, or community.

In addition to listening for these themes, we are working toward assessing four dimensions of disrupted spirituality using a pencil-and-paper self-report measure, the Life Orientation Inventory (Neumann & Pearlman, 1996).

Therapeutic Approaches to Spirituality

Therapeutic work to develop or restore spirituality often begins later in treatment, after the survivor client has dealt with disruptive trauma symptoms, addressed traumatic memories, and worked on developing relationships with self and others. At some point, the client begins to ask, "Is this all there is?" Not being plagued by symptoms is indeed an enormous relief, as is understanding one's past. But these processes do not constitute—rather they set the stage for—the development of one's full humanity. It is easy for the therapist to back away from this aspect of the work in the mistaken belief that the only path to spirituality is religion, which is not the therapist's bailiwick. In this work, as in every other realm, the therapist's stance is one of neutrality. We encourage the client to explore the meaning of life and of his or her life in particular, reasons for living and ways of living that would be rewarding, and ways of transcending self (such as acts of giving, helping or altruism; meditation; engagement with nature; or faith or religion). Again we must be sensitive to individual differences; each person's path to spiritual awareness is unique.

PROCESSES OF THERAPY WITHIN CONSTRUCTIVIST SELF DEVELOPMENT THEORY

I summarize below the processes that are at work throughout psychotherapy in the CSDT framework: These processes are discussed at greater length and in terms of specific clinical approaches in Saakvitne et al. (2000).

1. The relationship between the therapist and the client is the foundation of the work. It includes the use of the self of the therapist. We must be genuine without transgressing professional, ethical, or therapeutic boundaries. We must be willing to know ourselves and to grow with our clients. Throughout the work, we are attempting to learn what clients need and help them put it into words. It will not always be consistent with what the therapist needs. For example, a client may want to meet for longer sessions or more frequently than the therapist can manage. Or a client who fears opening up painful feelings may raise issues but not want to explore them. Conflict will emerge, as is inevitable in every intimate relationship. Both parties have a voice in the therapeutic relationship, and both should be heard and respected. Conflicting needs should be negotiated. Power differentials do not imply abuse.

2. Individual differences in what is traumatic and what is healing require that the client speak and the therapist listen. The client guides his or her own healing, with the therapist as witness, consultant, observer, and supporter.

3. Naming what is happening is extremely powerful for people who grew up in homes where silence or words were used as weapons. When denial or lying is part of children's contexts, it becomes difficult to trust their own perceptions. This is one source of people feeling as if they are "crazy":

they notice something important going on, but there is no external validation. When the client asks the therapist whether the therapist is annoyed (or
tired or distracted, etc.), the therapist must answer honestly (and sensitively).
Honest responses validate the client's perceptions.

4. Connecting the past and the present is essential. Many people find it
enormously helpful to understand how they got to be who they are today.
Another reason people feel "crazy" is that they believe their responses make
no sense or are disproportionate to the situation but they don't understand
why. Helping people trace the origins of their behaviors is healing and provides them with an effective tool.

5. Separating the past from the present helps disentangle clients from
their abusive contexts. Some clients will need to learn to distinguish between
feeling upset and being terrified, a distinction that may not be easy (van der
Kolk, 1994). When people are not currently in danger but are fearful, it is important to remind them gently that they can protect themselves now, that
they have resources they didn't have as children. There is a difference between one's spouse saying something hurtful in the present and a parent
abusing one in childhood. A mistake is not abuse.

APPLYING CONSTRUCTIVIST SELF DEVELOPMENT THEORY TO CLINICAL CASES

To illustrate the application of CSDT, I next briefly describe three psychotherapies. I focus here on aspects of the treatment that address dissociation, somatization, affect regulation, revictimization, relationship difficulties,
identity, and spirituality. All of these psychotherapies are long-term treatments with adult women who experienced sexual abuse in childhood or grew
up in chaotic homes. Because there is not a discrete traumatic stressor and
because the abuse and/or neglect began early for all three women, an assessment of premorbid functioning is not possible.

It is notable in all of these cases, as in those of many adult survivors of
childhood trauma, that they have functioned reasonably well in the world yet
their lives and relationships have been pervaded by the damage of childhood
abuse and neglect.

Treatment of an Adult Survivor of Childhood Sexual Abuse and Neglect

Kelly is a married Caucasian professional woman in her 40s, raised as a
Catholic. She has two teenaged children. Her couples therapist referred her
for treatment. Kelly was concerned about the dissociation she experienced
frequently (as a sense of a fine barrier coming between herself and the rest of
the world), as well as her inability to sense her feelings or tune in to others'

feelings. She also felt disturbed and confused by her intense involvement with a woman friend, which threatened her identity and esteem.

Traumatic Stressors

When Kelly was about 4 years old, her mother became ill and the family left Kelly with relatives. She did not know what was happening and felt worried and abandoned. When the family was reunited, there was an unspoken rule not to bother her mother. In addition, as the only child of older parents, she was often not noticed. Her father seemed perpetually absorbed in the newspaper. She would go off on her own for long hours at a very young age without being missed. When kindly neighbors took her home, her parents showed amusement or disinterest rather than concern. A neighbor sexually abused Kelly when she was a preschooler, and a priest abused her when she was a teen. Both of these experiences of ongoing sexual molestation took place in the context of relationships that Kelly described as otherwise warm and nurturing.

Clinical Picture

Kelly's difficulties trusting others, her enormous fear of interpersonal connection, her disconnection from her feelings, her compulsive habit of scratching herself until she bled, her low self-esteem, and her confusion about sexual feelings and intimacy all seemed to call for a relational therapy that would address issues of safety, trust, self-worth, affect tolerance, and identity. We assessed specific areas of schema disruption with the TSI Belief Scale. Her elevations were in the areas of other-intimacy, self-safety, and other-control. Her retrospective statement about what she was struggling with when she first came to treatment was low self-esteem, fear, vulnerability, self-righteousness, living with a "false face," hypersensitivity, hypervigilance, negativism, and being controlling. She thinks she was hypercritical of others as a means of compensating for her low self-esteem. Sexual arousal and connection with others were intertwined for Kelly.

Treatment

Before an assessment of Kelly's traumatic history could take place, she had to develop a sense of safety in the therapeutic relationship. This did not come easily. Kelly had been involved in a number of intense emotional relationships with women in the past. She was terrified of sexual feelings for women because such feelings signaled confusion about her sexual orientation and moral issues for her. In our first sessions, Kelly accused me of trying to seduce her and stated that she believed I was a lesbian. She remained in the treatment largely because she trusted the couples therapist who encouraged her to try to stay and work out her feelings with me. As we sorted through her intense reaction, it seemed to be connected to the fact that she had strong sexual feelings in response to my nurturing and supportive approach to her. Because these feelings were inexplicable and unacceptable to her, she attributed them to something I was doing to her, a painfully familiar path to meaning for Kelly. In my work on this issue with Kelly, I encouraged her to talk about and understand what she was feeling, beginning the work on affect tolerance. I did not respond directly to her questions about my sexual orientation, which I came to believe was a mistake on my part. In work with clients without a trauma history, I believe that their questions about me reflect something important about themselves that we need to understand which answering the questions immediately may not facilitate. However, I have found that a more open and direct approach is essential with trauma survivor clients. Kelly was unable to settle down and do the work she wanted to do without that information about me. This was in part a reflection of her other-control need and in part related to her need for self-safety. The reality of abuse elevates the need for safety in most trauma survivors (Pearlman, in press). Until safety is addressed, little else can be accomplished in therapies with survivors of early or severe abuse or neglect.

When survivor clients ask me personal questions (such as my sexual orientation or survivor status) in the first few sessions, I am now more likely to answer those questions. When such questions emerge later in the treatment, I find it more useful to express to the client my interest in why that question is coming up now. I may eventually decide to answer the question or not, as the client and I understand more about its meanings.

Issues of self-disclosure are complicated by (1) work-setting issues and norms, (2) the complexity of the answers, and (3) small communities. When one client asks for information in a milieu or group therapy context, answering it means providing information for the whole group which others may not want. A client may ask a therapist whether the therapist is married; if the therapist is in a long-term committed relationship but not married or if the therapist is the midst of a divorce or if the word "marriage" implies a heterosexual relationship but the therapist is gay, the answer may not be simple. If the treatment is taking place in a small community, answering the question may mean revealing more about oneself than one wants known in the community. If the therapist is a survivor but has not shared that information widely, he or she may not want to respond to the client's question. These complex issues deserve deeper attention than is possible here. We have discussed them elsewhere (Pearlman & Saakvitne, 1995) and encourage therapists to discuss them with colleagues.

With this client, this very difficult early interaction (which lasted for several months) revealed much that would be central to the treatment over time.

We learned that Kelly's feelings were mysterious to her; she usually located the source as outside herself. We learned that, for her, nurturance often led to sexual feelings. Saakvitne (1993) has written about the eroticized maternal transference, which aptly describes the process Kelly and I experienced. In many sessions, we also observed the dissociation that was plaguing Kelly. She used the phrase "the cheesecloth" to describe her sense of something porous but not transparent coming between herself and another person when anxiety began to emerge.

I saw Kelly in individual psychotherapy for 5 years, initially meeting once a week. After about 3 years, we reduced the frequency of sessions to once a month at Kelly's suggestion. In the first year, we talked a great deal about our relationship. Kelly's experience of me was that I was trying to harm her through what she perceived as my seductiveness. We worked for a long time trying to sort out what I was doing that contributed to this impression and what expectations Kelly was bringing from her past relationships that might contribute.

While we were doing this work, Kelly was also sharing her history with me. As she talked about those who had hurt her, shame emerged. She was surprised I did not hold her accountable for her abuse, that I thought the neglect she experienced was formative. Talking about her painful past with someone who did not pass judgment against her helped reduce her shame and eventually her dissociation. We talked about her relationships with her two teenaged daughters and with her husband. The therapeutic work entailed exploring the origins of Kelly's current difficulties, connecting her present struggles with the past, noticing and naming Kelly's experience (feelings or lack thereof, dissociation) during sessions and what went on between us, supporting Kelly in her efforts to create boundaries in relationships, and focusing on self-care. For a very long time, we ended every session with her response to my question, "What will you be needing over the hours and days ahead?" She wrote in a journal and read books about the effects of childhood trauma.

While there is not a one-to-one correspondence between the tasks of therapy and the growth of the self, some tasks contribute more specifically to particular realms. Naming interpersonal processes is the foundation of safety. Managing boundaries was also central to Kelly's ability to feel safe. Thinking about one's needs helps to develop a sense that one is entitled to need and therefore to feel, which is the beginning of affect tolerance. The naming of feeling states furthers the development of affect tolerance. Writing in a journal helps people put their feelings into words, develop self-awareness, and make sense of their experience. Connecting the past to the present develops identity. Self-care over time increases self-worth.

All of these tasks are undertaken in the context and service of developing a therapeutic relationship. In time, the client assimilates the therapist's respect. This respect eventually contributes to the client's sense of self-worth and, in this case, other-intimacy.

Treatment Outcomes

In time, Kelly began to believe that I had her best interest at heart. She gradually began to trust me. She and I developed frameworks for understanding her responses. I strongly emphasized self-care, which in her case meant not doing all of the housework along with her full-time job, setting limits and priorities with her family, and noticing her own needs and trying to meet them. The dissociation and scratching both lessened. Her relationships with her daughters improved as she demanded that they treat her more respectfully.

Kelly was underemployed when she first came to therapy. After a couple of years of treatment, she applied for and landed a job that demanded all of her many resources. Her new boss was high-strung, authoritarian, and somewhat unpredictable. She began to feel fearful, to dissociate at work, and to scratch herself again. We recontracted for weekly sessions. A year later, Kelly's daughters had left home. She was then working very long hours, leaving little time for the leisure and contemplative activities she had developed as part of her self-care plan. But the therapy relationship seemed to be holding her sufficiently; she dissociated and scratched herself far less often. Perhaps most important, Kelly was aware of her feelings for the first time. She stated that she felt "more authentic" and not as threatened by others. When I asked her what she found helpful about psychotherapy, she said, "feeling held and accepted."

Treatment of an Adult Survivor with a History of Emotional and Physical Neglect

Ms. C is a divorced professional woman in her 40s, mother of three adult children. She came to treatment at the suggestion of her physician after she had been through a debilitating bout of depression. She was aware of the impending deaths of her aging parents over the years ahead, losses that would be compounded by her youngest son leaving home to establish his own life. She felt quite alone in the world. Her work was unsatisfying.

Traumatic Stressors

Ms. C grew up in a rural area, the second of four children. Her father was a quiet, affectionate, retiring man. Her mother seemed tormented by her own demons; the nature of her difficulties is unclear, but she received psychiatric treatment for some years during her adulthood. Neither electroshock nor pharmacological treatment seemed to help her. Ms. C experienced her mother as unpredictable, inappropriate, paranoid, constantly angry, sometimes violent, and generally very unhappy.

When Ms. C was about 6 years old, she and her younger sister were left with neighbors without explanation. Apparently her mother was taken to a psychiatric hospital. She and her sister were left there for months, not knowing what had happened to their parents. One day, they were picked up and the family was reunited. Her mother's violent outbursts did not end, however, and her father became less and less available. The overall picture was one of emotional abuse and neglect. The result was that the children were in a fairly constant state of fear and hyperarousal, awaiting their mother's next flare-up or the next abandonment.

At age 15, Ms. C met and eventually married a young man who turned out to be quite troubled. From the outset of their marriage, he was involved with other women and sneered at Ms. C's requests that he come home in the evenings after work. He refused to share information about their financial situation. He generally treated Ms. C with contempt. The husband initiated a divorce while the children were young.

During the course of treatment, Ms. C lost her job in a downsizing.

Clinical Picture

As I became acquainted with Ms. C, it became clear that trusting others was a central difficulty for her. She had an increasingly crystallized identity as a toxic person whom others disliked. She felt hopeless about change, entrapped in her isolation by her fear of people. She stated, "There is no assumption of safety." She had experienced her husband's behavior as a revictimization. Her depression was evident.

Medication was unacceptable to Ms. C. When Ms. C was a child, her mother often threatened to take her to the doctor if she didn't behave. Despite her fears, Ms. C sought out psychotherapy because she felt desperate. She seemed to be a good candidate for a relational psychotherapy that would focus on self-worth, trust, identity, and the ability to notice, name, and meet her own needs.

I attempted to use pencil-and-paper measures to collect early assessment data, but Ms. C was unwilling to participate. She feared that I might violate her confidentiality or use the information obtained through the tests to hurt her in some way (as her mother had done with Ms. C's journal in adolescence). Eventually, several years into the treatment, Ms. C was interested in completing questionnaires. She experienced her ability to participate as sign both that she was beginning to trust me and that she was valuable and had something to contribute. The results at that time showed disruptions on the TSI Belief Scale in the areas of self-trust, other-trust, self-control, and other-control.

Treatment

I met with Ms. C for 50-minute weekly therapy sessions for about a year. Ms. C had difficulty settling in to a therapy session, reconnecting, working, and regrouping to leave. She requested longer sessions. After discussing her concerns and the possible ramifications of such a change, we began to meet for 1 hour and 15 minutes (1 ½ session) each week. The change was beneficial. It allowed Ms. C to reconnect, make sure I hadn't changed, do her work, and prepare to leave more comfortably. In addition, the fact that she had been able to formulate and verbalize a need and receive a positive response was very empowering, addressing her control needs.

The early months of the therapy were devoted to forming a therapeutic relationship. Ms. C was very clear that her trust would not come easily or quickly. I made many errors. Because of the warm humor we were able to share, I assumed at times we were further along in building trust than we were. When I made assumptions that weren't accurate, she struggled to name her concerns. I supported her in speaking, despite how difficult she found it, by responding as honestly and nondefensively as I could. During the first few years of this 8-year treatment, Ms. C's parents were both moved to a nursing home and then died. We spent much time during these early years trying to understand her childhood experiences and processing the intense feelings of anger, disappointment, hurt, longing, and grief that were connected to childhood for Ms. C.

Through intense commitment to change, Ms. C was able to keep coming back to therapy, able to keep trying to develop trust in another person. She wrote extensively in a journal along the way. She brought dreams to therapy sessions, which she mined successfully for important understandings of herself and her fears.

Treatment Outcomes

The therapy also focused on self-worth and identity, which are deeply intertwined for Ms. C. My positive regard for her, her ability to accept my invitation to participate in our research program and in developing this chapter, and her awareness of her value in the eyes and lives of her grandchildren helped her begin to build a sense of self as viable and benign, rather than toxic (self capacity and identity). Fortunately, Ms. C. was able to resolve much of her anger at her parents before they died. She mourned deeply for a few years, but with love and regret rather than rage and guilt. She is reemployed with her former employer, in a job she does not enjoy but tolerates. She continues to strive to feel entitled to speak her needs, with greater success than at the beginning of therapy, but still with difficulty. She continues to struggle to overcome her fears of betrayal and abandonment to connect with others. She has found new meaning in her own life through her connection with her grandchildren, who are devoted to her. When asked what she found helpful about the therapy, she replied it was my predictability, my constant acceptance of her, and my respect for her. She insisted on genuineness from me, which required overcoming my natural reserve as a therapist as well as some of my training about "being a therapist." To the extent that the therapy has been successful, I think it is because both of us have been willing to take risks, to grow, and to change.

Treatment of an Adult Survivor of Childhood Sexual Abuse and Adult Assault and Sudden Traumatic Loss

Ms. L is a divorced African-American woman in her mid-40s who is trained as an engineer. She has one adult daughter who, along with her daughter, lives with her. Her physician referred her to psychotherapy after a skiing accident that resulted in intense, prolonged pain and negative physical findings. Ms. L found herself unable to return to work or to function because of intense physical pain. She came to therapy with great skepticism, stating, "My doctor says it's all in my head."

Traumatic Stressors

Ms. L has a long history of traumatic experiences. Her biological father left home when she was 3 years old, and she had no contact with him until recently. When she was about 5, her mother and stepfather left her with her grandmother, without explaining why or whether they would return. They returned for her in a year, removing her again without notice from a home that had become the one safe haven that she had ever known.

The first sexual molestation she recalls took place when she was about 7 years old. She was sexually assaulted in childhood and adolescence by at least five perpetrators, including her stepfather, an older stepbrother and stepsister, one of their friends, and a shop owner. Her stepfather impregnated her when she was 12 years old; the family physician induced an abortion but did not intercede on her behalf. The sexual abuse by the stepfather ended when she was about 14.

Additional assaults and traumatic losses include being a victim in a physically abusive marriage, the death of her second child in childbirth, a marital rape which resulted in pregnancy and then abortion, and a skiing accident which resulted in chronic pain and an inability to work. More recent painful losses include the sudden, traumatic deaths of two close friends and her beloved younger sister.

Clinical Picture

When I first met Ms. L, she was incapacitated by physical pain. She was clinically depressed and reporting crying, feeling frustrated and disoriented, feeling "hollow inside," rapidly cycling thoughts, difficulty concentrating and sleeping, and nightmares. She contemplated suicide frequently and made some parasuicidal gestures ("tiny cuts" on her arm). She met the criteria for

PTSD. She was also quite dissociative, although it took us time to realize how extensive this problem was. When her physical pain worsened, her psychological difficulties intensified.

My early assessment was that she had impaired self-worth, difficulty tolerating feelings, and difficulty maintaining an inner sense of connection with benevolent others. She was accustomed to being very independent, having raised a child alone while working a very demanding job. She was used to a good deal of control in her life, and her identity was based in her role as "the person with the how-to book" in her large family. In other words, she experienced herself as the helper, not the recipient of help. Her inability to work and take care of her own needs strongly impacted her central need area, trust/dependency, as well as her self-esteem. She was a woman of action, not someone who had an active inner life. She was bright and creative. She had a fighting spirit and much determination. She had a strong faith in God, which was wavering when we first met. This diminution in her faith in turn affected her identity as a spiritual person.

Ms. L completed the TSI Belief Scale on four occasions over the course of our work together. One year into our work (the first administration), she showed disruptions in other-trust and other-intimacy relative to other outpatients who completed the scale. Three years later, none of her scores were elevated beyond the normal range, although these two areas remained her most sensitive.

Treatment

I initially saw Ms. L in weekly individual psychotherapy, which then increased to twice weekly as her suicidality increased. Initially, she talked primarily about the limitations she was experiencing as a result of her loss of mobility. The loss of work as a source of self-esteem and the need to rely on others to help her with daily chores were frustrating, enraging, frightening, and disorienting to her. In the second session, she alluded to a history of childhood sexual abuse. She had never discussed the abuse with anyone, using her capacity for denial and her high activity level to avoid thinking or feeling about it. The inactivity and anger about the accident and her subsequent immobility opened her to reflect upon her sexual abuse and to overwhelming rage. We used early sessions to help her begin to manage her pain through hypnotherapy. We talked about her safety in the face of suicidal longings (self-safety). We began to explore her reluctance to rely on others (other-trust). We talked about what it would be like to talk about the abuse (other-intimacy). Over the course of our work together, she confronted two of her perpetrators (a stepbrother and her stepfather). She was proud that she didn't feel frightened by these two men who once had overpowered her physically and continued to dominate her inner and interpersonal world for many years.

Ms. L eventually accepted a referral to a psychiatrist who runs a pain management center. In addition to helping her address and manage her pain, he prescribed antidepressant medication. This left us time and gave her essential support to work on helping her manage intrusive memories, develop her ability to soothe herself, and begin to build affect tolerance and self-worth. We experimented with returning to a once-a-week therapy schedule. In the early years of treatment, this led to a crisis; she needed more frequent sessions to remain stable. In later years, when we met only weekly, she would disconnect from her feelings and not think about the work of therapy between sessions.

She was able in time to organize friends and family to shop and clean her house. This raised issues about trust and dependency, which took her back to childhood. As her self capacities grew stronger, she was able to talk about the childhood abuse and neglect and to tolerate the rage and self-loathing that accompanied this work. The work also focused on our relationship, including her feelings about doing this work with a Caucasian woman ("fine"), about beginning to confide in and trust someone ("terrifying"), and about my various failures (e.g., forgetting to call when I had agreed to do so, not being able to help her get back to work, traveling a lot and not being there when she needed me; "fine" at first, "angry" in time). My job was to be constant, predictable, respectful, dependable, and honest.

Ms. L spoke often during this treatment about her faith and her relationship with God. When we were working on pain management through imagery, she created a very powerful image of "the hands of God soothing [her] pain." When she was actively working on traumatic memories, she experienced a great deal of fear. At this time, a huge, strong woman appeared one day in the "protected space" we created through imagery. Ms. L identified this woman as her protector, who made herself and her problems seem small yet still significant. Eventually Ms. L was able to recognize that the powerful guardian contained elements of herself, herself without her fears, herself with compassion both for her struggles and for her perpetrators.

Eventually I realized that Ms. L was hungry to make sense of her victimization within her own belief system. I responded with openness and interest when she raised questions like "Why did God choose me for this?" She found her own answers, which led her to a path of interpersonal forgiveness with one perpetrator; asking another perpetrator why he had harmed her, thereby opening a dialogue in which he was eventually able to apologize; and praying for another perpetrator whom she felt unable to encounter face-to-face.

Treatment Outcomes

In winding up this 8-year treatment, Ms. L reported that she has real friends, people who know her and whom she trusts, for the first time ever. She expressed interest in including men in her life and began to think about how she could let a man know her without feeling terrified (other-intimacy). She said she knows what feelings are and can tell the difference between feeling and logic. She doesn't always feel she has to move away from her feelings (affect tolerance). She started the practice of hugging her granddaughter, nieces, and nephews, and stated, "For the first time in our family, kids expect to be hugged." She said one of the biggest changes for her is that she is no longer afraid to admit that she's made a mistake (identity, self-esteem). About the therapy relationship, she said, "Laurie picked up the ball when I dropped it, something no one else in my life has ever done."

She has talked with family members about the sexual abuse and siblings have opened up about their own abuse by two of the same family perpetrators She stated that she was beginning to think people might like her for some reason other than what she could do for them (self-worth). She sees herself as creative and attractive for the first time (identity). She reconnected with her faith in God and found a new church. She felt she could say no (or not now) to requests for help from friends and family. When her physical pain feels overwhelming, she can think of reasons to live. She knows she can create meaning in her life.

CONCLUSION

I have presented a theoretical framework, CSDT, for understanding the impact of traumatic life experiences on survivors. This framework gives a theoretical context to the observed behavioral problems that constitute disorders of extreme stress, not otherwise specified, or complex PTSD. A theory, or an interrelated network of explicit assumptions, points to specific, systematic, interrelated treatment interventions and thus provides hope, perhaps the most important gift a therapist has to offer.

NOTES

1. For more approaches to building self capacities, see Deiter and Pearlman (1998), Pearlman (1998), Pearlman and Deiter (1996), and Saakvitne et al. (2000).
2. For more approaches to addressing disrupted schemas, see Rosenbloom, Williams, and Watkins (1999).

ACKNOWLEDGMENTS

I wish to thank Jeanne Folks, DMin., Kristin Hale, RN, Terri Haven, MSW, Sarah S. Nicholls, PhD, JoLynn Powers, PsyD, Anne C. Pratt, PhD, and other colleagues for comments on a draft of this chapter. I am also very grateful to the clients who collaborated with me in writing this chapter and who allowed me to write about our work in the hope of helping other survivors.

REFERENCES

American Psychiatric Association. (1994). *Diagnostic and statistical manual of mental disorders.* Washington, DC: Author.

Black, A. E., & Deiter, P. J. (1995). *An empirical investigation of self-other differentiation, beliefs about safety and control, and traumatic revictimization: An attachment theory perspective.* Paper presented at the annual meeting of the International Society for Traumatic Stress Studies, Boston, MA.

Black, A. E., & Pearlman, L. A. (1997). Self-esteem as a mediator between beliefs about self and beliefs about others. *Journal of Social and Clinical Psychology, 16*(1), 57–76.

Briere, J. (1984). *The long-term effects of childhood sexual abuse: Defining a post-sexual abuse syndrome.* Paper presented at the Third National Conference on Sexual Victimization of Children, Washington, DC.

Briere, J. N., & Elliot, D. M. (1994). Immediate and long-term impacts of child sexual abuse. *Future of Children, 4*(2), 54–69.

Briere, J., & Runtz, M. (1990). Symptomatology associated with childhood sexual victimization in a nonclinical adult sample. *Child Abuse and Neglect, 12,* 51–59.

Brock, K., Pearlman, L. A., & Deiter, P. J. (2001). *Reliability and validity of the Inner Experience Questionnaire.* Manuscript in preparation.

Connors, R. E. (2000). *Self-injury: Psychotherapy with people who engage in self-inflicted violence.* Northvale, NJ: Jason Aronson.

Courtois, C. A. (1979). The incest experience and its aftermath. *Victimology: An International Journal, 4,* 337–347.

Courtois, C. (1999). *Recollections of sexual abuse: Treatment principles and guidelines.* New York: W.W. Norton.

Curran, S., DeCou, K., Dusek-Gomez, N., Haven, T. J., & Rodriguez, M. F. (2000). *Fundamental fairness: Providing intermediate sanctions for women.* Ludlow, MA: National Institute of Corrections Project. Women in Intermediate Sanctions.

Dancu, C. V., Riggs, D. S., Hearst-Ikeda, D. E., Shoyer, B. G., & Foa, E. B. (1996). Dissociative experiences and posttraumatic stress disorder among female victims of criminal assault and rape. *Journal of Traumatic Stress, 9*(2), 253–267.

De Groot, J., & Rodin, G. M. (1999). The relationship between eating disorders and childhood trauma. *Psychiatric Annals, 29*(4), 225–229.

Deiter, P. J., Nicholls, S. S., & Pearlman, L. A. (2000). Self-injury and self capacities: Assisting an individual in crisis. *Journal of Clinical Psychology, 56*(9), 1173–1191.

Deiter, P. J., & Pearlman, L. A. (1998). Responding to self-injurious behavior. In P. M. Kleespies (Ed.), *Emergencies in mental health practice: Evaluation and management* (pp. 235–257). New York: Guilford Press.

DiPalma, L. M. (1994). Patterns of coping and characteristics of high-functioning incest survivors. *Archives of Psychiatric Nursing, 8*(2), 82–90.

Dutton, M. A., Burghardt, K. J., Perrin, S. G., Chrestman, K. R., & Halle, P. M. (1994). Battered women's cognitive schemata. *Journal of Traumatic Stress, 7*(2), 237–255.

Foa, E. B., Keane, T. M., & Friedman, M. J. (Eds.). (2000). *Effective treatments for PTSD: Practice guidelines from the International Society for Traumatic Stress Studies.* New York: Guilford Press.

Foa, E. B., & Meadows, E. A. (1997). Psychosocial treatments for posttraumatic stress disorder: A critical review. *Annual Review of Psychology, 48,* 449–480.

Ford, J. D. (1999). Disorders of extreme stress following war-zone military trauma: Associated features of posttraumatic stress or comorbid but distinct syndromes? *Journal of Consulting and Clinical Psychology, 67*(1), 3–12.

Fromm-Reichman, F. (1960). *Principles of intensive psychotherapy.* Chicago: University of Chicago Press.

Gelinas, D. J. (1983). The persisting negative effects of incest. *Psychiatry, 46,* 312–332.

Gonzalez, L. S. (1993). The relationship between child sexual abuse and adult functioning in men seeking psychotherapy. *Dissertation Abstracts International 54/10,* B:5387.

Green, A. (1978). Self-destructive behavior in battered children. *American Journal of Psychiatry, 135,* 579–582.

Grinker, R., & Spiegel, J. (1945). *Men under stress.* Philadelphia: Blakiston.

Herman, J. L. (1992a). Complex PTSD: A syndrome in survivors of prolonged and repeated trauma. *Journal of Traumatic Stress, 5*(3), 377–391.

Herman, J. L. (1992b). *Trauma and recovery: The aftermath of violence from domestic abuse to political terror.* New York: Basic Books.

Hilberman, E., & Munson, K. (1977/78). Sixty battered women. *Victimology: An International Journal, 2*(3/4), 460–470.

James, J., & Meyerding, J. (1977). Early sexual experience and prostitution. *American Journal of Psychiatry, 134,* 1381–1384.

Janoff-Bulman, R. (1992). *Shattered assumptions: Towards a new psychology of trauma.* New York: Free Press.

Jongedijk, R. A., Carlier, I. V. E., Schreuder, B. J. N., & Gersons, B. P. R. (1996). Complex posttraumatic stress disorder: An exploratory investigation of PTSD and DESNOS among Dutch war veterans. *Journal of Traumatic Stress, 9*(3), 577–586.

Kardiner, A., & Spiegel, H. (1947). *War stress and neurotic illness.* New York: Hoeber.

Kent, A., & Waller, G. (2000). Childhood emotional abuse and eating psychopathology. *Clinical Psychology Review, 20*(7), 887–903.

Klein, R. H., & Schermer, V. L. (Eds.). (2000). *Group psychotherapy for psychological trauma.* New York: Guilford Press.

Kohut, H. (1971). *The analysis of the self.* New York: International Universities Press.

Kohut, H. (1977). *The restoration of the self.* New York: International Universities Press.

Kuhn, T. S. (1970). *The structure of scientific revolutions* (2nd ed.). Chicago: University of Chicago Press.

Mahler, M. S., Pine, F., & Bergman, A. (1975). *The psychological birth of the human infant: Symbiosis and individuation.* New York: Basic Books.

Mahoney, M. J. (1981). Psychotherapy and human change process. In J. H. Harvey & M. M. Parks (Eds.), *Psychotherapy research and behavior change* (pp. 73–122). Washington, DC: American Psychological Association.

Mahoney, M. J., & Lyddon, W. J. (1988). Recent developments in cognitive approaches to counseling and psychotherapy. *Counseling Psychologist, 16*(2), 190–234.

Maltz, W. (1991). *The sexual healing journey: A guide for survivors of sexual abuse.* New York: HarperCollins.

Mas, K. (1992). *Disrupted schemata in psychiatric patients with a history of childhood sexual abuse on the McPearl Belief Scale.* Unpublished doctoral dissertation, California School of Professional Psychology, Fresno, CA.

McCann, I. L., & Pearlman, L. A. (1990). *Psychological trauma and the adult survivor: Theory, therapy, and transformation.* New York: Brunner/Mazel.

Miller, D. (1994). *Women who hurt themselves: A book of hope and understanding.* New York: Basic Books.

Miller, J., Moeller, D., Kaufman, A., Divasto, P., Pathak, D., & Christy, J. (1978). Recidivism among sex assault victims. *American Journal of Psychiatry, 135,* 1103–1104.

Nakashima, I., & Zakus, G. (1977). Incest: Review and clinical experience. *Pediatrics, 60,* 696–701.

Neumann, D. A., Houskamp, B. M., Pollack, V. E., & Briere, J. (1996). The long-term sequelae of childhood sexual abuse in women: A meta-analytic review. *Child Maltreatment, 1*(1), 6–16.

Neumann, D. A., & Pearlman, L. A. (1996). Review of the Life Orientation Inventory. In B. H. Stamm (Ed.), *Measurement of stress, trauma, and adaptation* (pp. 192–193). Lutherville, MD: Sidran Press.

Neumann, D. A., & Pearlman, L. A. (1994). *Toward developing a psychological language for spirituality.* Unpublished manuscript.

Newman, E., Riggs, D. S., & Roth, S. (1997). Thematic resolution, PTSD, and complex PTSD: The relationship between meaning and trauma-related diagnoses. *Journal of Traumatic Stress, 10*(2), 197–213.

Nicholls, S. S., Deiter, P. J., & Pearlman, L. A. (2001). *Self-harming behaviors and reasons for self-harm.* Unpublished manuscript.

Pearlman, L. A. (1996). Review of the TSI Belief Scale. In B. H. Stamm (Ed.), *Measurement of stress, trauma, and adaptation* (pp. 415–417). Lutherville, MD: Sidran Press.

Pearlman, L. A. (1998). Trauma and the self: A theoretical and clinical perspective. *Journal of Emotional Abuse, 1,* 7–25.

Pearlman, L. A. (in press). *TSI Belief Scale Manual.* Los Angeles, CA: Western Psychological Services.

Pearlman, L. A., & Deiter, P. J. (1996). *The impact of psychological trauma on self capacities: Theoretical and research perspectives.* Paper presented at the Symposium on Long-Term Correlates of Childhood Trauma: Theoretical Models and Reecent Empirical Findings, conducted at the annual meeting of the International Society for Traumatic Stress Studies, San Francisco, CA.

Pearlman, L. A., & MacIan, P. S. (1995). Vicarious traumatization: An empirical study of the effects of trauma work on trauma therapists. *Professional Psychology: Research and Practice, 26*(6), 558–565.

Pearlman, L. A., & McCann, I. L. (1994). Integrating structured and unstructured approaches to taking a trauma history. In M. B. Williams & J. Sommer, Jr. (Eds.), *Handbook of post-traumatic therapy* (pp. 38–48). Westport, CT: Greenwood Press.

Pearlman, L. A., & Saakvitne, K. W. (1995). *Trauma and the therapist: Countertransference and vicarious traumatization in psychotherapy with incest survivors.* New York: Norton.

Pelcovitz, D., van der Kolk, B. A., Roth, S. H., Mandel, F. S., Kaplan, S. J., & Resick,

P. A. (1997). Development of a criteria set and a Structured Interview for Disorders of Extreme Stress (SIDES). *Journal of Traumatic Stress, 10*(1), 3–16.

Piaget, J. (1971). *Psychology and epistemology: Towards a theory of knowledge.* New York: Viking.

Polusny, M. A., & Follette, V. M. (1995). Long-term correlates of child sexual abuse: Theory and review of the empirical literature. *Applied and Preventive Psychology, 4*(3), 143–166.

Richters, J. E. (1997). The Hubbell hypothesis and the developmentalist's dilemma. *Development and Psychopathology, 9,* 193–229.

Rosenbloom, D. J., Williams, M. B., & Watkins, B. (1999). *Life after trauma: A workbook for healing.* New York: Guilford Press.

Roth, S., & Cohen, L. J. (1986). Approach, avoidance, and coping with stress. *American Psychologist, 41,* 813–819.

Roth, S., Newman, E., Pelcovitz, D., van der Kolk, B. A., & Mandel, F. S. (1997). Complex PTSD in victims exposed to sexual and physical abuse: Results from the DSM-IV field trial for posttraumatic stress disorder. *Journal of Traumatic Stress, 10*(4), 539–555.

Rothschild, B. (2000). *The body remembers: The psychophysiology of trauma and trauma treatment.* New York: W.W. Norton.

Rotter, J. B. (1954). *Social learning and clinical psychology.* Englewood Cliffs, NJ: Prentice-Hall.

Saakvitne, K. W. (1993). Eroticized maternal transference in psychoanalytic treatment of female incest survivors. In M. C. Buttonheim (Chair), *Sexuality and intimacy in the adult relationships of childhood incest survivors.* Symposium conducted at the 101st annual meeting of the American Psychological Association, Toronto, Ontario, Canada.

Saakvitne, K. W., Gamble, S. J., Pearlman, L. A., & Tabor Lev, B. (2000). *Risking connection: A training curriculum for working with survivors of childhood abuse.* Lutherville, MD: Sidran Press.

Schauben, L. J., & Frazier, P. A. (1995). Vicarious trauma: The effects on female counselors of working with sexual abuse survivors. *Psychology of Women Quarterly, 19,* 49–64.

Sedney, M. A., & Brooks, B. (1984). Factors associated with a history of childhood sexual experience in a nonclinical female population. *Journal of the American Academy of Child Psychiatry, 23,* 215–218.

Solomon, S. D. (1997). Psychosocial treatment of posttraumatic stress disorder. *In session: Psychotherapy in practice, 3*(4), 27–41.

Steele, K., van der Hart, O., & Nijenhuis, E. R. S. (in press). Phase-oriented treatment of complex dissociative disorders: Overcoming trauma-related phobias. In A. Eckhart-Henn & S. O. Hoffman (Eds.), *Dissoziative Storungen des Bewusstseins* [Dissociative disorders of consciousness]. Stuttgart, Germany: Schattauer-Verlag.

Stolorow, R. B., Brandchaft, B., & Atwood, G. (1987). *Psychoanalytic treatment: An intersubjective approach.* Hillsdale, NJ: Analytic Press.

Sullivan, H. S. (1953). *The interpersonal theory of psychiatry.* New York: Norton.

Turner, K., DeRosa, R. R., Roth, S. H., Batson, R., & Davidson, J. R. T. (1996). A multi-modal treatment for incest survivors: Preliminary outcome data. *Clinical Psychology and Psychotherapy, 3*(3), 208–219.

van der Kolk, B. A. (1994). The body keeps the score: Memory and the evolving psychobiology of posttraumatic stress. *Harvard Review of Psychiatry, 1,* 253–265.

van der Kolk, B. A., & Pelcovitz, D. (1999). Clinical applications of the Structured Interview for Disorders of Extreme Stress (SIDES). *National Center for PTSD Clinical Quarterly, 8*(2), 21, 23–26.

van der Kolk, B. A., Pelcovitz, D., Roth, S., Mandel, F. S., McFarlane, A., & Herman, J. L. (1996). Dissociation, somatization, and affect dysregulation: The complexity of adaptation to trauma. *American Journal of Psychiatry, 153*(7), 83–93.

van der Kolk, B. A., & van der Hart, O. (1989). Pierre Janet and the breakdown of adaptation in psychological trauma. *American Journal of Psychiatry, 146,* 1530–1540.

van der Kolk, B. A., & van der Hart, O. (1991). The intrusive past: The flexibility of memory and the engraving of trauma. *American Imago, 48,* 425–454.

Walker, L. E. (1985). The battered woman syndrome study. In D. Finkelhor, R. J. Gelles, G. T. Hotaling, & M. A. Strauss (Eds.), *The dark side of families* (pp. 31–48). Beverly Hills, CA: Sage.

White, M. T., & Weiner, M. B. (1986). *The theory and practice of self-psychology.* New York: Brunner/Mazel.

Yalom, I. D. (1975). *The theory and practice of group psychotherapy* (3rd ed.). New York: Basic Books.

Zlotnick, C., Zakriski, A. L., Shea, M. T., Costello, E., Begin, A., Pearlstein, T., & Simpson, E. (1996). The long-term sequelae of sexual abuse: Support for a complex posttraumatic stress disorder. *Journal of Traumatic Stress, 9*(2), 195–205.

10

Dual Diagnosis and Treatment of PTSD

ALEXANDER C. McFARLANE

Why do some traumatized individuals get better with treatment but others remain with a chronic and relapsing disorder? This chapter will focus on the question as to whether dual diagnosis alters the treatment necessary in post-traumatic stress disorder (PTSD) and to what extent the outcome of the primary disorder is influenced by the presence of these comorbid conditions. A related question is whether each diagnosis requires a specific treatment or whether a trauma-focused treatment will resolve the PTSD and associated disorders. Hence one of the challenges for treatment is to ascertain what are the effective components and what is a result of specific interventions in contrast to nonspecific factors such as the evocation of hope and the provision of support. This begs the question as to whether a healer requires an underlying streak of faith which is imparted to the patient, an idea which is anathema to most scientific inquiry. Definite opinions and controversy tend to surround the treatment of any psychiatric disorder.

The existence of a sole psychiatric disorder in a clinical setting is the exception rather than the rule. Large epidemiological studies indicate that a range of other disorders, particularly affective disorders, panic disorder, and alcohol and substance abuse frequently emerge in conjunction with PTSD and that this is not isolated to treatment-seeking populations. The extent of comorbidity is a challenge to most researchers, who tend to avoid the contradiction this presents to the claimed specificity of treatment approaches. The effectiveness of any treatment program in PTSD is often discussed with little reference to the specifics or effectiveness of any treatment provided for these comorbid disorders. Thus, high levels of comorbidity pose a challenge to specificity of the treatments proposed for PTSD and should always be addressed in a treatment plan. The patients with a number of comorbid disorders are likely to have a worse long-term outcome than those with PTSD alone and may require chronic maintenance therapy.

These studies have also broadened attention as to the range of psychiatric disorders which can arise as a consequence of traumatic exposure. The question arises as to whether these disorders respond to a treatment which is primarily designed for PTSD or whether a specific intervention should be aimed at their core. The converse argument is that some of the treatments adopted for the PTSD are effective because they treat the comorbid disorder, which has an indirect effect on the PTSD symptoms. This has been addressed in some psychopharmacological trials where it is important to ensure that antidepressants do not simply exert their effect because they improve mood.

The adherents of particular schools of therapy are keen to cite the evidence which supports their approach but are defensively dismissive of any negative findings. These inclinations make the exploration of issues of treatment a topic which is destined to please only the most eclectic of clinicians. This is particularly the case when the issue of dual diagnosis is discussed. The origins of the current treatments used for treating PTSD are important in any consideration of the specificity of treatment effect.

THE NATURE OF COMORBIDITY

The fundamental question to be considered here in regard to the issue of treatment is the nature of the comorbidity between PTSD and a range of other disorders. Answering this question is difficult because studies have been conducted in a number of different settings. First, there are large-scale epidemiological studies which have examined this question in combat-related PTSD and non-combat-related PTSD treatment-seeking populations. Using a retrospective lifetime diagnostic method, these studies have attempted to examine the onset and course of these disorders. In reviewing the literature, Deering, Glover, Ready, Eddleman, and Alarcon (1996) have suggested that the question of whether different types of traumatic events cause different patterns of comorbidity should be examined. They concluded that while there were significant similarities between different traumas, different profiles did exist according to the different types of trauma. They also suggested that the evidence showed that these disorders were interwoven with PTSD rather than being truly comorbid conditions.

The Vietnam Experience Study suggested that 66% of those veterans with current PTSD had either an anxiety disorder or a depressive disorder and a further 39% had substance abuse (Keane & Kaloupek, 1997). Kulka et al. (1990) used a more sensitive methodology in an examination of 3,016 veterans for the National Vietnam Veterans' Readjustment Study (NVVRS). They found 73% comorbidity with substance abuse, 31% with antisocial personality disorder, and 28% with major depression.

The National Comorbidity Survey of Kessler et al. (1995) showed that among males with PTSD 88% had a comorbid disorder. Major depression accounted for 48% of this and 52% also were suffering from alcoholism. Of the subjects with PTSD, 59% had more than three diagnoses. Significant differences were identified in women with PTSD, some 79% having an accompanying disorder; 30% had alcoholism. These data also suggested that, at least among women, substance abuse tended to be the consequence of the disorder rather than preceding it. These results were somewhat different from those of the epidemiological catchment area study cohort in St. Louis, where Cottler, Compton, Mager, Spitznagel, and Janca (1992) suggested that in a significant percentage of people, drug and alcohol abuse preceded the development of PTSD and therefore could contribute to traumatic events.

In a study of bushfire victims, McFarlane and Papay (1992) demonstrated in disaster victims similarly high rates of comorbid disorder in a community sample. These findings are important because they demonstrate that comorbidity is not simply an issue relevant to treatment seeking. While comorbidity is an important predictor of treatment, it does not indicate that those with more severe disorders are emerging in clinical settings.

Skodol et al. (1996) demonstrated the relevance of this finding beyond U.S. veterans. Similar rates and types of PTSD comorbidity were found in a variety of groups, particularly if these disorders had already preceded PTSD. This suggested that they were significant risk factors. Long, MacDonald, and Chamberlain (1996) also found that Vietnam veterans in a New Zealand setting had high rates of comorbidity, on the order of 73%.

Several epidemiological studies have examined samples of trauma victims prospectively. For example, Shalev et al. (1998) found that both major depression and PTSD should be seen as independent sequelae of traumatic events, which have similar prognoses and interact if they exist simultaneously to increase distress and disability. The authors found that the rates of comorbidity were similar between depression and PTSD at 1 month after the traumatic event in 44.5 and 43.2 subjects, respectively. In a similar study of motor accident victims, Blanchard, Buckley, Hickling, and Taylor (1998) suggested that PTSD and depression are independent but correlated responses to trauma. The group of patients who have a combination of these disorders finish up being more distressed and more disabled and also tend to have a more chronic disorder.

Clinical Studies

The prevalence of comorbidity has been examined in a range of clinical studies of both Vietnam veterans and non-veteran populations (e.g., Keane &

Kaloupek, 1997). It is difficult to draw any general conclusions on the basis of these studies other than to note that comorbidity is highly prevalent. For example, Bleich, Koslowsky, Dolev, and Lerer (1997) found that 95% of PTSD subjects in a sample of Israeli war veterans seeking treatment had a comorbid major depressive disorder. The different courses of these disorders suggested that depression is not simply the sharing of common symptoms, but should be viewed as a separate diagnosis. Bremner, Southwick, Darnell, and Charney (1996) suggested that PTSD begins soon after exposure, with hyperarousal symptoms emerging first, and that the natural course of alcohol and substance abuse parallels that of PTSD. The clinical relevance of comorbidity was examined by Dansky, Roitzsch, Brady, and Saladin (1997), who found that even in a research setting where high rates of comorbidity had been identified, clinicians continued to underdiagnose PTSD when the clinical focus of a unit was substance abuse. It seems that there is a general conclusion that the importance of comorbidity is frequently missed in clinical settings. This is a finding which has important implications for research studies. Other studies examined specific disorders such as social phobia. For example, Orsillo, Heimberg, Juster, and Garrett (1996) found that social anxiety and social phobia are important problems that are again frequently unrecognized in Vietnam veterans with PTSD in clinical settings.

Keane and Kaloupek (1997) concluded that the overwhelming majority of patients presenting for treatment with PTSD have a wide range of symptoms which go beyond the specific diagnostic criteria of the disorder. This conclusion would emphasize the importance of addressing these issues in any discussion of PTSD treatment.

Substance-Abusing Populations

An alternative interest has emerged in the last decade, namely, the prevalence of trauma among substance abusers. These studies have essentially looked at treatment-seeking substance abuse groups and identified the rates of comorbidity. Among different samples, there has been significant variability. For example, in a sample of inner-city methadone maintenance patients, Villagomez, Meyer, Lin, and Brown (1995) found 20% rates of PTSD in women and 11% in men. Dansky, Saladin, Brady, Kilpatrick, and Resnick (1995) suggested that rates of traumatization in an epidemiological sample of women who had received treatment for substance abuse disorders were extremely high, on the order of 80%, and approximately one quarter had current PTSD. Brown, Recupero, and Stout (1995) approached the question from a different perspective. They looked at an inpatient substance abuse treatment program and found that approximately one-quarter of the sample had significant PTSD symptomatology. Women had higher rates of traumatic events and were more likely to be diagnosed. Brown et al. found that among substance abusers the PTSD group tended to have higher rates of admission for treatment.

Clark et al. (1997) examined this issue in an adolescent sample. They found that depression and PTSD symptoms were more strongly associated with alcohol dependence in females than in males. They also found that conduct disorder frequently coexisted with the depressive disorders in this population.

Wasserman, Havassy, and Boles (1997) suggested that in cocaine abusers, women experienced more PTSD than men, even when exposed to the same event. They suggested that, generally speaking, the PTSD preceded the cocaine abuse and proposed a self-medication hypothesis. In the cocaine treatment population, those with PTSD tended to have more additional diagnoses than patients with other psychiatric disorders. In addressing these subjects comparatively, Deykin and Buka (1997) suggested that adolescents in the treatment setting tended to have five times the reported rates of PTSD in adolescents from a community sample, highlighting the importance of considering this issue in substance abuse populations.

In considering this evidence from a theoretical perspective from both epidemiological and clinical samples, McFarlane (1998a) highlighted that trauma alone is an important issue in increasing the risk of alcohol abuse. When combined with psychiatric disorder, this significantly increased the rates. Hence, there does appear to be important evidence from longitudinal studies investigating the role of substance abuse as a self-medication issue in PTSD. This possibly is a major challenge to the conventional wisdom that it is best to attempt to control the substance abuse before treating the PTSD symptoms.

A variety of hypotheses have been entertained to explain the degrees of comorbidity. In particular, the high degree of overlap of symptoms has suggested that this might be artifactual. If this were the case, the treatment of PTSD should address the coexisting issues of the treatment of anxiety and depression. This epiphenomenon issue has also been suggested as a possibility because of the reporting behavior of some subjects when interviewed, who tend to give high rates of positive responses. If this is an issue of overreporting, again it suggests that treatment of the primary PTSD should address the comorbidity issues.

Another issue is that comorbidity, such as depression and substance abuse (Kessler et al., 1995), may be a predisposing factor for PTSD. This is clearly the case in some individuals, but in many individuals these two disorders emerge simultaneously. A significant group of individuals do carry a variety of risk factors for general psychiatric morbidity, and their major disorder emerged following traumatic stress as well as PTSD. The challenge for researchers is to determine whether the onset of disorders other than PTSD in the setting of the trauma do predict a different course and treatment response. Given the underdeveloped state of the treatment literature, this question has not been answered.

Furthermore, another interesting perspective has emerged that PTSD can emerge in chronically mentally ill populations (McFarlane, Shaw, & Bookless, 1997; Mueser et al., 1998). Psychiatric patients generally demonstrate very high rates of traumatization. Mueser et al. (1998) found that 43% of their sample had PTSD, but only 3 of 119 had this recognized in their charts. Childhood sexual trauma was particularly common. Hence, another possibility exists that PTSD may be an antecedent of a variety of severe mental disorders. Thus, the treatment of PTSD may be an important factor in limiting later emergence of a general range of psychopathologies. To further complicate the issue, Lundy (1992) and McFarlane et al. (1997) have examined the question of psychosis-induced PTSD. In other words, can the experience of a psychotic illness be sufficient to trigger the emergence of full blown PTSD as a consequence of the experience of the illness? This raises some additional challenging questions about how the fear response to the illness of schizophrenia should be addressed and what impact this would have on the course and phenomenology of the schizophrenic illness. Thus, particularly in the chronically mentally ill, trauma may predispose a person to severe mental illness or may be a consequence of it. Given the low rates of recognition of these phenomena in critical settings, it is impossible to make any informed statements about how this should be addressed in treatment.

Treatment Literature and Dual Diagnosis

In general, the treatment literature in psychiatry has not adequately addressed the whole problem of comorbidity. The issue either is not discussed in the subject selection or is minimized by the authors. Clinical reality would tend to suggest that there is an oversimplification of the true nature of this problem in clinical settings. Furthermore, studies which have been done examining pure clinical populations have very little relevance to the general clinical setting, as the patient with PTSD alone is relatively less likely to seek treatment and is not in the general mainstream of patients.

The treatment literature is characterized by studies with samples of subjects who, first, are willing to volunteer for treatment studies and, secondly, are able to contain their distress within the protocol of the investigation. In countries such as Australia and the United Kingdom, which have free health care systems, there is little incentive for subjects to become involved in treatment research, in contrast to a system where the user pays, such as the United States. In the United States, this also can cause significant biases because it means the treatment outcome studies are not conducted on the more informed and socially advantaged segment of the population, which may again raise some important questions as to the generalizability of the data. Given that avoidance is a central element of this disorder, those who are more phobic (e.g., people with social phobia) are likely to have significant difficulties coping with the social interactions necessary to contain their distress in clinical settings. Clinical studies can only be completed on those who can cope with the direct confrontation of their avoidance through structured clinical interviews. Trauma-focused treatment such as cognitive-behavioral therapy and EMDR (eye movement desensitization and reprocessing) therapy are only acceptable treatments for those patients who do not have high levels of avoidance. Those with depression and related difficulties, overrepresented in the most chronically and severely ill and particularly those with associated substance abuse, are patients who have been least addressed in the available treatment literature. Therefore the demands of clinical trials have the potential to diminish the value of the information obtained and also give false impressions about the ease of treatment.

Childhood and interpersonal trauma are likely to be disruptive of an individual's attachment behavior. The individual comes to live in a state of survival vigilance where even relatively gentle interpersonal approaches can be construed as interpersonal threats. The treatment relationship becomes severely impeded by its capacity to provoke a variety of trauma-related behaviors. The individual can become locked into a linear and defensive pattern of communication. In the content of depressive symptomatology, the individual's nihilism can further permeate the therapeutic relationship and inhibit his or her capacity to sustain any interpersonal involvement

ISSUES OF COMORBIDITY IN TREATMENT

Concurrently Emerging Disorders

In some individuals who have been exposed to extreme traumatic events, the comorbid disorder, rather than the PTSD, can be the dominating clinical feature. The individual can present with severe depressive symptomatology, and the traumatic ruminations are an important but relatively secondary component. This is in contrast to the individual whose intrusive and distressing recollections and associated hyperarousal are the immediate difficulties for which the person seeks treatment. A critical clinical question is whether treating the associated disorder, rather than the PTSD, has a differential effect on general psychiatric measures to treating the PTSD and not the associated disorder. The general wisdom is that the primary disorder should be identified and treated vigorously while the symptoms are monitored and appropriate strategies are devised for management of the associated disorder, whether they be psychotherapeutic or pharmacological. Again, while not referred to in the majority of the literature, a significant percentage of people who have been involved in psychotherapeutic studies would have also tried medication. Hence, we know very little about the longitudinal interaction of these treatments. Is it best to place somebody on medication before psychotherapy or visa versa?

Clinical wisdom would generally indicate that highly distressed individuals can be placed on the appropriate medication, such as a selective serotonin reuptake inhibitor (SSRI), to assist in controlling their distress. In particular, their nihilism and sense of hopelessness may make it difficult for such patients to involve themselves in a psychotherapeutic intervention. Extreme hyperarousal can trigger dissociative reactions. For this reason, the management of such individuals' distress before they begin trauma-focused treatments, especially in the form of an associated anxiety disorder or depression, may significantly improve the outcome from the psychological treatment.

The value of addressing diagnoses simultaneously has been suggested by Brady, Sonne, and Roberts (1995). In an open-labeled trial of sertraline for comorbid PTSD and alcohol dependence, they were able to show that despite the limitations of the study the medication assisted the PTSD symptoms and decreased alcohol consumption. Similarly, Hien and Levin (1994) found that female patients on methadone who were not given treatment for their PTSD tended to be hindered in their treatment response and had complications such as dropping out, depression, and new polysubstance abuse. Kofoed, Friedman, and Peck (1993) concluded that PTSD and substance abuse must be treated simultaneously as coprimary illnesses, and that the effectiveness of drug and alcohol treatment is decreased by the existence of extreme psychological symptoms. Appropriate management of these symptoms tends to improve the outcome.

In a population of adolescents, Goenjian et al. (1997) examined the effect of a brief trauma/grief-focused psychotherapy program following the 1988 earthquake in Armenia. In a follow-up 1½ and 3 years after the earthquake, they found that psychotherapy had significantly decreased the posttraumatic stress symptoms. While there had been no change in the severity of the depressive symptoms in subjects given psychotherapy, the depressive symptoms among those not treated had significantly worsened with time. This is an interesting population-based study emphasizing that a trauma-focused treatment may not have a generalized effect, stressing the necessity of providing a primary-based treatment for both disorders.

The essence of addressing the traumatic memory comes from Breuer and Freud's (1962) first lecture, "Psychical Mechanisms of Hysterical Phenomena: A lecture." They argued that the trauma does not simply act as a releasing mechanism for symptoms. Rather, they proposed that psychic trauma, or more precisely "the memory of the trauma," acts like "a foreign body which long after entry must continue to be regarded as the agent that is still at work" (p. 56). They discussed the process of treatment where the "individual hysterical symptom immediately and permanently disappears when we succeeded in bringing clearly to light the memory of the event by which it was provoked and in arousing the accompanying affect and when the patient has described the event in greatest possible detail and put the affect into words" (p. 57). This could really be an account of the aim of cognitive-behavioral approaches. The important issue is that posttraumatic depression, social phobia, or substance abuse may not be effectively managed until these trauma-based memories have at least been dealt with in some way in the course of treatment.

For example, a Clyde, young man in his early 20s who had been exposed to a major natural disaster during his developmental years, presented for treatment some 14 years after the event. Prior to the traumatic experience, it seemed that he was a talented and engaging child. In the ensuing years, his difficulties increasingly emerged as intense separation anxiety. When he was required to attend boarding school, he was intensely homesick for a pro-longed period of time. He became highly successful in his chosen field of study and won a scholarship to a major university in the capital. Although he had coped with study away from home, moving to a distant city in which he had no social contacts led to a severe episode of depression which required him to return home. Prior to his referral, the depression had been treated with electroconvulsive therapy (ECT).

His clinical history indicated that this young man's mind was intensely preoccupied by memories of the disaster. When away from his family in the city, Clyde was constantly frightened that bushfires would engulf the city Similarly, when at home he would be transfixed by memories of what had transpired during the disaster, when several friends at the neighboring school and an entire neighbor's family had been incinerated; his family's farm had also been devastated, with many livestock killed and others having to be sub-sequently destroyed.

This case demonstrates the importance of treating the depression and the posttraumatic symptoms simultaneously. A year's psychiatric treatment of the depression had led to little resolution of the individual's distress. A com-bination of treatment with a monoamine oxidase inhibitor (MAOI) together with specific cognitive-behavioral therapy focusing on the memory of the fires, as well as a psychodynamic approach by a different therapist exploring separation issues and the way that relationships tended to cause a constant recapitulation of the trauma, was applied. This led to a significant and emerging pattern of improvement, which generalized between outcome measures of PTSD and depressive disorder.

Primary Disorder Not the PTSD

For some individuals, the primary symptoms of depression or anxiety can be so overwhelming that they prevent any psychotherapeutic approach to the traumatic memories because of the intensity of the consequent distress and dissociation. In such an individual, it is necessary first of all to gain control of the primary symptoms before the patient can accept a direct approach to the underlying PTSD. In general, such patients are relatively readily accepting of psychotropic medications because of the degree of loss of control which they feel.

Comorbid Disorder Following the Onset of PTSD

In a significant percentage of cases, the comorbid disorder does not simply follow the course of the PTSD. For example, the impact of the PTSD on the individual's life, including the disruption of relationships at work, can lead to the onset of a variety of symptoms, particularly of major depression and substance abuse. In clinical settings, chronic pain syndromes in those who have been physically injured can often become a major focus of the person's treatment. This requires a formulation of the nature of pain as a type of memory. The aversive nature of pain is in part to do with its associations. If an injury occurs at the time of the traumatic event, pain can act as a major and repetitive trigger for the traumatic memory. The use of sophisticated physical rehabilitation, where the nature of the link between the person's fear and the pain is highlighted, can significantly assist the psychotherapeutic process. On occasions, depressive symptoms can emerge as the traumatic memory is addressed. With such individuals, the introduction of antidepressant medication can sometimes assist the maintenance and continuation of the trauma-exposure program.

Because of disorders which can emerge following the traumatic event, it is important to closely examine the impact of PTSD on the individual's self-esteem and well-being. Some patients claim that the sense of lack of control and the recurrence of the traumatic memories is worse than the primary experience. It significantly undermines their resources and capacity to address and deal with daily life.

There may be situations where an individual presents with a severe psychiatric illness and in the course of treatment a prior PTSD is identified. There are neurobiological reasons (McFarlane, 1997) why PTSD may lead to significant dysregulation that can predispose to other psychiatric disorders. For example, following traumatic events, there is a significant turnover in frontal lobe dopamine. In a vulnerable individual, this may lead to the emergence of schizophrenia (McFarlane, 1998b). In the absence of outcome research, it is difficult to provide objective data to suggest that treating the PTSD in this instance can contribute to improving the prognosis of the schizophrenia. However, many of the symptoms of schizophrenia have a significant overlap with PTSD, including the flattened affect and withdrawal (Stampfer, 1990). This would argue for the importance of looking at the role that underlying PTSD can play in the maintenance of the psychiatric disorder which later emerges. PTSD in this situation can be particularly difficult to identify, as the frequency and dominance of the intrusive memories may have diminished as the trauma has receded into the past.

PTSD Following a Major Psychiatric Disorder

Mueser et al. (1998), McFarlane et al. (1997), and Lundy (1992) have focused on how PTSD is common among those with mental illness, which can be a consequence of the experience of the extreme distress of the disorder. To date there is no treatment literature addressing these symptoms, and few clinical anecdotes. However, it would make sense that assisting an individual to cope with the distress and the meaning of an experience is critical, particularly in an illness associated with psychotic symptoms where there is primary disruption of the internal facility for language. The inability to use language to control and maintain one's sense of reality is central to one's self esteem and humanity. PTSD possibly can be seen as a disorder where external reality disrupts the individual's capacity for language. Thus, a situation where the terror of the illness disrupts this capacity for self-organization, as well as this capability being disrupted through the underlying neurobiological change of the illness, presents a major challenge to treatment. It begs the question as to the extent to which schizophrenia is a stress-related disorder. Hence one could argue that assisting individuals with stress inoculation techniques, as was found by Foa (1997) to be effective in controlling posttraumatic symptoms, may be more helpful than focusing on the primary experience of the psychosis, which clearly has the capacity to lead to further delusional elaboration.

BROADER ISSUES

If dual diagnoses require specific or additional interventions, an important issue is to define what are the general or nonspecific elements of treatment which are of benefit, independent of the exact clinical picture. Attention to a range of other issues apart from the specific therapeutic interventions can be extremely important in determining an effective outcome. These factors should be explicitly addressed in both clinical and research settings. They are seldom addressed in the treatment literature.

Issues of Safety

More specific psychological interventions cannot begin until a range of other issues have been addressed. The greatest need of any traumatized individual is to feel safe, and this often requires attention to various practical dimensions. For example, the victims of a natural disaster may have to secure their physical safety and protect their possessions. The victims of torture may have a variety of resettlement issues that are paramount in their mind. Perhaps one of the greatest challenges is to deal with the family in which sexual abuse or domestic violence is ongoing. Here there may be a relatively limited range of options open to the clinician. The immediate physical protection of the client and associated legal issues may take precedence. The initial aim of treatment must be to restore a modicum of safety and control (van der Kolk, 1987). Similarly with rape victims, assisting them with any criminal prosecution and addressing the immediate concerns about their safety will be essential before considering any form of psychological intervention. The loss of self-regulation and risk-taking behavior can further compound the individual's suffering by further exposure to trauma and loss.

There is no research which has addressed the questions as to whether the available treatments are effective either for PTSD or comorbid disorders in individuals who are still exposed to risk. This is particularly important in cases where the treatment usually aims to desensitize the person to the threat. Equally, addressing the cognitive schemas which organize the person's protection should be addressed with caution, as the predictions about the dangerousness of the world may be well founded and critical to survival.

Education

Giving traumatized individuals a psychological map to enable them to explore and understand their reactions does much to contain their distress and allow them to institute a series of self-regulatory processes. The past persistently and subtly intrudes into the attempt that the traumatized person makes to organize current experience. The nature of traumatic memory and its molding of present perception and affect is strangely not apparent to many patients, nor to therapists unfamiliar with the importance of trauma as a determinant of psychopathology. Patients are often confused by their symptoms and are uncertain as to the best ways to adapt to their current distress. Education can provide a simple but effective language which allows people to begin to feel that they are not the helpless victims of a mute past which haunts them and which they struggle to express.

Provision of information is essential in prevention of PTSD but equally important in treatment. This allows individuals to develop a cognitive structure in order to begin to pursue the issues of meaning as well as have a greater sense of control over their intrusive and avoidant symptoms. The initial assessment of a patient is part of this process. Often it will be the first occasion where there has been a conscious linking of the trauma-related cognitions and affects. A detailed behavioral analysis may explain the range of triggers to memories of the trauma as well as the individual's autonomic, cognitive, and behavioral responses

Education needs to focus on explaining how the physiological accompaniments of arousal can lead to a somatic focus of the trauma, particularly in conjunction with the residual effects of an injury sustained at the time of the trauma. These residual symptoms can act as a subtle symbolic trigger of traumatic images. Often patients come to treatment with specific ideas about causation, particularly if physical symptoms are a prominent feature. This preoccupation tends to be more common among people from Asian cultures. The physical symptoms experienced by sufferers of PTSD can complicate the development of the therapeutic alliance with a psychological focus unless these symptoms are assessed carefully and adequately explained (Shalev, Bleich, & Ursano, 1990). These patients often have a complex set of attributions and beliefs to explain their physical distress, which need to be understood (as in the case of the Agent Orange controversy; Hall, 1986). Education is equally relevant to the range of affective and anxiety symptoms which emerge in these settings.

Nonspecific Factors

Much of what is written in the area of PTSD emphasizes the specific ingredients of each treatment approach. To date, there has been no study which independently assesses the therapeutic process to ensure that the specific ingredients of treatment are as specific as claimed. Although the Temple University psychotherapy study is many years old, its conclusions remain relevant today; the data suggested that it was unclear whether behavioral therapists and psychotherapists did actually use fundamentally different approaches (Sloane, 1975). Jackson (1992) has emphasized that the act of listening both in depth and with empathy may be the critical element in healing, and this is likely to be the case particularly with traumatized people. Giving hope and rebuilding trust should not be undervalued. An investigation of the importance of these nonspecific factors in PTSD is important for the further progress of treatment in this area. Even with manualized treatments, it is difficult to control for such nonspecific elements.

The indirect impact of any intervention on other family members is also an issue which requires ongoing assessment. Trauma does not occur in a vacuum, and often a number of family members may be similarly traumatized, for example, by the events of a natural disaster, sexual abuse, or torture. The success of any treatment intervention may be influenced by whether there are other traumatized family members. In addition, the effects of providing treatment in the context of a litigation have not been investigated and may require the patient to develop ways of retelling the trauma with an active distancing of the affect so as to cope with the legal process.

The Management of Disabilities and Handicaps

Increasingly, it is becoming apparent in a range of disorders that while treatment may be effective in lessening the symptoms, it may have relatively little effect or a delayed impact on the associated disabilities and handicaps, such as involvement in intimate relationships and the fulfillment of work and parental roles. Often, these issues are inadequately assessed in PTSD treatment literature, although the National Vietnam Veterans' Readjustment Study (Kulka et al., 1990) provides an unusually rich account of the effects of war trauma on people's functioning. There is a need to develop psychotherapeutic interventions in PTSD and associated disorders that have specific strategies not only to overcome symptoms but also to improve the functional capacity of patients. This should be one of the outcome criteria when we are assessing the relative value of any form of psychotherapy in PTSD and a matter constantly kept in mind with individual patients.

Dissociation

One of the most disabling sets of symptoms associated with PTSD and co-morbid diagnoses are the dissociative symptoms. These also pose a particular therapeutic dilemma, as often they are triggered by attempts to focus on the meaning or affect associated with the trauma. This state can emerge in the course of treatment with little warning and is easy to miss. Patients who are prone to dissociation need to be taught how to anticipate the emergence of this state and to have strategies to orientate themselves to their immediate environment. To date, there is little systematic outcome literature demonstrating the most effective way of dealing with these symptoms. Increasingly, it is becoming apparent that major characterological adaptions become part of the trauma response, particularly when this occurred in early childhood. The most appropriate psychotherapeutic management of these issues needs further investigation (Herman, 1992).

CENTRAL ASPECTS OF TREATMENT IRRESPECTIVE OF DIAGNOSIS

The aim of therapy with traumatized patients is to help them move from being haunted by the past and interpreting subsequent emotionally arousing stimuli as a return of the trauma, to being present in the here and now, capable of responding to current exigencies to their fullest potential. In order to do that, people need to regain control over their emotional responses and place the trauma in the larger perspective of their lives, as a historical event, or series of events, that occurred at a particular time and in a particular place, and that can be expected to not recur if the traumatized individual takes charge of his or her life. The key element of the psychotherapy of people with PTSD is the integration of the alien, the unacceptable, the terrifying, the incomprehensible. Life events initially experienced as alien, imposed from outside upon passive victims, must come to be personalized and integrated as aspects of one's history and life experiences (van der Kolk & Ducey, 1989). The massive defenses, initially established as emergency protective measures, must gradually relax their grip upon the psyche, so that dissociated aspects of experience do not continue to intrude into one's life experience and thereby threaten to retraumatize an already traumatized victim.

Psychotherapy must address two fundamental aspects of PTSD: (1) deconditioning of anxiety, and (2) altering the way victims views themselves and their world by reestablishing a feeling of personal integrity and control. In only the simplest cases will it be sufficient to decondition the anxiety associated with the trauma. In the vast majority of patients, both aspects need to be treated. This means the use of a combination of procedures for deconditioning anxiety, for reestablishing a personal sense of control (which can range from engaging in physical challenges to reestablishing a sense of spiritual meaning), and forming meaningful and mutually satisfying relationships with others (often by means of group psychotherapy).

The therapeutic relationship with these patients tends to be extraordinarily complex, particularly since the interpersonal aspects of the trauma, such as mistrust, betrayal, dependency, love, and hate, tend to be replayed within the therapeutic setting. Dealing with trauma confronts all participants with intense emotional experiences ranging from a sense of helplessness to an intense longing for revenge, from vicarious traumatization to vicarious thrills (van der Kolk, 1994). The devastating effects of trauma on affect modulation, attention, perception, and the giving and taking of pleasure bring us face to face with the full range of human emotions, from the desire to love and feel safe to the wish to dominate, use, and hurt others (Wilson & Lindy, 1994).

CONCLUSION

To date, there is little information about the treatment of dual diagnoses in PTSD. It is an issue of central relevance to service provision, particularly in a day of evidence-based research. Much of the current research practice argues against acknowledging the existence of comorbidity. In general, dual diagnoses argue for the importance of eclectic treatment of the traumatized patient. The clinician needs to acknowledge the value of a range of different treatment approaches which may be used in different sequences according to the individual clinical picture. The relative dominance of the hyperarousal, mood disorder, avoidance, and intrusive symptoms will be important in determining the sequence and nature of the treatments chosen.

It is important not to have unreasonable expectations of patients that they will easily cope with their distress, especially those who have been abusing substances. Increasingly, as we have seen above, the literature is pointing to the value of conjoint treatment approaches.

REFERENCES

Blanchard, E. B., Buckley, T. C., Hickling, E. J., & Taylor, A. E. (1998). Posttraumatic stress disorder and comorbid major depression: Is the correlation an illusion? *Journal of Anxiety Disorders, 12*(1), 21–37.

Bleich, A., Koslowsky, M., Dolev, A., & Lerer, B. (1997). Post-traumatic stress disorder and depression: An analysis of comorbidity. *British Journal of Psychiatry, 170,* 479–482.

Brady, K. T., Sonne, S. C., & Roberts, J. M. (1995). Sertraline treatment of comorbid posttraumatic stress disorder and alcohol dependence. *Journal of Clinical Psychiatry, 56*(11), 502–505.

Bremner, J. D., Southwick, S. M., Darnell, A., & Charney, D. S. (1996). Chronic PTSD in Vietnam combat veterans: Course of illness and substance abuse. *American Journal of Psychiatry, 153*(3), 369–373.

Breuer, J., & Freud, S. (1962). On the psychical mechanism of hysterical phenomena: A lecture. In J. Strachey (Ed. and Trans.), *The Standard edition of the complete psychological works of Sigmund Freud* (Vol. 33, pp. 53–69). New York: Hogarth Press. (Original work published 1893)

Brown, P. J., Recupero, P. R., & Stout, R. (1995). PTSD substance abuse comorbidity and treatment utilization. *Addictive Behaviours, 20*(2), 251–254.

Clark, D. B., Pollock, N., Bukstein, O. G., Mezzich, A. C., Bromberger, J. T., & Donovan, J. E. (1997). Gender and comorbid psychopathology in adolescents with alcohol dependence. *Journal of the American Academy of Child and Adolescent Psychiatry, 36*(9), 1195–1203.

Cottler, L. B., Compton, W. M., Mager, D., Spitznagel, E. L., & Janca, A. (1992). Posttraumatic stress disorder among substance abusers from the general population. *American Journal of Psychiatry, 149,* 664–670.

Dansky, B. S., Roitzsch, J. C., Brady, K. T., & Saladin, M. E. (1997). Posttraumatic stress disorder and substance abuse: Use of research in a clinical setting. *Journal of Traumatic Stress, 10*(1), 141–148.

Dansky, B. S., Saladin, M. E., Brady, K. T., Kilpatrick, D. G., & Resnick, H. S. (1995). Prevalence of victimization and posttraumatic stress disorder among women with substance abuse disorders: Comparison of telephone and in-person assessment samples. *International Journal of Addictions, 30*(9), 1079–1099.

Deering, C. G., Glover, S. G., Ready, D., Eddleman, H. C., & Alarcon, R. D. (1996). Unique patterns of comorbidity in posttraumatic stress disorder from different sources of trauma. *Comprehensive Psychiatry, 37*(5), 336–346.

Deykin, E. Y., & Buka, S. L. (1997), Prevalence and risk factors for posttraumatic stress disorder among chemically dependent adolescents. *American Journal of Psychiatry, 154*(6), 752–757.

Foa, E. B. (1997). Psychological processes related to recovery from a trauma and an effective treatment for PTSD. *Annals of the New York Academy of Sciences, 821,* 410–424.

Goenjian, A. K., Karayan, I., Pynoos, R. S., Minassian, D., Najarian, L. M., Steinberg, A. M., & Fairbanks, L. A. (1997). Outcome of psychotherapy among early adolescents after trauma. *American Journal of Psychiatry, 154*(4), 536–542.

Hall, W. (1986). The Agent Orange controversy after the Evatt Royal Commission. *Medical Journal of Australia, 145,* 219–255.

Herman, J. (1992). *Trauma and recovery.* New York: Basic Books.

Hien, D., & Levin, F. R. (1994). Trauma and trauma-related disorders for women on methadone: Prevalence and treatment considerations. *Journal of Psychoactive Drugs, 26*(4), 421–429.

Jackson, S. W. (1992). The listening healer in the history of psychological healing. *American Journal of Psychiatry, 149,* 1623–1632.

Keane, T. M., & Kaloupek, D. G. (1997). Comorbid psychiatric disorder in PTSD: Implications for research. *Annals of the New York Academy of Sciences, 821,* 24–34.

Kessler, R. C., Sonnega, A., Bromet, E., Hughes, M., & Nelson, C. B. (1995). Posttraumatic stress disorder in the National Comorbidity Survey. *Archives of General Psychiatry, 52,* 1048–1060.

Kofoed, L., Friedman, M. J., & Peck, R. (1993). Alcoholism and drug abuse in patients with PTSD. *Psychiatric Quarterly, 64*(2), 151–171.

Kulka, R., Schlenger, W. E., Fairbank, J. A., Hough, R. L., Jordan, B. K., & Marmar, C. R. (1990). *Trauma and the Vietnam War generation: Report of the findings from the National Vietnam Veterans' Readjustment Study.* New York: Brunner/Mazel.

Long, N., MacDonald, C., & Chamberlain, K. (1996). Prevalence of posttraumatic stress disorder, depression and anxiety in a community sample of New Zealand Vietnam War veterans. *Australian and New Zealand Journal of Psychiatry, 30*(2), 253–256.

Lundy, M. S. (1992). Psychosis-induced posttraumatic stress disorder. *American Journal of Psychotherapy, 46*(3), 485–491.

McFarlane, A. C. (1997). The prevalence and longitudinal course of PTSD. *Annals of the New York Academy of Sciences, 821,* 10–23.

McFarlane, A. C. (1998a). Epidemiological evidence about the relationship between PTSD and alcohol abuse: The nature of the association. *Addictive Behaviours, 23*(6), 813–825.

McFarlane, A. C. (1998b). Post-traumatic stress disorder and schizophrenia. *Directions in Psychiatry Forum, 4*(14th–15th November 1997), *Hayman Island, Queensland, Australia.* Chatswood, New South Wales, Australia: Excerpta Medica Communications.

McFarlane, A. C., & Papay, P. (1992). Multiple diagnoses in posttraumatic stress disorder in the victims of a natural disaster. *Journal of Nervous and Mental Disease, 180,* 498–504.

McFarlane, A. C., Shaw, K., & Bookless, C. L. (1997). The phenomenology of traumatic reactions to psychotic illness. *Journal of Nervous and Mental Disease, 185,* 434–441.

Mueser, K. T., Goodman, L. B., Trumbetta, S. L., Rosenberg, S. D., Osher, F. C., Vidaver, R., Auciello, P., & Foy, D. W. (1998). Trauma and posttraumatic stress disorder in severe mental illness. *Journal of Consulting and Clinical Psychology, 66*(3), 493–499.

Orsillo, S. M., Heimberg, R. G., Juster, H. R., & Garrett, J. (1996). Social phobia and PTSD in Vietnam veterans. *Journal of Traumatic Stress, 9*(2), 235–252.

Shalev, A., Bleich, A., & Ursano, R. J. (1990). Posttraumatic stress disorder: Somatic comorbidity and effort tolerance. *Psychosomatics, 31,* 197–203.

Shalev, A. Y., Freedman, S., Peri, T., Brandes, D., Sahar, T., Orr, S. P., & Pitman, R. K. (1998). Prospective study of posttraumatic stress disorder and depression following trauma. *American Journal of Psychiatry, 155*(5), 630–637.

Skodol, A. E., Schwartz, S., Dohrenwend, B. P., Levav, I., Shrout, P. E., & Reiff, M.

(1996). PTSD symptoms and comorbid mental disorders in Israeli war veterans. *British Journal of Psychiatry, 169*(6), 717–725.

Sloane, R. B. (1975). Short-term analytically oriented psychotherapy versus behavioural therapy. *American Journal of Psychiatry, 132*, 374–377.

Stampfer, H. G. (1990). "Negative symptoms": A cumulative trauma stress disorder? *Australian and New Zealand Journal of Psychiatry, 24*(4), 1–2.

van der Kolk, B. A. (1987). *Psychological trauma.* Washington, DC: American Psychiatric Association Press.

van der Kolk, B. A. (1994). Foreword. In J. P. Wilson, & J. D. Lindy (Eds.), *Countertransference in the treatment of posttraumatic stress disorder* (pp. vii–xii). New York: Guilford Press.

van der Kolk, B. A., & Ducey, C. P. (1989). The psychological processing of traumatic experience: Rorschach patterns in PTSD. *Journal of Traumatic Stress, 2,* 259–274.

Villagomez, R. E., Meyer, T. J., Lin, M. M., & Brown, L. S. (1995). Posttraumatic stress disorder among inner city methadone patients. *Journal of Substance Abuse Treatment, 12*(4), 253–257.

Wasserman, D. A., Havassy, B. E., & Boles, S. M. (1997). Traumatic events and posttraumatic stress disorder in cocaine users entering private treatment. *Drug and Alcohol Dependence, 46*(1/2), 1–8.

Wilson, J. P., & Lindy, J. D. (Eds.). (1994). *Countertransference in the treatment of posttraumatic stress disorder.* New York: Guilford Press.

11

Cross-Cultural Treatment of PTSD

J. DAVID KINZIE

CASE STUDIES

The following cases represent the challenges and complexities of treating patients with posttraumatic stress disorder (PTSD) from other cultures.

Case Study 1: Ven

Ven represents a woman with severe and prolonged trauma from the concentration camp experience and the difficulties of being a refugee and subjected to ongoing stress of a new country. The patient has now been in continuous treatment for more than 13 years.

History

When first seen, Ven was a 49-year-old Cambodian female who talked in a rambling, pressured, somewhat preoccupied manner. Her primary symptoms at the first interview were difficulty sleeping, trembling, startle reaction, pain in her legs, and total numbness up to the knees. She had nightly occurring nightmares and multiple somatic complaints. She had very poor concentration, loss of appetite, decreased interest in her environment, and suicidal thoughts. Because of her Buddhist beliefs and a need to take care of her children, she felt she would not take her own life. In addition to these symptoms, she felt sad and depressed most of the time.

She had no formal education, had lived on a farm in Cambodia, and was one of three girls in her family. Her father died in Cambodia before the Pol Pot regime took over. When Pol Pot's Khmer Rouge seized power in 1975, her husband was killed, and later she saw his corpse with bullet wounds and his legs cut off. About a year later, one of her sons was killed and she saw his decapitated body the next day. The visions of these two corpses come back to her daily. Two of her children died of starvation, and she endured many hours of hard labor, malnutrition and the threat of dying much of the time. She saw many corpses during the 4 years of the Pol Pot regime. In 1979, she fled from Cambodia to Thailand with two of her children, leaving three other children behind. She stayed in Thailand for 3 years, then went to the Philippines for a year, and finally came to the United States in 1983.

Ven appeared very disheveled and had pressured speech and was almost incoherent when telling her story. She looked uncomfortable, had poorly combed hair and was missing several front teeth. She had a stocking anesthesia on both legs up to her knees. Ven became quite visibly depressed and quite shaken throughout the interview. Although, there was no thinking disorder, there was a frantic attempt to guard against talking about these tragic events. The clinical impression of this very unfortunate woman was PTSD and major depressive disorder; her anesthesia, which did not follow an anatomic pattern, was probably a sympathetic conversion reaction related to seeing her husband with both his legs cut off.

Treatment

Treatment for Ven has been consistent for 13 years. This has involved regular visits to the psychiatrist and medication to reduce the primary symptoms of depression and PTSD. She originally was treated with the antidepressant doxepin and the adrenergic-blocking medicine clonidine. This resulted in reduction of her insomnia and nightmares. She also has been in a socialization group with other Cambodians led by a Cambodian social worker who also served as case manager and interpreter. The socialization groups decreased Ven's sense of isolation and provided a social environment that helped her reconnect with her compatriots.

Over the next 13 years, several problems arose which led to the return of posttraumatic stress symptoms. About 4 years after she started treatment, her elderly mother died of what was probably lung cancer. There was a great deal of grief involved, with some reactivation of her symptoms, but she was able to do the appropriate Buddhist ceremonies which seemed to help. Later, she developed severe hypertension that was treated in the clinic by adjusting the antidepressant and the clonidine.

Several years ago, a daughter moved in with a new boyfriend, which caused Ven much stress, social embarrassment, and increased her PTSD symptoms. At that time, she stopped going to group and became more isolated and alone. She was switched from doxepin to fluoxetine, and she began to lose a great deal of weight probably due to this medicine. In addition, her sleep deteriorated. She became somatically preoccupied, and indeed it did appear that she might have a serious illness. She was referred to family medicine to undergo various studies that turned out to be normal. However, she was found to be having some menopausal symptoms and was placed on hormonal medications. The negative examinations made her feel better.

After the children married, Ven lived alone, which seemed to cause further isolation and increased symptoms. She moved back with her son which helped somewhat, but she became worried about possible welfare cuts and was very afraid that she would not have enough money or food to live on.

At this time, she had increased hypertension; propranolol was added to the clonidine and doxepin, which brought the blood pressure down and helped the hyperarousal symptoms.

Ven reestablished connections with her children in Cambodia, and this caused an increase in nightmares due to the memories raised when she talked with them by phone, as well as increased stress as they asked continuously for money which she was not able to provide.

She became worried about welfare cuts and not becoming a U.S. citizen which greatly increased her symptoms. She received classes in this and was eventually able to pass the citizenship test.

Over this time, sleep, appetite, and concentration have improved. Her nightmares have reduced to about two a month and she has reestablished a relationship with her children, with whom she now lives. She has returned to group and has become an active participant and has been quite stable medically for the past 6 months. Ven remains extremely vulnerable to any new stressors, as demonstrated previously.

Formulation

This is a patient who had a severe traumatic experience in Cambodia with the death of her husband and children and ongoing threats of her own death, starvation, forced labor, and witnessing of corpses and murder while in the Khmer Rouge concentration camps. These experiences provided the original trauma leading to the posttraumatic stress and depression symptoms. The symptoms were aggravated by her refugee status in a foreign county, ongoing stress related to the death of her mother, physical problems, conflicts and unsettling relationships with her children, the perceived threat of not being able to become a U.S. citizen, and reestablishing contact with her children in Cambodia which reactivated her trauma.

The patient had a good premorbid function, given a lack of literacy and living in a rural society. There is no evidence of any prior stress with the exception of the death of her father when she was still a teenager.

The patient had several problems which required clinical intervention. These included the symptoms of depression and PTSD, the need for social support and contact with other members of her society, and the need to reduce stress related to her relationships with her family, possible loss of income, and poor physical health. In regard to her health, it was deemed useful to have the psychiatrist do some of the medical management, such as monitoring the blood pressure, supervising the treatment, ordering necessary lab tests, and making appropriate referrals. Other interventions included supportive psychotherapy with the psychiatrist and ethnic social worker, who have worked with her continually for the last 13 years. In addition, the socialization group therapy was aimed at reducing the isolation, developing contact with other refugees in a similar situation, sharing experiences, continuing the traditions of their culture, and learning how to live in the United States.

Over time, the patient has had marked reduction in her symptoms. Her mood is mostly euthymic, and the nightmares have greatly decreased. She is less socially isolated and works well in the group. She continues to have ongoing stresses which can be easily monitored by both her own statements and her blood pressure. She has greatly benefited socially from treatment but has a need for ongoing therapy to treat the chronic conditions traumatized refugees often develop.

Case Study 2: Phong

Phong suffered the severe trauma of 12 years of "reeducation" in communist concentration camps and had come to the United States as part of a program designed to bring over ex-government officials and military personnel from Vietnam. At the initial clinic visit, the patient, a single Vietnamese male in his mid-60s who was living by himself, came in with the chief complaint of depression and nightmares. He has been in continuous treatment for 3 years.

History

The patient had been a high military official reaching the rank of colonel who served until the last day of the South Vietnamese government's existence in 1979. Subsequently, he was captured by the communists and sentenced to the "reeducation camp" and was incarcerated for 12 years. He tried to escape at least once but was captured. He was beaten often by his guards, mostly at the beginning phase of his incarceration. He had to engage in harsh labor, working in the hills and forests with long periods of starvation, and witnessed the deaths of many fellow inmates. He suffered from infectious diseases and was not given any medical treatment. After his release, he was on probation and was not able to hold any jobs or seek employment.

He now complains of headaches occurring constantly and of not being able to sleep because of nightmares that frequently awaken him. This often results in him screaming at night. These nightmares usually deal with his time as a POW and are about people who died around him in the camp or previously during combat.

He has been virtually isolated socially since coming to the United States. He had no network in this country. He feels people are following him and is quite vigilant about people walking around him and has made no contact with others. He describes himself as being sad all the time, having poor memory, and frequent plans to kill himself.

The patient was born in North Vietnam and went to South Vietnam in 1954. He had a high level of education, was considered upper class, and was dedicated to the South Vietnamese regime. He was married with two children. During an escape attempt in 1979, his wife and children were killed, and he did not hear about their deaths until 3 years after their death.

He was a well-dressed, dignified looking Vietnamese with a very reduced affect who was easily irritated. He answered questions with brief comments, and although he was not friendly he was trying to cooperate. He described paranoia and hypervigilance as well as suicidal but not homicidal thoughts. There was some mild impairment in his memory.

This man clearly was suffering from major depression and severe PTSD that was related to 12 years in a concentration camp. The trauma has left him with nightmares, intrusive memories, social isolation, numbing, hypervigilance, and suspicion which have crossed over to paranoia. An additional loss has been the death of his wife and daughters, adding to his sense of frustration and isolation. Although in the past he was quite resilient, able to survive unimaginably difficult times, he is now nonfunctioning in his new country.

Treatment

The primary treatment was led for 3 years by a Vietnamese-speaking psychiatrist and a Vietnamese case manager. Phong was started on medications – fluoxetine, trazadone, and clonidine twice a day. He continued to have frequent nightmares and screaming at night for several years, although the medicine greatly helped relieve his headaches and resulted in a reduction of nightmares and startling reactions. The patient also attended Vietnamese socialization groups and a specifically designed socialization center experience which would help with job training and reintegration in the United States. He was noted in both groups to be somewhat distanced from others, quite reserved, presented a somewhat superior attitude and was very sensitive about associating with those of a lesser social class. The socialization center exposure facilitated English communication, which proceeded at a very good rate. In one group, the patient had developed tolerance of others, and even though his angry outbursts continued periodically, he showed less bitterness and intensity. The patient was cooperative in individual therapy and in some groups, but after 2 years dropped out of socialization groups partly due to his inability to relate to the other Vietnamese members. His nightmares have disappeared over the last 3 years, and he has had a decrease in his depressive mood; however, he remains worried and irritable and his concentration remains a problem. He has developed very few new social relationships and prefers to be by himself and engage in solitary activities such as reading and painting.

Formulations

This man, with severe PTSD of long-standing trauma and isolation in Vietnam, came to the United States and experienced depression and severe PTSD as well as social isolation, numbing, and even paranoia. The plan was to decrease the major symptoms of PTSD and depression with medication and to provide continuity of ongoing treatment with a Vietnamese-speaking psychiatrist and a Vietnamese case manager along with group therapy. The primary trauma related was the incarceration, although it was implied by the patient (but never elaborated on) that he had seen a great deal of combat and the death of others, which may have contributed to his PTSD. He had additional anguish when he later found that his wife and two children had died during an escape attempt. The intervention of individual therapy with the psychiatrist and the medication proceeded smoothly, with gradual reduction of depressive symptoms and the arousal symptoms of PTSD. His irritability and suspiciousness made it hard for him to engage in an ongoing socialization group experience even though it reduced his sense of isolation. Despite the social isolation, numbing, and avoidance behavior, which has been very difficult to treat, he has cooperated in most aspects of the treatment program.

Case Study 3: Christina

This patient represents the problems in treating a traumatized asylum seeker whose legal status remained undetermined.

History

The patient, Christina, was referred by a local minister because of multiple symptoms including depression relating to traumatic events she suffered in Africa. She is a Congolese refugee in her mid-20s who was previously a university student. During the Civil War in the Congo (formerly Zaire), her family was involved in some local politics; and when she and her husband were at the university, troops captured her parents and burned their house. Their status was unknown, but they were presumed dead. She, her husband, and other students in a very crowded truck traveled for many days trying to get

out of the country. In the forest, troops surrounded them, the men were sep-
arated from the women, and the women were then raped. When Christina's
husband came to her rescue, he was beheaded. All the men were killed, the
women and some of the children were raped, and several of the women were
also killed. Eventually, the remaining women and children escaped in the
truck and returned to the capital. She was hidden by a relative who helped
her get onto a boat on which she stowed away for a considerable time until it
arrived in the United States and she was able to sneak into the country. She
eventually found other people from her country and became a refugee spon-
sored by a Christian organization. Her primary symptoms have been poor
sleep, very poor appetite, no enjoyment in life, and at times suicidal ideation.
Because she was a Catholic, she said she would not kill herself. She had
nightmares of the events, intrusive thoughts of her time in Africa, and has
felt on guard and vigilant most of the time.

The patient came from a professional family where all the children were
professionals or attending the university. She describes no trauma until the
outbreak of the Congolese Civil War. She has not had any contact with her
family and feels very lonely. In the few calls she made to Africa, she found out
that her grandparents also were killed and her life would be in danger if she
returned. She asked for political asylum here in the United States.

The patient was an attractive young African woman who was well com-
posed and well dressed. Although reluctant to speak, she told her story in
halting but direct English with quite graphic details of her life. She appeared
sad and overwhelmed and cried during the interview. She often asked why so
much could happen to her at such a young age.

Treatment

The patient was initially treated for depression and PTSD with imipramine;
later clonidine was added. She was seen in individual supportive psychotherapy over the next 6 months, keeping all of her appointments. Her primary
thoughts were of loneliness, isolation, poor concentration, and sometimes
poorly defined pain. Surprisingly, in all the sessions she never mentioned her
husband again but frequently commented about the loneliness she felt from
the absence of her parents, whom she felt she would never see again. The
headaches were treated with propranolol, and the clonidine was stopped. She
applied for political asylum and the treating psychiatrist wrote a letter of support. She was eventually given political asylum, which did reduce her stress a
great deal and gave her more of a sense of permanency about her residency.
She was able to begin taking classes at a local university and could legally get
a job. She established contact with other African students, got her own apartment, and began to get comfortable although she missed Africa. Her nightmares decreased but did not totally diminish. She felt comfortable enough to
stop treatment after 8 months.

Formulation

This was a well-adjusted, intelligent highly successful African woman coming from an upper-middle-class family. Her family was caught up in a bloody Civil War which resulted in the the death of her husband, her grandparents, and probably her parents. She was smuggled out of the country and had indeterminate refugee status in the United States until she received asylum. Her own Christian religion led to contacts in the religious community here in the United States which provided some support, particularly in food, lodging, and aid in obtaining the necessary legal support for her to stay in the country. Her premorbid adjustment was quite good, and there is no history of trauma prior to the catastrophic events of the Congolese Civil War. The intervention involved continuing the support of the religious community and being instrumental in helping seek political asylum, which allowed her to continue in school and obtain employment. This gave her a measure of independence, which seemed to give her a great deal of personal self-esteem. The medication also reduced her symptoms of depression, nightmares, poor sleep, and headaches. She seemed comfortable in the presence of a white American psychiatrist and the supportive, confidential, and perhaps nonreligious focus of the relationship gave her an outlet to recount some of the more disturbing events of her life. Under this therapy, she was able to mobilize her own considerable skills and move ahead with adjustment to the United States.

Treating psychiatric patients when the clinician and the patient are from different cultures is a difficult task. The barrier to treatment can involve differences in language, status, understanding about the cause of mental illness, or even the goals of treatment. When the patient has been severely traumatized, the issues are even more difficult since humiliation, shame, avoidance behavior, and exaggerated physiological response may make the patient even more reluctant or unable to engage in treatment. While approaches to cross-cultural psychiatry have made remarkable advances recently with the publication of several sophisticated new books, the role of trauma in the cross-cultural setting has been minimized. This despite the accumulating evidence that members of some ethnic groups have suffered a catastrophic amount of trauma and consequently have developed PTSD. The goals of this chapter are to review some of the evidence regarding traumatized ethnic groups, summarize the approaches to cross-cultural psychiatric treatment, and offer treatment approaches that help overcome the cultural barriers.

BACKGROUND

The American clinician is likely to encounter three broad types of PTSD patient from other cultures or minorities: the minority American citizen, the foreign refugee, and the asylum seeker, who is often an illegal immigrant.

Minority Americans

The most heavily studied group of PTSD patients have been the Vietnam conflict veterans (Kulka et al., 1990) where racial/ethnic differences were found. The current prevalence was 29.9% among Hispanics, 20.6% among African-Americans, and 13.7% among white males. When adjusted for predisposing factors, the difference between blacks and whites became insignificant, but the Hispanic prevalence rate remained significant. Although in civilian populations exposure to trauma may differ by ethnic groups, once exposed the rate of PTSD usually does not differ between ethnic groups (Norris, 1992; Kilpatrick et al., 1989; Breslau, Davis, Audreski, & Petersen, 1991; Cottler, Compton, Mager, Spitznagel, & Janca, 1992).

The Refugees

The number of refugees with forced migration worldwide has risen to 16 million people, not including 2 million displaced people of the former Yugoslavia region (Leopald & Harrell-Bond, 1994). Some 15 to 25 million internally displaced persons who have not crossed over political borders are not classified as refugees. The Vietnam War resulted in 700,000 refugees from Vietnam, Cambodia, and Laos (Mollica, 1994) and the civil wars of Nicaragua, El Salvador, and Guatemala displaced 2 million people (Farias, 1994).

More recent studies of refugees began with the arrival of Indo-Chinese refugees to the United States after 1975. With the introduction of the DSM-III diagnostic criteria (American Psychiatric Association, 1980), reliable psychiatric diagnoses became possible. Depression and then PTSD among Southeast Asian refugees began to be documented more systematically (Bochnlein, Kinzie, Rath, & Fleck, 1985; Kinzie & Manson, 1983; Kinzie, Frederickson, Rath, & Fleck, 1984; Kroll et al., 1989). Research following the terrible plight of Vietnamese refugees, as well as of refugees from the brutal regime of the Cambodian Pol Pot from 1975 to 1979, resulted in a number of studies on the effect of severe trauma. In a clinic for Indo-Chinese refugees, PTSD was found to be present in 92% of Cambodians, 93% of the Mein, and about 54% among the Vietnamese (Kinzie et al., 1990). In community samples of Cambodian refugees, rates of PTSD have ranged from 12% (Cheung, 1994), to 50% (Kinzie, Sack, Angell, & Manson, 1986), to 86% (Carlson & Rosser-Hogan, 1991).

In a longitudinal study of Cambodian adolescent refugees, rates of both depression and PTSD were also at about 50%. However, depressive symptoms diminished over time, while PTSD symptoms were more persistent and episodic (Kinzie et al., 1986; Kinzie, Sack, Angell, & Clarke, 1989).

Psychological problems and symptoms have been reported in other refugee studies. One study on San Salvador refugees described men as having problems with nightmares, alcohol abuse, and losing control, while the women reported angry feelings, somatic complaints, and crying (Farias, 1991). Of 30 children exposed to warfare in Central America, 10 had PTSD (Arroyo & Eth, 1985). Among Chilean and Salvadorian migrants, those who had experienced torture had higher rates of PTSD than those who had neither torture nor trauma (Thompson & McGarry, 1995). Of the 87 Ethiopian Jews making the long trek to Israel, 27% had moderate-to-severe psychological symptoms (Arieli & Aycheh, 1992). Among 38 young Afghan refugees, 13 had PTSD, depression, or both (Mghir, Raskin, Freed, & Katon, 1995). Reports of Afghan refugees in Pakistan indicated that many had been subjected to severe trauma and torture, with the most common psychological symptoms being anxiety and depression, which was more often found among the torture survivors. Substance abuse had also increased in this group (Dadfur, 1994).

Studies of the Bosnian refugees are just beginning to be published. A first study of the Bosnian survivors of "ethnic cleansing" found that 65% had PTSD and 35% had depression (Weine et al., 1995). The disruption of Bosnian family life because of massive trauma has recently been described (Weine, 1997).

Asylum Seekers

Asylum seekers arrive in a country on a temporary visa and request refugee status. During a prolonged waiting period, their refugee status claims are reviewed, basic services are not allowed, and they live under threat of forced repatriation (Silove, Sinnesbrink, Field, Manicavasagan, & Steel, 1997). In a study of 104 Burmese political dissidents who escaped to Thailand and survived without legal protection, the number of traumatic events experienced was very high—an average of 30 (Allden et al., 1996). Of the 104 individuals, 38% had elevated depressive symptoms and 23% met criteria for PTSD. Symptoms of avoidance and increased arousal were positively related to the cumulative trauma exposure; and the unclear future and legal status of these asylum seekers contributed to their ongoing symptoms. In a study of Tamil migrants in Australia, it was found that asylum seekers had trauma and psychiatric symptoms similar to those of other refugees, but they had increased postmigration stress related to their insecure residency status (Silove, Steel, McGarry, & Mohan, 1998). These authors concluded that premigration trauma accounted for 20% of the variance in PTSD, while postmigration stress, including loss of culture and support, problems with health care and welfare, and adjustment difficulties, contributed 14% of the variance. Among Cambodian adolescents, war trauma was found to relate to PTSD symptoms, while postmigration stress related to depression (Sack, Clarke, & Seeley, 1996).

CROSS-CULTURAL THERAPY

The treatment of psychiatric disorders across cultures begins with the complex issue of assessment. The complexity develops because each culture (itself an elusive concept) can define normality and psychopathology differently from other cultures. In the clinical interview, the patient's culture may determine what are appropriate problems to present to the clinician and the clinician's culture (medical and or psychological) determines how problems are understood and classified (Tseng, 1997) This process is further complicated by problems in communication, the degree of cultural sensitivity of the clinician, and the use of appropriate psychological instruments (Westermeyer, 1993). Appropriate sensitive evaluation proceeds as a dynamic process. The patient's culture may influence the help-seeking behavior, but further behavior in the interview will often be determined by the patient's interpretation of the clinician as an individual. The "style" of the clinician determines the amount and type of information gathered. His or her sensitivity and understanding of the ongoing relationship can greatly improve the intervention and the accuracy of the information (Tseng & Streltzler, 1997).

Clearly, cross-cultural therapy itself requires special approaches. The therapist needs to be flexible, appreciate the patient's culture, explore the patient's expectations, and openly negotiate the goals. Often, the patient expects the therapist to be active and to take the lead and reduce symptoms (Kinzie, 1985). This is consistent with the role of a Western-style physician, perhaps the model most patients have when they come forward with symptoms. Generally the use of medication is very acceptable. In most non-Western cultures, there is no analogy to the one-to-one self-exploration that occurs in dynamic psychotherapy. This cross-cultural psychotherapy often takes on a unique aspect. Yamamoto, Selva, Justice, Chang, and Leong (1993) used the broader term "intervention" instead of "therapy" and emphasized education, medical treatment, and community follow-up. These authors emphasized the importance of the family in treatment and that empathy and transference issues involve both the individual and his or her family. There needs to be an activity that involves helping the family cope with the patient's illness.

There are specific problems in refugee populations that have large psychosocial impact. The patient often experiences marginalization and minority status, poor physical health, head trauma injuries, collapse of social support, and the difficulties of adapting to a host country (Ekblad, Kohn, & Jansson, 1998). With psychological trauma, the adjustments are even more difficult. The symptoms of PTSD such as nightmares, startle reaction, avoidance behavior, irritability, and poor concentration probably represent a psychological state unknown in the patient's premigraton life and for which traditional healing does not exist. Although it has been suggested that some massive loss and personal reactions represent a cultural bereavement (Eisen-bruk, 1991), it is clear that the symptoms do cross linguistic and cultural bar-riers (Boehnlein & Kinzie, 1993; Sack, Seeley, & Clarke, 1997). How the pa-tient interprets the symptoms and approaches the losses certainly depends to some extent on values, religious beliefs, and the remaining social contacts.

The symptoms themselves—avoidance behavior, numbing, and amne-sia—can clearly prevent many traumatized survivors from seeking help. Many refugees stated it was often difficult to talk about the past: "Better to forget about it" was a common statement. Those having Buddhist beliefs in Karma may feel that they had been bad in a previous life or lives and that the severe trauma is their fate which must be accepted; therefore, they do not need or deserve treatment. Other factors such as rape may be so culturally shameful that it cannot be discussed even in the confidential setting of a physician's office (Young, 1998). A particularly disturbing event is domestic violence, which is seen as very shameful and a failure of the family—or even as the right of a man to punish his wife. These social taboos may prevent these topics from being divulged or discussed.

> A Vietnamese patient was interviewed by an American psychiatrist with a fe-male Vietnamese interpreter. She spent most of the time describing her somatic complaints, which began when her husband was killed in the Vietnam War. When the interpreter left the room, the patient spoke in fair English describing severe domestic abuse and her subsequent relief when her husband was killed. She returned to somatic complaints when the interpreter came back in the room.

All of the above factors, in addition to some clinicians' problems with their own avoidance, not taking a trauma history, and their difficulty in ap-proaching some shameful events with patients, make formulating the diagno-sis very difficult. Indeed, when patients already in treatment at an Indo-Chinese clinic were reinterviewed, a high percentage of PTSD was found to be present (Kinzie et al., 1990). Much of this had been missed in previous in-terviews, thus demonstrating how difficult it is to thoroughly evaluate patients in the cross-cultural setting.

STUDIES ON THE TREATMENT OF TRAUMATIZED INDIVIDUALS IN TRANSCULTURAL SETTINGS

Several well-developed programs have emerged in the United States to treat refugees, many who have experienced severe trauma. Among them are the Harvard Refugee Clinic in Boston, the International Mental Health Pro-gram of the Department of Psychiatry at St. Paul/Ramsey Mental Health Center in St. Paul, Minnesota, and the Indo-Chinese Psychiatric Program at

Oregon Health Science University in Portland, Oregon. These have all utilized psychiatrists trained in cultural psychiatry and ethnic mental health professionals to bridge language and cultural barriers. These programs have been successful in treating a large number of patients and providing a wealth of clinical data on approaches to the psychiatric care of this difficult population. A lack of specific studies on the effects of treatment leaves unanswered how best to treat PTSD among refugees.

Another series of reports have come from the literature of survivors of torture (Chester & Jaranson, 1994). Note that the primary treatment has often been psychotherapy, but no controlled outcome studies have been completed. Others have described treatments which have been useful for victims of torture. These have included "insight" therapy (Sommier & Genefke, 1986; Vesti & Kastrup, 1992), relational therapy (Varvin & Hauff, 1998), and short-term treatment for depression and torture survivors (Drees, 1989). Cognitive therapy (Basoglu, 1992, 1998) and psychodynamic therapy (Bustos, 1992; Allodi, 1998) have been frequently employed. Other approaches include supportive therapy, desensitization, family groups (Fischman & Ross, 1990), and giving testimony (Vesti & Kastrup, 1992). Although cognitive therapy has been effective in treating PTSD (Keane, Albano, & Blake, 1992), most experienced clinicians feel that severely traumatized individuals require much longer treatment than the relatively short-term approach of behavioral therapy.

The common ingredients of most treatments involve telling the trauma story with reframing and reworking (Mollica, 1988). Clearly, this needs to be done in a safe setting with appropriate timing. Even the retelling of the trauma story is dependent upon the patient's cultural experience. For example, South American refugees seem more willing to retell the trauma stories, and perhaps are even helped by often retelling them. Indochinese are reluctant to tell the trauma story and often have an exacerbation of symptoms after such therapeutic attempts (Morris & Silove, 1992). Drug therapy has been used for refugee victims of extreme trauma, and Jaranson, (1991) stressed the importance of starting medication for highly symptomatic patients even if evaluation is still in progress. There have been studies to indicate that different doses are needed in non-Caucasians versus Caucasians, and pharmacokinetic (metabolic) and pharmacodynamic brain receptor influences have been demonstrated (Lin, Poland, & Nagasaki, 1993). The issue is complicated by studies which show very poor compliance among Indo-Chinese patients (Kroll et al., 1989; Kinzie, Leung, Boehnlein, & Fleck, 1987). Among refugees tricyclic antidepressants (TCAs), selective serotonin reuptake inhibitors (SSRIs), and clonidine have been found useful for some symptoms. The antidepressant effects of TCAs and SSRIs have treated depression and sleep disorder (Kinzie, 1998) Clonidine has been particularly useful for hyper-arousal and nightmare symptoms (Kinzie & Leung, 1989; Kinzie, Sack, & Riley, 1994)

Most therapies have been useful for reexperiencing hyperarousal symptoms but rather ineffective in avoidance and numbing symptoms. There have been some evidence that long-term socialization group therapy with emphasis on supportive environment, redoing cultural rituals, education about this disorder and medication, and learning to live in a North American society have helped with social isolation and some avoidance behavior (Kinzie et al., 1988).

A most disturbing aspect of PTSD is its tendency to recur when there are real or symbolic threats resembling the original trauma. The patients described increasing anxiety, nightmares, poor sleep, and irritability when viewing war or disaster stories on television or experiencing an accident or an assault. It recently has been shown that there are ethnic differences to this reactivity. On viewing videotapes of various accidents or disasters, many more Cambodians with PTSD experienced an increased heart rate than did American Vietnam War veterans with PTSD (Kinzie et al., in press). This reactivity may be useful in monitoring relapse during therapy.

CLINICAL GUIDELINES FOR OPTIMAL CROSS-CULTURAL TREATMENT OF PTSD

In this section guidelines are suggested for the optimal cross-cultural care of patients with PTSD. These guidelines are often impossible to put totally into practice and should represent an ideal which must be adjusted as the clinical setting, practical matters, finances, availability of interpreters, medical services, and legal pressures dictate. Since optimal treatment requires a fully developed program, I describe that first, with individual therapeutic considerations to follow.

A PRACTICAL PROGRAM FOR THE CROSS-CULTURAL TREATMENT OF PTSD: STRUCTURE AND STAFFING ISSUES

To be fully responsible for the psychiatric care of traumatized patients from diverse culture, a comprehensive program needs to incorporate the following key elements (Kinzie, 1991):

1. The program needs to be able to treat the major psychiatric disorders in the population in addition to PTSD. Many studies have indicated that depression and other anxieties are comorbid with PTSD. Additionally, schizophrenia occurs in traumatized patients (Kinzie & Boehnlein, 1989) and is a very complex and disruptive condition. Alcohol and substance abuse is low in Asian refugees but has been found to be higher in Hispanic males. The implication is that a psychiatric program, although having a special focus on trauma, must in fact be a general psychiatric clinic which is prepared for a variety of different psychiatric disorders.

2. The program must address the language needs of the patients. This means having well-trained interpreters or better yet bilingual mental health workers who are familiar with basic mental health concepts.

3. There needs to be easy access to the program. Minorities and refugees often feel stigmatized by the implications of a mental illness, so to reach a point of entry with minimal barriers is essential to establishing contact. Appointments need to be made without long waiting lists or complex screening procedures. Crises need to be met by workers with the appropriate language and clinical skills.

4. The program needs to establish credibility within the refugee or minority community. The success of the program depends upon the reputation within the served communities of being competent and committed to a long-term relationship with them.

5. The program needs linkages and continuity with all services. Ideally, if all services—outpatient, day treatment, hospitalization, and crisis intervention—can be located in one setting with the same providers, the patients will receive more comprehensive service with minimal disruption of support.

6. The program needs to integrate both physical and mental disorders. Refugees, as well as much of the general population, do not distinguish between psychiatric and physical symptoms and clearly wish to have the physical diseases evaluated. Also, there is much overlap between disorders and ongoing evaluation is indicated. The staff, especially psychiatrists who are comfortable with physical exams and laboratory studies, can facilitate this evaluation. A close relationship with the clinic's department of family medicine or internal medicine makes referrals much easier.

7. There needs to be a mechanism for the patients to give feedback regarding the program and advice for future direction. The program can not exist separate from the community it serves and needs frequent interaction to provide appropriate sensitive service.

8. The staffing needs are crucial. It is important that psychiatrists be broad-based competent clinicians who can handle a wide variety of clinical conditions. They must be able to diagnose in a transcultural setting and have a thorough knowledge of the culture of the patient being treated. A knowledge of trauma and its treatment is important.

9. Bilingual medical mental health workers, to be effective, need to have training in mental health and counseling. These are the bridges between the patient and the professional staff. With training, they can provide case management, group therapy, and individual as well as interpretive services.

The Treatment Process

The central therapeutic factor within this program-based treatment is the doctor–patient relationship. This, even more than in traditional therapy, depends on the personality of the therapist (Kinzie & Fleck, 1987). Traumatized minorities are very sensitive to rejection or symbolic threats, and certain personal qualities of the therapist are crucial in establishing this relationship. These qualities include genuineness, warmth, empathy, interest in and knowledge about the patient's culture, understanding of the likely traumas that the patient faced, and calmness and acceptance on hearing the trauma story. In short, the therapist needs to like and appreciate the patient. The specific approaches are listed below:

1. *Establish safety.* The interview must be safe, with absolute confidentiality (an important issue with interpreters), and with no pressure to tell or not to tell the story and clear respect for the cultural values such as shame for rape or family disgrace at having left behind sick or elderly parents.

2. *Promote continuity of care.* It is important that psychiatrists or therapists taking the history provide an ongoing relationship. There is no place for separation of evaluation and treatment. There is no safety in telling a difficult story to one provider only to be switched to another. The therapist must be central and consistent throughout the treatment. Also, treatment must be committed to the long-term goal and needs of the patient. This is particularly true for traumatized refugees for whom overcoming trauma in a new country is a long and difficult process. Expectation to get well in a prescribed time frame (e.g., 10 sessions) is too great a pressure, is generally unrealistic, and leaves the patient with the possibility of being abandoned (perhaps as in previous trauma experiences).

3. *Take seriously patients' symptoms, which usually are somatic, and respect their subjective complaints.* Patients rarely come with a trauma story or even full PTSD symptoms. They come because of perceived distress—often such as aches and pains, poor sleep, difficulty concentrating, loss of energy, a sense that something is altogether wrong with their body, and occasionally a feeling that they are going to die. Physical symptoms need to be seriously explored. Some physical exam and lab studies need to be done to reassure both the doctor and the patient.

4. *Take a complete history, including events before and after the trauma.* This helps both the therapist and patient to put the patient's life in perspective and provide credibility to the relationship with the patient. The trauma needs to be addressed as part of the history in the degree of detail the patient can (and wants to) tolerate. It is important for the therapist to be patient, empathetic, and not overwhelmed. There are major cultural differences in expression of grief and anguish, and one should not be surprised by restrained affect or apparent exaggerated behavior.

5. *Give an explanatory model appropriate to the patient's culture and symptoms.* The symptoms are often confusing to the patients, and many even feel that they are "going crazy." Most patients are helped by a clear statement enumerating the stressful pressures resulting from the trauma and explaining that the mind and body are reacting to these pressures. It helps to further explain

that everyone, even a strong person like the patient, has a breaking point, which is the way the body reacts to too much pressure. This helps to place the symptoms in a normal stress reaction frame of reference. Although this seems appropriate for many patients, some are unable, at least initially, to relate the trauma or traumas to the symptoms and models (Karma or even spirit possession) which fit their worldview. A clear statement may need to be made by the therapist showing his or her understanding of the evilness of the traumatic event and that he or she understands that a reprehensible act has occurred.

6. *Establish a treatment contract and goals.* To refugees and some members of minorities who are depressed and have low self-esteem, negotiations with a Western-style professional may not be easy or even completely appropriate. A useful approach is to state the likely early goals—improved sleep, reduced nightmares, and better mood— and ask if there are other aspects that need to be worked on. Patients will sometimes describe physical symptoms which bother them, and these may need to be helped with symptomatic relief or a later evaluation when the psychiatric symptoms improve. The contract implies an ongoing relationship, symptomatic reduction, and the expectation that the patient will improve with no termination point determined at this stage.

7. *Provide relief of symptoms.* In the first session, it is usually necessary to start medication and provide relief even if the evaluation is not complete. Medicine not only provides help with distressing symptoms and fits with the role of the Western-style physician but provides a sense of competency to treat the patient's needs. This treatment is usually not difficult as a variety of medications are fairly effective. It is the author's experience in treating more than 300 members of minorities and refugees that the antidepressants are very useful. If the patient has difficulty sleeping as well as depression, the tertiary tricyclics, such as imipramine or doxepine, often provide rapid improvement in sleep and mood. The SSRIs have been extensively used and have a different side effect profile, less sedation, less constipation, more agitation, and more sexual dysfunction. With one or the other, some effective relief can be achieved. If nightmares or hyper-arousal symptoms persist, clonidine (usually in a daily dose of 0.1 mg a.m and 0.2 mg at bedtime) can be added. The realistic goal is to provide good sleep for 8 hours each night with a reduction in the occurrence of nightmares to once per week.

8. *Provide environmental safety.* For refugees and asylum seekers, there are multiple ongoing problems which need to be addressed and which an effective clinic through the physician and case managers can provide. This includes contacting social agencies regarding welfare income, housing, and medical assistance. It may be necessary to write letters to attorneys regarding the patient's request for asylum or to the U.S. Immigration and Naturalization Service (INS) to provide information for language wavers in the citizenship examination.

9. *Develop therapeutic themes.* In the ongoing contact, the patient and therapist develop a steady, safe relationship based on issues and themes. Often for refugees, these continue around losses from their previous country, such as deaths in the family, loss of their homeland and society, and frequently financial losses. In addition, there are ongoing problems in adjusting to the new country, dealing with unfamiliar laws and customs, and sometimes more disturbing issues of raising children with problems of drugs and gangs. For some issues, the therapist listens and supports, and for others he or she offers practical advice and suggestions and even information about living in this country.

10. *Listen to and share in the trauma story.* How to handle the trauma story is a difficult clinical decision. The stories are often told in an incomplete, disconnected, and emotionally charged manner. Patients may feel relieved and unburdened by telling their stories and having been listened to and understood. However, many will find that the interview will stimulate memories and that there may be an exacerbation of nightmares and intrusive thoughts for a time. Some ethnic groups, either by exploring internal problems or by confronting the cruelty and torture inflicted by political opponents, may gain intellectual mastery and integration in their lives. Others may find acceptance and avoidance as the most adaptive approach. In that case, the best clinical strategy is to follow the patient's lead, avoiding extensive trauma discussion. When the patient has marked nightmares and hyperarousal symptoms, further stimulation may need to be postponed for a time. The most important aspect is to clearly recognize that the effects of massive trauma, deaths, torture, brutality in concentration camps, and loss of home and country can never be fully understood or integrated. Life will never be the same. The losses are real, permanent, and bring into question the meaning of life, suffering, and even death. There is no quick fix, and a promise of a rapid cure will ring false and hollow. Sometimes the authentic position is to stay with the patient through the pain. The sharing of the experience decreases isolation and brings two people of markedly different backgrounds and experiences closer. There may be no better therapy than this.

SPECIAL ISSUES IN CROSS-CULTURAL TREATMENT

Group Therapy

Many ethnic groups consider psychological distress very private and personal matters and are very reluctant to open up in group therapy. A useful method is to organize groups for socialization that emphasize social interactions, education about illness and medication, and adjustment to the new country (Kinzie et al., 1988). Following traditional ceremonies and celebrations in the group maintains ties to the old culture. Overall, the primary goal of group is to greatly decrease isolation and avoidance behavior and consolidate ethnic identity.

Western-style focused psychotherapy when led by treating psychiatrists who provide authority and safety can be performed. In our experience, with a psychiatrist leading group therapy one time a month with Cambodians, it required 2 years before the patients could discuss trauma without being totally consumed. The patients felt the therapy was helpful but usually took one week afterward to recover from the effects of intrusive shared memories.

Detection of Relapse

The nature of chronic PTSD is to wax and wane over time. The major symptoms can be reactivated by stress or actual threats. The early symptoms are not always verbalized by patients. From much clinical data with traumatized Indo-Chinese, we found that physiological changes such as increased pulse and blood pressure mark the beginning of activation of PTSD. When exposed to traumatic videotapes, Cambodians had a frequent increase in pulse rate (Kinzie et al., in press). In our clinic, we have checked blood pressure and pulse on all Cambodian patients for more than 10 years and found that the cardiovascular signs correlate very strongly with current stress. In addition, 43% have developed hypertension. The change in pulse and blood pressure are valuable markers of stress, and treatment by beta-blockers or clonidine can reduce the hyperarousal symptoms as well as the hypertension.

REFERENCES

Allden, K., Poole, C., Chantavanish, S., Ohmar, K., Aung, N., & Mollica, R. F. (1996). Burmese political dissidents in Thailand: Trauma and survival among young adults in exile. *American Journal of Public Health, 86,* 1561–1569.

Allodi, F. (1991). Assessment and treatment of torture victims: A critical review. *Journal of Nervous and Mental Disease, 179,* 4–11.

Allodi, F. (1998). The physician's role in assessing and treating torture and the PTSD syndrome. In J. Jaranson & M. Popkin (Eds.), *Caring for victims of torture* (pp. 89–106). Washington, DC: American Psychiatric Press.

American Psychiatric Association. (1980). *Diagnostic and statistical manual of mental disorders* (3rd ed.). Washington, DC: Author.

Arieli, A., & Aycheh, S. (1992). Psychopathology among Jewish Ethiopian immigrants to Israel. *Journal of Nervous and Mental Disease, 180,* 465–466.

Arroyo, W., & Eth, S. (1985). Children traumatized by Central American warfare. In S. Eth & R. S. Pynoos (Eds.), *Posttraumatic stress disorders in children* (pp. 101–120). Washington, DC: American Psychiatric Association Press.

Basoglu, M. (1992). Behavioural and cognitive approach in the treatment of torture-related psychological problems. In M. Basoglu (Ed.), *Torture and its consequences: Current treatment approaches* (pp. 402–429). Cambridge, UK: Cambridge University Press.

Basoglu, M. (1998). Behavioral and cognitive treatment of survivors of torture. In J.

Jaranson & M. Popkin (Eds.), *Caring for victims of torture* (pp. 131–148). Washington, DC: American Psychiatric Press.

Boehnlein, J. K., & Kinzie, J. D. (1993). Commentary–DSM diagnosis of posttraumatic stress disorder and cultural sensitivity: A response. *Journal of Nervous and Mental Disease, 180,* 597–599.

Boehnlein, J. K., Kinzie, J. D., Rath, B., & Fleck, J. (1985). One-year follow-up study of posttraumatic stress disorder among survivors of Cambodian concentration camps. *American Journal of Psychiatry, 142,* 956–959.

Breslau, N., Davis, G. C., Andreski, P., & Petersen, E. (1991). Traumatic events and posttraumatic stress disorder in an urban population of young adults. *Archives of General Psychiatry, 48,* 216–222.

Bustos, E. (1992). Psychodynamic approaches in the treatment of torture survivors. In M. Basoglu (Ed.), *Torture and its consequences: Current treatment approaches* (pp. 333–347). Cambridge, UK: Cambridge University Press.

Carlson, E. B., & Rosser-Hogan, R. (1991). Trauma experiences, posttraumatic stress, dissociation, and depression in Cambodian refugees. *American Journal of Psychiatry, 148,* 1548–1551.

Chester, B., & Jaranson, J. (1994). The context of survival and destruction: Conducting psychotherapy with survivors of torture. *National Center for Post Traumatic Stress Disorder [Palo Alto, CA], Clinical Newsletter, 4*(1), 17–20.

Cheung, P. (1994). Posttraumatic stress disorders among Cambodian refugees in New Zealand. *International Journal of Social Psychiatry, 40,* 17–26.

Cottler, L. B., Compton, L. B., Mager, D., Spitznagel, E. L., & Janca, A. (1992). Posttraumatic stress disorder among substance users from the general population. *American Journal of Psychiatry, 149,* 664–670.

Dadfur, A. (1994). The Afghans: Bearing the scars of a forgotten war. In A. Marsella, T. Borneman, S. Ekblad, & J. Orley (Eds.), *Amidst peril and pain* (pp. 125–140). Washington, DC: American Psychological Association.

Drees, A. (1989). Guidelines for a short-term therapy of a torture depression. *Journal of Traumatic Stress, 2*(4), 549–554.

Eisenbruk, M. (1991). From post-traumatic stress disorder to cultural bereavement: Diagnosis of Southeast Asian refugees. *Social Science Medicine, 3,* 673–680.

Ekblad, S., Kohn, R., & Jansson, B. (1998). Psychological and cultural aspects of immigration and mental health. In S. O. Okpaku (Ed.), *Clinical methods in transcultural psychiatry* (pp. 42–66). Washington, DC: American Psychiatric Press.

Farias, P. J. (1991). Emotional distress and its socio-political correlates in Salvadoran refugees: Analysis of a clinical sample. *Culture, Medicine and Psychiatry, 15,* 167–192.

Fischman, Y., & Ross, J. (1990). Group treatment of exiled survivors of torture. *American Journal of Orthopsychiatry, 60*(1), 135–142.

Jaranson, J. (1991). Psychotherapeutic medication. In J. Westermeyer, C. L. Williams, & A. N. Nguyen (Eds.), *Mental health services for refugees* (DHHS Publication No. ADM 91-1824, pp. 132–145). Washington, DC: U.S. Government Printing Office.

Keane, T. M., Albano, A. M., & Blake, D. D. (1992). Current trends in the treatment of posttraumatic stress symptoms. In M. Basoglu (Ed.), *Torture and its consequences: Current treatment approaches* (pp. 363–401). Cambridge, UK: Cambridge University Press.

Kilpatrick, D. G., Saunders, B. E., Amick-McMullan, A., Best, C. L., Veronen, L. J., & Resnick, H. S. (1989). Victim and crime factors associated with the development of crime-related posttraumatic stress disorder. *Behavior Therapy, 20,* 199–214.

Kinzie, J. D. (1985). Cultural aspects of psychiatric treatment with Indochinese refugees. *American Journal of Social Psychiatry, 5*(1), 47–53.

Kinzie, J. D. (1991). Development, staffing and structure of psychiatric clinics. In J. Westermeyer, C. L. Williams, & A. N. Nguyen (Eds.), *Mental health services for refugees* (DHHS Publication No. ADM 91-1824, pp. 146–156). Washington, DC: U.S. Government Printing Office.

Kinzie, J. D., & deRi, T. (1998). Ethnicity and Psychopharmacology: The experience of Southeast Asians. In S. O. Okpaku (Ed.), *Clinical methods in transcultural psychiatry* (pp. 171–190). Washington, DC: American Psychiatric Press.

Kinzie, J. D., & Boehnlein, J. K. (1989). Posttraumatic psychosis among Cambodian refugees. *Journal of Traumatic Stress, 2,* 185–198.

Kinzie, J. D., Boehnlein, J. K., Leung, P., Moore, L., Riley, C., & Smith, D. (1990). The prevalence of posttraumatic stress disorder and its clinical significance among Southeast Asian refugees. *American Journal of Psychiatry, 147,* 913–917.

Kinzie, J. D., Denny, D., Riley, C., Boehnlein, J. K., McFarland, B., & Leung, P. (1998). A cross-cultural study of reactivation of PTSD symptoms. *Journal of Nervous and Mental Disease, 186,* 670–676.

Kinzie, J. D., & Fleck, J. (1987). Psychotherapy with severely traumatized refugees. *American Journal of Psychotherapy, 41*(1), 82–94.

Kinzie, J. D., Fredrickson, R. H., Rath, B., & Fleck, J. (1984). Post-traumatic stress disorder among survivors of Cambodian concentration camps. *American Journal of Psychiatry, 141,* 645–650.

Kinzie, J. D., & Leung, P. (1989). Clonidine in Cambodian patients with post-traumatic stress disorder. *Journal of Nervous and Mental Disease, 177*(9), 546–550.

Kinzie, J. D., Leung, P., Bui, A., Ben, R., Keopraseuth, K. O., Riley, C., Fleck, J., & Ades, M. (1988). Cultural factors in group therapy with Southeast Asian refugees. *Community Mental Health Journal, 24,* 157–166.

Kinzie, J. D., & Manson, S. M. (1983). Five-years' experience with Indochinese refugee patients. *Journal of Operational Psychiatry, 11*(2), 105–111.

Kinzie, J. D., Sack, W. H., Angell, R. H., & Clarke, G. (1989). A three-year follow-up of Cambodian young people traumatized as children. *Journal of the American Academy of Psychiatry, 28,* 501–504.

Kinzie, J. D., Sack, W. H., Angell, R. H., & Manson, S. (1986). The psychiatric effects of massive trauma on Cambodian children: I. The children. *Journal of the American Academy of Child Psychiatry, 25,* 370–376.

Kinzie, J. D., Sack, R. L., & Riley, C. M. (1994). The polysomnographic effects of clonidine on sleep disorders in posttraumatic stress disorder: A pilot study with Cambodian patients. *Journal of Nervous and Mental Disease, 182,* 585–587.

Kinzie, J. D., Leung, P., Boehnlein, J., & Fleck, J. (1987). Antidepressant blood levels in Southeast Asians: Clinical and cultural implications. *Journal of Nervous Mental Disease, 175,* 480–485.

Kroll, J., Habenicht, M., Mackenzie, T., Yang, M., Chan, S., Vang, T., Nguyen, T., Ly, M., Phommesouvanh, B., Nguyen, H., Vang, Y., Souvannasoth, L., & Cabugao, R. (1989). Depression and posttraumatic stress disorder in Southeast Asian refugees. *American Journal of Psychiatry, 146,* 1592–1597.

Kulka, R. A., Schlenger, W. E., Fairbanks, J. A., Hough, R. L., Jordan, B. K., Marmar, C. R., & Weise, D. S. (1990). *The National Vietnam Veterans Readjustment Study*. New York: Brunner/Mazel.

Leopold, M., & Harrell-Bond, B. (1994). An overview of the world refugee crisis. In A. Marsella, T. Bornemann, S. Ekblad, & J. Orley (Eds.), *Amidst peril and pain* (pp. 17–32). Washington, DC: American Psychological Association.

Lin, K., Poland, R., & Nagasaki, G. (Eds.). (1993). *Psychopharmacology and psychobiology of ethnicity*. Washington, DC: APA Press.

Mghir, R., Freed, W., Raskin, L., & Katon, W. (1995). Depression and posttraumatic stress disorder among a community sample of adolescent and young Afghan refugees. *Journal of Nervous and Mental Disease, 183*, 24–30.

Mollica, R. (1988). The trauma story: The psychiatric care of refugee survivors of violence and torture. In F. M. Ochberg (Ed.), *Post-traumatic therapy and victims of violence* (pp. 295–314). New York: Brunner/Mazel.

Mollica, R. (1994). Southeastern Asian refugees migration, history and mental health issues. In A. Marsella, T. Bornemann, S. Ekblad & J. Orley (Eds.), *Amidst peril and pain* (pp. 83–100). Washington, DC: American Psychological Association.

Morris, P., & Silove, D. (1992). Cultural influences in psychotherapy with refugee survivors of torture and trauma. *Hospital and Community Psychiatry, 43*, 820–824.

Norris, F. (1992). Epidemiology of trauma: Frequency and impact of different potentially traumatic events on different demographic events. *Journal of Consulting and Clinical Psychology, 60*, 409–418.

Sack W. H., Clarke, G. N., & Seeley, J. (1996). Multiple forms of stress in Cambodian adolescent refugees. *Child Development, 67*, 107–116.

Sack, W. H., Seeley, J. R., & Clarke, G. N. (1997). Does PTSD transcend cultural barriers? A Study from the Khmer adolescent refugee project. *Journal of the American Academy of Adolescent Psychiatry, 36*, 49–54.

Silove, D., Sinnesbrink, I., Field, A., Manicavasagan, V., & Steel, Z. (1997). Anxiety, depression and PTSD in asylum-seekers: Associations with pre-migration trauma and post migration stressors. *British Journal of Psychiatry, 170*, 351–357.

Silove, D., Steel, Z., McGarry, P., & Mohan, P. (1998). Trauma exposure, post-migration stressors and symptoms of anxiety, depression and posttraumatic stress in Tamil asylum seekers: Comparison with refugees and immigrants. *Acta Psychiatrica Scandanavica, 97*, 175–181.

Somnier, F., & Genefke, I. (1986). Psychotherapy for victims of torture. *British Journal of Psychiatry, 149*, 323–329.

Thompson, M., & McGarry, P. (1995). Psychological sequelae of torture and trauma in Chilean and Salvadorean migrants: A pilot study. *Australia and New Zealand Journal of Psychiatry, 29*, 84–95.

Tseng, W. S. (1997). Overview: Culture and psychotherapy. In W. S. Tseng & J. Streltzer (Eds.), *Culture and psychopathology: A guide to clinical assessment* (pp. 1–27). New York: Brunner/Mazel.

Tseng, W. S., & Strelzer, J. (1997). Integration and conclusions. In W. S. Tseng & J. Streltzer (Eds.), *Culture and psychopathology: A guide to clinical assessment* (pp. 241–252). New York: Brunner/Mazel.

Varvin, S., & Hauff, E. (1998). Psychotherapy with patients who have been tortured. In J. Jaranson & M. Popkin (Eds.), *Caring for victims of torture* (pp. 117–129). Washington, DC: American Psychiatric Press.

Vesti, P., & Kastrup, K. (1992). Psychotherapy for torture survivors. In M. Basoglu (Ed.), *Torture and its consequences: Current treatment approaches* (pp. 348–362). Cambridge, UK: Cambridge University Press.

Weine, S. (1997). *Bosnian survivors: Memories and witnessing—After Dayton.* Paper presented at the annual meeting of the American Psychiatric Association, San Diego.

Weine, S. M., Becker, D. F., McGlashan, T. H., Lamb, P., Lazrove, S., Vojuoda, D., & Hyman, L. (1995). Psychiatric consequences of "ethnic cleansing": Clinical assessments and trauma testimonies of newly resettled Bosnian refugees. *American Journal of Psychiatry, 152,* 536–542.

Weine, S., Vojuoda, D., Hartman, S., & Hyman, L. (1997). A family survives genocide. *Psychiatry, 60,* 24–39.

Westermeyer, J. J. (1993). Cross-cultural psychiatric assessment. In A. C. Gow (Ed.), *Culture, ethnicity and mental illness* (pp. 125–144). Washington, DC: American Psychiatric Press.

Yamamoto, J., Selva, J. A., Justice, L. R., Chang, C. Y., & Leong, G. B. (1993). Cross-cultural psychotherapy. In A. C. Gow (Ed.), *Culture, ethnicity and mental illness* (pp. 101–124). Washington, DC: American Psychiatric Press.

Young, M. (1998). Psychological consequences of torture: Clinical needs of refugee women. In S. O. Okpaku (Ed.), *Clinical methods in transcultural psychiatry* (pp. 391–411). Washington, DC: American Psychiatric Press.

12

Treatment Methods for Childhood Trauma

KATHLEEN NADER

The possible long-term consequences of childhood traumatic exposure have been well-documented (see Table 12.1). This and an outbreak of school shootings over the last 15 years (sometimes perpetrated by individuals traumatized as children) have underscored the need for effective treatment interventions for traumatized children. It was not until the mid-1900s that we began to engage in a close examination of children's traumatic reactions (A. Freud , 1965; A. Freud & Burlingham, 1943; Carey-Trefzer, 1949; Bloch, Silber, & Perry, 1956; Lacey, 1972; Levy, 1945; Terr, 1979). In the last quarter of the 20th century we learned to interview and assist children directly regarding their traumatic responses (Terr, 1979; Eth & Pynoos, 1985; Nader, 1996a), and in the 1980s and 1990s we developed and adapted a number of treatment methods to address these reactions. Clinicians who have adapted methods or successfully used these adaptations for traumatized children have contributed to descriptions of these methods in this chapter.

Multiple issues affect a child's symptomatic presentation and needs in treatment. Field and laboratory studies have examined topics such as developmental issues, cultural issues, attachment styles, temperament, personality, and memory in children. A number of these issues are addressed by childhood trauma treatment methods discussed in this chapter. We have made great strides in reducing the symptoms of posttraumatic stress disorder (PTSD) and associated symptoms such as depression in children. In determining the long-term results of our interventions, however, it will be neces-

TABLE 12.1. Possible Results of Unresolved Trauma

Results	Some examples
Influenced life	Reasonably normal life influenced by experience (e.g., may affect expectations, attitudes, interactions, choices, and behaviors; may create vulnerabilities)
Changes in personal traits	Changes in cognitive ability, morality and/or normal mood; reduced confidence; inhibitions; increased aggression
Disturbances in interpersonal functioning	Choosing friends who have been or feel victimized; loss of friends; irritability/bullying; withdrawal; isolation
Cognitive dysfunction	Memory and concentration problems; inhibited imagination; confusion; delayed processing of information
Mental health disturbances	Chronic or complicated PTSD; substance-related disorders; conduct, mood, anxiety, somatoform, eating, sleep, impulse control, personality, and/or dissociative disorders
Attempts at numbing emotions	A style of confusion, self-distraction, or distracting others; substance or medication abuse; varying levels of dissociation
Compulsive repetition of traumatic behaviors and sequences	Dangerous risk taking; reenactments of aspects of the event such as promiscuity or prostitution after molestation, aggressive acts when dressed like an assailant, or feeling choked and exhausted any time adrenalin increases; provoking attacks
Attempts at self-punishment or warding off	Provoking attacks; poor self-care; repeated poor choices with problematic results; self-isolation; self-mutilation
Repetitive somatic complaints or general ill health	Aches and pains such as stomachaches, body aches, headaches; deficient immune response

Note. See Garbarino, Kostelny, and Dubrow (1991); Herman, Perry, and van der Kolk (1989); Nader (1996a, 1996b, 1997); Nader and Fairbanks (1994); Nader and Pynoos (1993); Pynoos and Nader (1988); Pynoos et al. (1987); Terr (1991); van der Kolk and Sapporta (1991); Nader, Blake, and Kriegler (1994).

sary to recognize, define, and measure components of a child's experience and response in addition to PTSD and associated disorders.

FACTORS INFLUENCING PRESENTATION, TREATMENT, AND OUTCOME

Treatment issues vary in response to the nature of the traumatic experience (Terr, 1991; Nader, 1997) and characteristics of the child (e.g., personality, experience, or age). A number of factors affecting presentation and treatment are discussed below. Examining the exact effect of any element is complicated by the interaction of elements. For example, abused children have increased aggression and conduct problems more often than do nonabused children (Dodge, Bates, Pettit, & Valente, 1995). Yet, multiple factors may contribute to aggressive behavioral development (e.g., genetic predisposition, social cognitions, temperament, neighborhood quality, neurochemical actions, conflict ridden attachments, coercive discipline, or chronic goal blocking) (Dodge et al., 1995).

Age and Developmental Issues

For children, those clinicians treating traumatic stress must consider the affect of age on traumatic experience and response as well as the effect of trauma on the child's continuing development. Developmental issues influence children's experience, symptomatic presentation, behavior in treatment, and course of recovery. These developmental influences affect children's appraisals of threat, meanings assigned to aspects of the event, emotional and cognitive coping, capacities to tolerate their reactions, and abilities to address secondary life changes (Pynoos & Nader, 1993). In addition to traumatic effects similar to those experienced by adults, children's catastrophic experiences can disrupt normal development including, for example, aspects of memory (Siegel, 1996), morality and conscience (Garbarino, Kostelney, & Dubrow, 1991), basic trust and interpersonal attachment (James, 1994), and cognitive and personality development. Age may not only influence perception and meaning attributed to aspects of the traumatic experience but may also affect the aspects of the event that take initial prominence. For example, the importance of a parent to survival (James, 1994, pp. 7, 24–27) may influence the initial focus of a young child's experience. When he was 3 years old, Donnie's mother was murdered in front of him by her boyfriend. The man put the gun in Donnie's mouth but removed it instead of shooting him. In his first session, Donnie's pictures and gestures were focused on the blood in his mother's hair. He twirled his finger as though around a curl when he told the therapist he had a picture of his mother when her hair was pretty. If he had been older, his initial focus might have been the gun in his mouth rather than the look of his dead mother.

Developmental/Age Groups

Because of trauma-induced regressions or precocious development and the interaction of age and other factors (e.g., culture, child traits, previous experience, and/or aspects of the trauma), the effects of age on traumatic experience and response (and vice versa) are complex. Moreover, the competence achieved in one phase affects each subsequent phase (Combrinck-Graham, 1991). The descriptions below generally apply to Western cultures and may vary somewhat within them.

Preschool.   Younger children may suffer more personality and behavioral changes following traumatic exposure (Kostelny & Garbarino, 1994; Terr, 1979). Young children are dependent upon adults for nurture and safety (Macksoud, Dyregrov, & Raundalen, 1993). Threats to caregivers as well as to loved ones or direct threats to children's lives may increase their risk for traumatization (Scheeringa & Zeanah, 1995; Rossman, Bingham, & Emde, 1997). In life and in treatment, youngsters may initially react with anxious attachment or with separation or stranger anxiety (Macksoud et al., 1993).

Young children are more concrete in their thinking (Lewis, 1995). For this age group, literal interpretations, animistic thinking, faulty hypotheses, and inaccurate associations are common (Murray & Son, 1998). For example, what occurs in proximity (space and time) may be seen as causal. Also, distinguishing "one" from "more" is problematic; the notion that one man is bad may be generalized to all men. Although interpretations may be literal, statements may not be. For example, "I hate you" may mean dislike of what you are doing (Murray & Son, 1998).

After the age of 2, children can show what did and did not happen. Preschoolers are better at identifying familiar people and details relevant to their lives (Murray & Son, 1998). Between the ages of 2 and 7, children can mentally represent information but not yet integrate the information in a logical manner (Piaget, 1952a). Between 18 months and 2 years of age, children begin to use symbolic play and language to represent experience (Piaget, 1956, pp. 335–338). Young children demonstrate, in their play, their perceptual memories in the absence of verbal memory for their experiences (Terr, 1985). Superpowerful and giant figures (e.g., dinosaurs, heroes/heroines) that represent perceived powerful and idealized human figures in their lives may be represented in their play (Lewis, 1991). Preschool children move easily from one focus of attention to another and are easily distracted. They may become frightened during traumatic play and stop. In this event children may be able to continue after being comforted or after distracting themselves temporarily. For example, Susie was traumatized at 18 months in a car accident. At age 2, she had the therapist move a toy car on one side of a road in her direction while she moved a car on the other side in the other direction. Every time the cars approached each other, Susie froze. After the therapist verbalized how scary it was for the cars to come close, Susie stopped and began play with dolls before returning to the car play. This pattern repeated for weeks until Susie could permit the cars to pass each other.

Between the ages of 3 and 9, children develop the ability to express their metacognitive thoughts (i.e., thoughts about thinking) (Siegel, 1996). These accomplishments are important to integrated personality development. Children learn that the appearance of something is distinct from its reality; that other people may think differently; that one person can experience simultaneously multiple emotions; that thoughts can change; that beliefs and desires are associated with emotions, and emotions influence behavior (Siegel, 1996);

and that more than one factor can influence an outcome (Murray & Son, 1998). For the preschool child at the beginning of these accomplishments, emotional and intellectual problems are still difficult to solve, fantasy and reality still poorly differentiated, and affects difficult to conceptualize (Lewis, 1991).

School Age.   In the stage of concrete operations (Piaget, 1962), children increase their objectivity and bring their thinking into line with others (Combrinck-Graham, 1991; see the preceding subsection). School-age children are becoming socialized and are trying to construct an orderly and lawful world (Lewis, 1991). They develop what Combrinck-Graham (1991) has called "interpersonally accountable, independent competence" (p. 258). This phase lacks sexuality, self-sufficiency, or the ability to assume complete care of others. Under ideal circumstances, the family environment remains important; children move between family and peer milieux, bringing back input while still holding family in esteem (Combrinck-Graham, 1991). Some clinicians have suggested that during the period in which the sexes dislike each other, same sex groups may be more advantageous than mixed groups (Murray & Son, 1998).

At this age, children can readily depict, in thought and in play, the intense wishes that may have occurred during or after a traumatic event (e.g., fantasized interventions or escapes). They are able to focus on more than one aspect of a situation at a time, are able to grasp changes throughout a sequence of events (not just the beginning and end), can form mental pictures and describe sequences of events without performing them, and are aware that some actions can be reversed by subsequent actions (Brodzinsky, Gormly, & Ambron, 1986, pp. 220–223).

Adolescence.   Issues of dependence/independence, invulnerability/ vulnerability, real/ideal, competence/incompetence, relationship of self to others, and the transition to adulthood are of particular importance for adolescents. These issues may manifest in a variety of ways. If one or both parents have been killed, an adolescent may unconsciously seek to replace the relationship with one or both parents with a girlfriend or boyfriend or with a peer or an adult. This may occur whether the relationship was cherished or conflicted. Factors of adolescence and the event may change the relationship with either or both parents and may complicate development. For example, in a conflicted situation an adolescent may avidly defend an offending parent against the other. In a depressive fugue-like state, Cindy's father stabbed her mother and brother and then stabbed Cindy several times in the head. Her need to defend and support him (and protect her ability to keep him in her life) against an angry mother, a court charged with protecting the children, and others made it difficult for her to process other feelings related to her experience. It placed this previously well-behaved child in stronger opposition against her disciplinarian mother and in staunch defense of an absent mild-mannered and depressed father. Children of any age may need acceptance and facilitation of intense and opposing emotions and attitudes.

Although image is important to adolescents, with a good therapeutic relationship and a safe and private setting, adolescents can and do participate fully in treatment, and they may regress. For example, between ages 14 and 16, John started every session by either protesting that he did not need treatment or reporting his friends' similar comments about him. After a few or many minutes, he described the painful details of a public shooting in which he and a friend were multiply wounded and other friends were killed. Frequently, while demonstrating events, he took toys or used imaginary people in war zones as he lapsed into symbolic play. On a few occasions, he engaged in play with toys as though he were a very young child—the play appeared unrelated to the trauma but represented a progression of previously delayed developmental phases that had occurred in the absence of his estranged father.

Interaction of Age and Other Factors

When treatment is tailored to the youth's evolving needs, the youth's current presentation rather than age takes prominence in setting the tone and focus of treatment. The influence of age upon traumatic response becomes intertwined with other factors (e.g., personality; role in family; aspects of the experience, or the reawakening of earlier developmental issues). The following three cases illustrate this interaction. At 16 years old, Isabel and Susan each experienced the traumatic deaths of their fathers. Ann was sexually molested between the ages of 3 and 12. Isabel and Ann were each the eldest child with one younger brother. Both were responsible, intelligent, and had leadership qualities. Although other ongoing responses for the two were linked to specific aspects of their very different individual traumatic experiences, despite age differences, Isabel and Ann exhibited some similar qualities. Both became extremely independent, took on parenting responsibilities in the family, became distressed if not in charge or control of a situation, but were fatigued and otherwise affected by so much responsibility, became a "one-person show," and exhibited specific traumatic symptoms when stressed. In contrast, Susan's father was shot when she was 16. She was the middle child of three (two brothers), was close to her father, and felt protected and cherished by him. Unlike Isabel, she became overly dependent upon her mother after her experience.

Issues that may be important to the development of character and personality and that may be prominent at one age or phase may still be significant at other ages. For example, issues of trust and protection that are important for infants and preschoolers may become factors for older children, adolescents, and adults. These issues may take prominence in the course of treatment as previously unresolved aspects of trust and protection or because the traumatic experience has challenged faith in normal/harmless human responses or a sense of safety. Attendance to physical needs, restoration of a sense of safety, and issues related to trust are important to trauma survivors of all ages.

Precocious Development

A loss of innocence or a precocious development may occur in a variety of forms for traumatized children. Children have premature concerns about the world (Terr, 1991), and if exposure has been ongoing they may even be able to describe emotions (e.g., responses to ongoing violence) unfamiliar to children who have enjoyed a normal sense of safety (Nader, 1996a). Traumatic experiences result in premature knowledge (e.g., sexual; vulnerability of adults) and atypical characteristics. For example, normally, between ages 3 and 7, children report few dreams upon being awakened from REM (rapid eye movement) sleep; dreams contain few human characters (animals are more often present) (Foulkes, 1990; Foulkes, Hollifield, Sullivan, Bradley, & Terry, 1990). At ages 11 to 12, dreaming begins to approximate that of adulthood and children are able to construct a dream narrative (Westerlund & Johnson, 1989). Some traumatized preschool children have dreams more like those described by older children. Following a long series of hospital procedures, a 3-year-old girl dreamed of "cutters"coming to cut her and her efforts to get away. A 5-year-old boy with relapsed leukemia began to dream of space men coming to take him to their planet. In his early dreams he was afraid of them. He died a few months after he developed a comfortable relationship with them in his dreams (Nader, 1996b).

Regression

Following traumatic experiences, individuals may be regressed much of the time or may regress spontaneously, for example, in response to traumatic reminders or in the safety of the therapeutic setting. Even adolescents and adults may function at more primitive levels, for example, more concrete and literal levels of processing information and/or easier distraction. Traumatized children may indulge in play at older ages than nontraumatized youth (Nader, 1997; Terr, 1989).

It is important that clinicians, parents, and teachers learn to identify specific regressive tendencies. Childlike behaviors are common under some normal circumstances (e.g., during anger, playfulness, or endearment). Moreover, regression may be as subtle as a reawakened desire for a person, place, or situation that signifies good or safe feelings. Regressions (e.g., loss of skills) may be complicated or exaggerated by other symptoms (e.g., changed biochemistry, lack of sleep, cognitive difficulties, or preoccupations). Consequently, regression may be difficult to recognize. In children, it may be interpreted as laziness, sloppiness, defiance, or attention-getting behavior.

Moral Development

Single or multiple childhood traumatic experiences may challenge moral development in a number of ways. In response to L. Kohlberg's three major proposed stages of moral development and C. Gilligan's suggestion of gender differences (Lewis, 1991; Wolff, 1991; Yates, 1991), Stillwell, Galvin, and Kopta (1991) constructed an empirical model of conscience through analysis of normal children (see Table 12.2). This model traces children's moral development from a conscience in which they trust the knowledge and power of adults to a mature conscience with flexibility.

Even one traumatic experience may challenge a child's belief in adult (and/or divine) wisdom and ability and may challenge belief in reasons for "being good" (Nader & Pynoos, 1993). Ongoing familial violence (e.g., abuse, molestation, domestic violence) disrupts these aspects of morality and engen-

TABLE 12.2. An Empirical Model of the Development of Conscience in Normal Children

Conscience	Description
External (before age 6)	"Big people know best;" accept limits and punishments; find badness or goodness in actions/objects as defined by external authority; fail to abstract moral rules from experiences
Brain or heart (modal age 7)	Rules derived from experiences; child consults brain or heart (and often authority figures for certainty); imitation, identification, and obedience to avoid punishment or to be found pleasing
Heart/mind or personified (modal age 12)	As early as age 9, rule-governed moral experience mastered; more attention focused on affective aspects; choices generally remain right or wrong; desire to respond to others' emotions; grown-ups not always right; someone older and wiser—like God—might know better; desire to please and be found pleasing by adults; personified conscience may develop as an internal representation with capacity for relationship, argumentation, inspiration, or generation of fear, shame, and guilt
Confused (modal age 15)	Characterized by confusion, indecisiveness, and struggles with "gray" areas of good and evil; challenges of peer culture and the popular culture; competition between adult and peer authority
Integrated (modal age 17)	Characterized by flexibility, recognizing more than two options; understanding the overlap of good and evil; a return of confidence regarding moral issues; increased modulation of moral emotions; understanding, benevolence, and optimism

Source: Data from Stillwell et al. (1991).

ders issues of betrayal, modeling, identification, and reenactment (Zeanah & Zeanah, 1989). In addition to what is learned by ongoing witnessing/experiencing of violence, children in inner cities and in war zones across the world are exposed to and drawn into ongoing confrontations that, when devoid of an ideological interpretation, may result in a hopelessness and despair that lead to within-group violence, depression, and self-hatred (Garbarino et al., 1991).

Noting that most people justify killing if it is necessary (e.g., in war, or to protect someone from danger), Garbarino (1999) suggests that inner-city children exposed to ongoing violence who kill may do so based on a moral code dominated by a troubled emotional life and an intense personal need for justice as well as a different idea of what is necessary for survival. For example, after retrieving with a gun his own stolen chain from another boy, Calvin shot the boy in the head, later explaining that he did so to avoid being in danger of reprisal from the boy in the future (Garbarino, 1999).

Children's Memories

Memories contribute to an individual's sense of identity, continuity, and predictability in life (Lewis, 1995). They are key to many methods of intervention for traumatized children. Many treatment methods include verbal review (sometimes repeatedly) of traumatic events or episodes (Pynoos, Nader, & March, 1991). Even young children can and do accurately recall, over considerable time, participatory and nonparticipatory (e.g., witnessing), single-incident or ongoing traumatic experiences (Howe, 1997; Lewis, 1995). A study of initial and 6-month recall of preschoolers (30, 36, and 48 months old) has indicated an increase in memory with age and their ability to recall considerable information about their traumatic experiences, whether or not they had initial intrusive thoughts (Howe, Courage, & Peterson, 1995). In a study of children 18 months to 5 years old who had undergone emergency room treatments, there was little decline in memory of central aspects of events although decline in memory of peripheral issues was substantial (Howe, 1997). Even when there is a tendency to "dissociate" during an experience (e.g., see Lindsay & Read, 1995), memory for the experience as well as the dissociated object (e.g., a spot on the ceiling) may be well preserved. Although there is some evidence with abuse cases that the probability of remembering can increase as a function of the number of abuse incidents (Goleman, 1992; Howe, 1997), repeated exposure to similar events may result in memories that blend or solidify into a single script-like representation. Individual incidents may lose their uniqueness, details may become blurred (Lindsay & Read, 1995; Howe, 1997; Terr, 1994), and modulation of cortisol output may occur (Gunnar et al., 1996).

Children under the age of 6 have more difficulty distinguishing fact from fantasy and may confound what they did with what they thought of doing. They are, however, able to distinguish their thoughts from other people's actions (Lewis, 1995). Distortions of time and space have been observed in children following traumas (Terr, 1983; Pynoos & Nader, 1989). Some researchers have found that children try to fill in gaps in their memories by confabulating; however, if given prompts or cues, children remember quite well (Lewis, 1995; Johnson & Foley, 1984). Pynoos and Nader (1989) found that children incorporate their wishful thinking into their unassisted retelling of a traumatic event. However, they were able to report their experiences accurately when assisted to begin at a specific point and proceed through the details of the event.

Although children can accurately recall and retain memories of an event, faulty pre- and postevent information can result in distortions in recall (Siegel, 1996). It is important that clinicians avoid introducing these confusions. For nontraumatic events, children aged 3 and 4 are more suggestible than 5- and 6-year-olds. By the age of 4, children usually resist attempts to suggest a history of abuse. Children may have difficulty challenging their parents' perceptions of events, however, and if repeatedly told something did not occur will come to doubt their own perceptions. Studies of small samples of adults suggest that individuals with higher scores on measures of creative imagination or dissociation are more likely to recover false or previously unavailable true events when asked to form a mental image of an event (International Society for Traumatic Stress Studies [ISTSS], 1998).

Under normal circumstances, distinctive, unique, and personally consequential experiences are best remembered and distinctive items are the easiest to learn and hardest to forget (Howe, 1997). In studies of children in stressful situations, there is evidence that corticosterone (an adrenal stress hormone) impairs memory (McEwen, 1982). In contrast to this is a wealth of evidence that traumatic experiences produce detailed memories that are etched in and long lasting (Terr, 1991; Koss, Figueredo, Bell, Tharan, & Tromp, 1996, p. 421; Nader, 1997; Pynoos & Eth, 1985). In fact, memories for highly emotional episodes contain information not found in other recall narratives, including a focus on beliefs that have been violated due to the nature of the event (Howe, 1997; Stein, Wade, & Liwag, 1996). There is evidence that, in addition to PTSD and comorbid symptomatology, these intense traumatic impressions can result in troublesome ongoing patterns of behavior (see below).

State of mind at the time of encoding information or events may determine their accessibility to later retrieval (Siegel, 1996). For example, if one is presently sad, it can be easier to recall events experienced when one was sad in the past. A state of mind can include dominant emotional tone, perceptual biases, behavioral response patterns, and increased accessibility of particular (explicit or implicit) memories. Activation profiles may include clusters of emotional tones, associated sensations, memories, and mental models. For dissociatively disordered patients, shifts in state of mind can be accompanied by various degrees of memory barriers (Siegel, 1996).

One hypothesis suggests that experiences that deviate too much from the prevailing knowledge and context may be harder to encode and retain (Howe, 1997). This has been posed as an explanation for traumatic experiences not remembered. Moreover, when reactivity levels are lower (perhaps due to temperamental predispositions, better coping skills, or sensitivity in support from caregivers) children may, in fact, encode, store, and elaborate more about unique and stressful situations than individuals with high reactivity (Howe, 1997; Murray & Son, 1998). Physicians have sometimes told children that they would never regain specific memories of injuries—especially head injuries. Nevertheless, these "lost memories" have been regained in a process of step-by-step review and re-review (Nader & Mello, 2000). Creating a therapeutic environment is conducive to remembering (McCann & Pearlman, 1990, p. 23; Parson, 2000). For example, while an 8-year-old girl was sitting on a bench in a laundromat, a car drove through the glass wall of the laundromat, propelling her headfirst into the corner of a washing machine. The doctor told her she would never regain memory of the time surrounding hitting the washing machine because of her head injury. In the course of therapy, she was able to regain memory of the moments preceding, during, and after the impact, relieving an ongoing sense of confusion and separateness from her family members and enabling additional trauma work. Similarly, a girl regained memories of being hit by a flying table during a tornado. Her self-esteem improved in realizing aspects of her response, and her readiness to tackle other aspects of traumatic response improved.

The Child's Personality and Experience

Recognizing the uniqueness of an individual and his or her experience is essential. Even if in the same room for the same trauma, each person's experience will have variations in description, focus, perspective, meaning, and impact. Qualities such as culture (Heras, 1992; Marsella, Friedman, Gerrity, & Scurfield, 1996; Nader, Dubrow, & Stamm, 1999), temperament, and previous experience all play a part in children's responses to traumatic experience and to treatment. Gender, race, and locus of control have been associated with differences in children's traumatic responses (Joseph, Brewin, Yule, & Williams, 1991, 1993; March, Amaya-Jackson, Terry, & Costanzo, 1997; Shannon, Lonnigan, Finch, & Taylor, 1994). Some of these findings may have been confounded by their coexistence with other factors. For example, some of the effects of ethnicity on response may be accounted for by ecological factors (Dodge, Bates, Pettit, & Valente, 1995) or exposure levels (March, Amaya-Jackson, et al., 1997).

Temperament

We have a great deal more to learn about how children's temperaments and styles interact with traumatic reactions, treatment presentation, and long-term results. Moreover, theorists define temperament differently (Brodzinsky et al., 1986, pp. 111–120). Nevertheless, disparate theorists underscore the importance of treating the child as an individual and respecting behavioral style (Berens, 1985; Chess & Thomas, 1991; Keirsey & Bates, 1978).

One theoretical view focuses on the infant's unique way of responding to the world. For many infants, the 9 main criteria—activity level, rhythmicity or regularity of biological functions, approach or withdrawal to new stimuli, adaptability, threshold of responsiveness, intensity of reaction, quality of mood, distractibility, and attention span/persistence—cluster into three types: the easy baby, the difficult baby, and the slow-to-warm baby (Chess & Thomas, 1991; Thomas & Chess, 1977). There is evidence that, in Western culture, the difficult baby is more prone to develop a behavior disorder by age 9. However, children studied who did not develop the disorder had been given opportunities to adapt at their own slow pace and were not denigrated for their negative moods. For this 20-year study, the lack of persistence of temperament clusters suggests increasing environmental and perhaps biological influences on temperament over time (Chess & Thomas, 1991).

Another theoretical view is based on Carl Jung's idea that people favor one of different combinations of four mental functions: sensation versus intuition (focus on concrete vs. abstract realities) and thinking versus feeling (objective vs. subjective judgment criteria). Jung described eight types, each characterized by the predominance of one of the functions expressed in either an extraverted or introverted way (Berens & Nardi, 1999; Berens, 1985, 1998; Jung, 1971; Myers & McCaulley, 1985). Myers (1980) added judging versus perceiving (wanting things settled vs. keeping options open) (see also Myers & McCaulley, 1985). Keirsey and Bates (1978) outlined four main temperaments and related them to Myers' 16 types (see also Keirsey, 1987). Following Keirsey's lead, Delunas (1992) suggests that, in addition to its influence on the way individuals approach life and treatment, temperament makes an individual prone to specific psychological difficulties.

Even when a child's preexisting temperament can be identified, trauma changes aspects of temperament. For example, children may become more concrete in focus and/or more difficult behaviorally. It is essential to approach a child at her or his current level and manner of functioning, recognizing her or his own rhythm and posttrauma needs (Nader, 1997).

Attachment

A number of treatments for childhood trauma focus wholly or in part upon assisting the development of secure attachments or healing trauma-related attachment problems (Culbertson & Willis, 1998; James, 1994; Parson, 2000). A secure attachment is adaptive and derives from the infant's confidence that his or her help-seeking signals will receive prompt and appropriate adult response. If quality of care is inconsistent, sporadic, or regularly insensitive, infants develop insecure attachments (Ainsworth, 1973; Bowlby, 1969, 1973; Thompson, 1991). Several theorists believe that early attachment styles become "working models" governing significant social ties or interactions throughout life (Bowlby, 1973; Bretherton, 1990; Main, Kaplan, & Cassidy, 1985). Moreover, a secure attachment fosters the gradual and appropriate self-reliance that leads to mastery and autonomy (James, 1994, p. 24). Thus, attachment styles may affect expectations and interactions with the treating clinician and others as well as the development of specific difficulties.

Childhood traumas (e.g., sexual abuse) have affected adult attachment styles and psychological development (Roche, Runtz, & Hunter, 1999). Attachment insecurity has been associated with distress, depression, and personality disorders beyond any effects of abuse severity (Alexander et al., 1998). Adults with a history of childhood abuse have reported—more than others—relationship problems during childhood and adult life (Styron & Janoff-Bulman, 1997). Although the results are mixed, behavior problems have been found in preschool children with insecure attachments (Thompson, 1991).

Parental attachment style may also affect children's memory capacity and their responses to stressful or novel situations (Howe, 1997). Children whose parents had an avoidant or anxious/ambivalent attachment style made more errors than other children did in recalling stressful medical procedures (Goodman & Quas, 1996). Toddlers with insecure attachments had elevated cortisol levels in response to stressful or novel situations, in contrast to children with secure attachments (Gunnar, Brodersen, Krueger, & Rigatuso, 1996; Nachmia, Gunnar, Mangelsdorf, Parritz, & Buss, 1996). In studies of rhesus monkeys, reactive monkeys' elevated cortisol levels were inherited by their offspring and continued to be elevated even when monkeys were placed in foster care (Suomi, 1995; Suomi & Levine, 1998).

In addition to the normal attachment bonds between infants and parents are the bonds that occur under traumatic circumstances. One form of this is the increased attachment to those with whom children endure a traumatic experience (Nader & Pynoos, 1993). Another form is often described as the hostage syndrome. According to James (1994, pp. 24–27), abused children are hostages—held captive by their dependence and lack of alternatives. Trauma bonds occur when attachment-seeking behaviors increase during traumatic events: the child victim perceives outside help as unavailable; a dominant person alternates terroristic and nurturing behaviors, thus strengthening the bonds; responses such as dissociation, numbing, or self-blame, among others, lead to a confusion of pain and love; the victim's need for attachment overcomes fears. Trauma bonding is based on terror. Trauma-bonded persons commonly feel that their lives are in danger and their abuser is in total control. Relief over survival is often expressed as gratitude toward the perpetrator.

Features of the Traumatic Experience

Experience influences and is influenced by traumatic response. Previous experience may heighten attention to specific aspects of a traumatic experience (Pynoos & Nader, 1989). For example, the child whose sister had drowned when the paramedics arrived too late to revive her was preoccupied with the arrival of the paramedics and issues of resuscitation in a school shooting. Moreover, details of the traumatic experience may influence subsequent attention and behavior:

> After breaking up with her boyfriend, an adolescent girl shot herself in the head. The girl could not speak but was cognizant enough to slowly move her hand up her body toward the wound when asked where it was. She lay basically nonresponsive for days before dying in the hospital. Although she remained quiet when other family members entered, she became agitated, apparently trying to move, upon the periodic entrance of the sister who had found her, called the paramedics, and stayed with her. Subsequently, the sister accidentally slit her wrist on a sharp container at work. The sister increased her risk-taking behaviors, including rock climbing without the proper equipment. She told a psychiatric resident that she had become very curious about what it felt like to die and had wondered about it while looking down from the rocks. She was tempted to allow herself to fall to find out.

CHOOSING A TREATMENT METHOD

Effective treatment is more likely when the clinician, the method, and the child are a good fit with each other. A clinician's skill may be primarily a combination of training, knowledge, experience, and fit. For effective use, each treatment method described in this chapter requires a period of training and supervision. Knowledge of children, psychotherapeutic principles, and trauma are prerequisites.

Primary treatment methods (group or individual) for childhood trauma are often combined with adjunct treatments (e.g., parent and/or child groups). Treatment methods described in this chapter are not appropriate for children who are developmentally delayed, mentally retarded, or otherwise cognitively compromised. There are often general adaptations made in methods of intervention for different age groups. For example, often (1) for preschoolers, there is more focus on play, sometimes with a clinician verbalizing reactions and sequences for the child; (2) for younger school-age children, play and drawing are combined with cognitive review and discussion; and (3) for adolescents, the focus is often more on discussion, perhaps with some role play. The method and amount of comfort given differs for different age groups.

Most of the treatments described below include the following: (1) repeated review of the event, (2) reprocessing or redefinition of memories, (3) restoration of a sense of competence and relative sense of safety, and (4) increase in sense of control. Methods developed primarily for treatment of children exposed to single incidents of trauma, sexually or physically abused children, or special populations have sometimes been adapted and used for more than one population. For some populations, the primary goals of treatment are those other than or in addition to reduction of PTSD. For example, the primary goals for children with dissociative disorders may be reintegration of parts of self and assisting the child to take responsibility for and/or own all of his or her own emotional states and actions. For children exposed to ongoing violence (e.g., inner cities; war zones), issues such as moral code and despair may be among the priorities.

Some relief is provided for traumatized children by a caring adult's preliminary interventions or comforting contacts (Nader, 1996a). Methods described in this chapter have helped to reduce and/or relieve PTSD symptoms. Many of them have helped to improve the child's self-esteem and quality of life. These accomplishments are of utmost importance. Nevertheless, in determining the effectiveness of treatments over time, it is essential to examine the factors in addition to PTSD symptoms that produce future psychological problems, vulnerabilities, and undesirable behavior patterns.

Beyond PTSD

We have become fairly adept at measuring the symptoms of PTSD in children (Carlson, 1997; Stamm, 1996; Nader, 1996a). We have successfully reduced PTSD symptoms simply by skillfully interviewing children about their traumatic reactions (Nader, 1996a) and with massage therapy (Field, Seligman, Scafidi, & Schanberg, 1996). Prevention of future difficulties, however, may include more than resolving the symptoms of PTSD and symptoms associated with PTSD. For example, in addition to a loss in impulse control, abused children may develop qualities such as defensive hypervigilance to hostile cues and inattentiveness to relevant nonhostile cues; perceptual readiness to attribute hostility to others; a large repertoire of highly accessible aggressive responses to interpersonal problems; and knowledge that aggressive behaviors can lead to positive consequences for the attacker (Dodge et al., 1995). Some of these symptoms may abate with the resolution of PTSD symptoms (March, Amaya-Jackson, Foa, & Treadwell, 1999); others may require additional measures.

There is evidence that children of traumatized individuals have increased vulnerability to, for example, future traumatization, psychological difficulties, and increased symptoms when exposed to traumatic events (Danieli, 1998; Nader, 1998; Soloman, Moshe, & Mikulincer, 1988). Trauma may result in increased readiness to arousal or increased reactivity (van der Kolk & Sapporta, 1991). Studies of primates under stress suggest that reactivity may be biochemically inherited, resulting in highly reactive offspring whose reactivity remains constant even when they are placed with foster mothers (Suomi & Levine, 1998). This finding suggests that a traumatized person's tendency toward heightened reactivity may be passed on to off-spring.

When all goes well, we take forward with us qualities that have become prominent and undergone maturation at various stages of our youth (e.g., curiosity, playfulness, conscience, and independence). An ability to play may become part of a well-rounded life, or a well-chosen profession may include the youthful joy of creative play. We have not examined carefully whether a profession chosen as a result of traumatic experience may also include the full range of desirable traits. Qualities such as an adolescent's sense that anything is possible can be very useful in accomplishing the seemingly impossible. In most cases, it is hoped that in adulthood this quality will include a realistic understanding of one's vulnerability. Trauma can induce inhibition related to a heightened sense of vulnerability or may result in dangerous risk taking.

There is some evidence that initial suppression of reexperiencing may result in increased arousal symptoms (Nader & Fairbanks, 1994). When, over time, traumatic reexperiencing declines, it may be translated into traumatic play or behaviors (Nader & Pynoos, 1991). As has already been discussed, even "lost memories" can be regained. Murray and Son (1998) suggest that forgetting is as important as remembering after traumas and that clinicians should ignore irrelevant memories. The question becomes "Which memories are irrelevant?" If, in fact, special meaning is embedded in the details of the event and/or some memories are blocked from consciousness because they are too painful to face, then some of these lost memories will be important to resolve.

If, at the end of treatment, the clinician and the child have not uncovered and resolved specific traumatic moments or emotions, these emotions may translate into repeated complexes of behavior and emotions. For example, clinical evidence (see Nader, 1997; Nader & Pynoos, 1993) has shown us that (1) unexpressed depression over not assisting an injured child across the room may result in the repeated need to rescue others, an ongoing depression over a sense of ineffectualness, or a sense of hurting others somehow; (2) unresolved anger that a friend hindered escape from injury may result in perpetual unspecific angry feelings at those who are close, in choosing friends who endanger others including oneself, or in a tendency to endanger friends; and (3) the unrecognized desire to remove oneself from harm may result in a style of running away in response to stress, an ongoing sense of failure or ineffectualness, or in a repeated sense of inescapable endangerment. If the cause of these scripts, patterns, or disorders has been undiscovered in relation to the event, it may remain unrecognized and go untreated. A girl molested by her father and others until age 12 remembered only his rubbing against her body. Under stress she experienced tightness of the throat, nausea, fatigue, and a sense of aloneness, being trapped, and being caretaker to everyone else, but she did not remember the forced oral copulation until treatment sessions in her 50s (Nader, 1996b, p. 20). Even unresolved curiosity may become a part of reenactments (e.g., curiosity about what death feels like).

We have many questions to answer regarding the vulnerabilities and patterns of behavior engendered by traumatic experiences. For example, how does personality style (e.g., compulsive vs. narcissistic) or temperament influence the long-term results of trauma? One of the main concerns in the debate between therapies that advocate reprocessing traumatic memories versus those that condition response to the memories or condition behavior is what happens to the memory impressions over time. When response and behavior are reconditioned, do the memory impressions become suppressed? If so, might they later be expressed in patterns of behavior (e.g., disguised reenactments), life scripts (e.g., stress leads to disguised reexperiencing or reenactment), psychological difficulties (e.g., disturbances in conduct, depression), or even violence? How much more difficult is it to transform patterns of behavior that have become ingrained over years? Does the return of a sense of competence and control modulate or counteract the patterns and problems through adulthood? What vulnerabilities stay dormant until triggered by the right set of circumstances and the right set of reminders?

Measuring Outcomes

Measuring outcomes is fraught with difficulties including issues of time, contamination, selection, and identifying true measures of effectiveness. We can only know the true efficacy of our treatment methods by examining children over years into adulthood. Over periods of years, however, individuals are affected by numerous influences. In most cases, treatment programs include adjunct methods considered important to full recovery; any one component is difficult to assess over years. For methods used with children identified from a large population, if small numbers agree to treatment, we do not know how the larger group would have fared in the treatment (or whether only those who would benefit from the treatment agree to it).

Symptom reporting may fluctuate with treatment, self-knowledge, and maturity. There is evidence that, after 1–2 years, children report fewer symptoms for themselves than trained parents, teachers or clinicians report for them (Nader, 1991)—perhaps related to awareness of expectations of others, desires to be pleasing, and immaturity. Over additional years, symptoms may be better recognized and reported or, no longer overt, may become embedded in symbolic play/activity (Nader & Pynoos, 1991), personality, interactional styles, and patterns of behavior, or they may exist as vulnerabilities. It is essential that we learn to fully identify and assess the results of trauma in addition to PTSD and associated features.

INDIVIDUAL TREATMENT METHODS

Because children can be strongly influenced by what they think others expect of them, and because some aspects of traumatic experience and response are very personal, some issues that can be thoroughly addressed in the privacy of an individual session may not be addressed in a group.

Cognitive-Behavioral Therapy

Behavioral therapists strive to change behaviors and thereby reduce distressing thoughts and feelings. Cognitive therapists first change thoughts and feelings, thereby improving functional behavior (March et al., 1999). How events are cognitively appraised and what one already knows can influence reactions to stressful, novel, or traumatic situations (e.g., Howe, 1997). Behavioral techniques have been adapted, individually or in combination, to treat traumatized children (e.g., Odom & Strain, 1984; Fantuzzo, 1990; Saigh, 1992). An individual trauma-focused cognitive behavioral therapy (CBT) method, described below by Judith A. Cohen of MCP–Hahnemann, University School of Medicine, Allegheny General Hospital, Pittsburgh, PA, focuses on the treatment of sexually abused children. Parallel approaches for children exposed to other traumatic stressors have had positive clinical results (Cohen, Berliner, & Mannarino, 2000; Cohen, Mannarino, Berliner, & Deblinger, 2000).

History and Precursors

Empirical research regarding the symptoms of sexually abused children (Mannarino, Cohen, & Gregor, 1989; Deblinger, McLeer, Atkins, Ralph, & Foa, 1989; Friedrich, Grambsch, et al., 1992; Wozencroft, Wagner, & Pellegrini, 1991; Briere, 1992, 1995) and the factors that mediate symptom formation (Mannarino, Cohen, & Berman, 1994; Mannarino & Cohen, 1996, Friedrich, Luecke, Beilke, & Place, 1992) have led to the development of trauma-focused CBT interventions (Deblinger & Heflin, 1996; Cohen & Mannarino, 1993). Symptoms such as depression, anxiety, and inappropriate behaviors responded to CBT interventions when used with nonabused children. Furthermore, CBT techniques seemed a logical approach to cognitive distortions (e.g., responsibility for the abuse) (Mannarino et al., 1994). The belief that PTSD symptoms were derived in part from fear conditioning also suggests that exposure techniques may be helpful in decreasing PTSD symptoms (Cohen, Berliner, et al., 2000; Cohen, Mannarino, et al., 2000).

Although Cohen and Mannarino (1993) placed somewhat greater emphasis on cognitive components and Deblinger and Heflin (1996) focused more on exposure techniques, these treatment models contain overlapping components. They have since been integrated into a single treatment for both the child and the nonoffender parent (Cohen, Deblinger, & Mannarino, 1997).

Methods

Treatment includes exposure, cognitive restructuring, behavior management, psychoeducation, stress management, and safety skills (Cohen, Berliner, et al., 2000; Cohen, Mannarino, et al., 2000; Cohen, 1999).

Child Interventions.   "Gradual exposure" techniques encourage the child to describe abusive episode(s) repeatedly and with increasing detail over the course of several sessions. Initially the child discusses sexual abuse in general (e.g., the definition of sexual abuse, the kinds of children it happens to, and how it might make a child feel). Then, the child describes any episode or aspect of the sexual abuse—in a variety of ways (e.g., writing a book or drawing a picture). Gradually, the child provides increasing details about what occurred and his or her thoughts and feelings about what happened. Over the course of several sessions, the child reviews and adds to his or her book or other artwork. The goal is to decrease PTSD avoidant symptoms, as well as to unpair thought or discussions of the abuse from negative emotions such as fear (Cohen, Berliner, et al., 2000; Cohen, Mannarino, et al., 2000).

Cognitive restructuring regarding responsibility or causation of the abuse occurs through the identification of cognitive errors, exploration of alternative explanations, and replacing inaccurate cognitions. The child first is given a variety of scenarios not related to sexual abuse, then progresses to questions about sexual abuse scenarios different than the child's, and finally is asked about his or her own abuse experience. In all of these scenarios, the child is asked to identify who was responsible for making a particular event occur. The concept of regret versus responsibility is also explored (e.g., doing something regrettable that increased vulnerability to abuse such as taking a ride with a stranger is different from being responsible for the perpetration of the abuse).

Behavioral management strategies are used for children who are exhibiting inappropriate behaviors, including sexualized behavior problems. Contingency reinforcement programs help the child develop more appropriate alternative behaviors and rewarding adaptive behaviors.

Psychoeducational interventions include providing the child with information about sexual abuse, typical reactions to the experience, and good outcomes possible following therapy. Safety skills are taught and reinforced through the use of board and card games; the child is encouraged to use problem-solving methods to select the safest course of action. Care is taken to avoid making the child feel responsible for past abuse due to previous lack of safety skills.

Stress management techniques such as deep breathing, progressive muscle relaxation, thought stopping, and positive imagery are taught to the child in order to give the child a sense of control over negative thoughts and emotions, especially when they occur at times such as bedtime, during school, or with friends, when it would not be appropriate to use exposure or cognitive restructuring techniques. These stress management techniques may also be used during exposure sessions if the exposure exercises produce overwhelming negative emotions (Cohen, Berliner, et al., 2000; Cohen, Mannarino, et al., 2000).

Parent Interventions. Caretaking adults other than perpetrators of abuse (unless the offender has received counseling and acknowledges appropriate responsibility) may benefit from a number of treatments. Exposure techniques with the parent in individual session include hearing the parent's description of the abuse and then sharing (with the child's permission) the child's descriptions of what happened. Book/artwork is shared with the parent in progressive sessions, until the parent can tolerate direct discussion of the child's experiences without overwhelming negative emotions. After adequate progress by the parent and child in therapy, joint sessions (Deblinger & Heflin, 1996) permit the child and parent to directly discuss the child's experience, and the parent to model adaptive coping and provide appropriate emotional support. The goal is to enhance communication between the parent and child, so that the child will feel able to go to the parent if future symptoms or traumatic events occur.

Cognitive restructuring is used to correct distortions that the parent may have about why the abuse occurred, why the child did not tell about it right away, and what sexual abuse means for the child's future normal adjustment. Cognitive distortions are identified and corrected using standard cognitive reframing techniques. Role playing a "best friend" scenario ("What would you tell your best friend if she was blaming herself because her child had been abused?") is often helpful.

Parents learn behavioral management techniques (if needed) including positive attention, active ignoring, time-out procedures, and contingency reinforcement programs. Parents are encouraged to maintain normal familial rules and roles. Stability and predictability at home help the child to feel safe and suggest that the child is not "damaged" from having been abused.

Psychoeducational information about sexual abuse, including how often it occurs, how often children delay disclosure, common emotional and behavioral reactions, and positive outcomes following sexual abuse, is helpful in normalizing both the child's and the parent's reaction to the abuse, as well as in helping parents to be optimistic about their children's future.

Stress management techniques are taught for parents' own use and to allow them to instruct the child in their use at home. Efforts are made to enhance parental safety skills and problem-solving techniques not only to adequately protect the child from future exposure but also to prevent future over-protection (which might delay age-appropriate independence) (Cohen, Berliner, et al., 2000; Cohen, Mannarino, et al., 2000).

Population

These techniques have been used for school-age children and adolescents and adapted for sexually abused preschool children (Cohen & Mannarino, 1993). This treatment approach is appropriate only after abuse allegations have been independently validated; it (exposure components in particular) should *not* be used to elicit information for forensic purposes. Gradual exposure may result in a transient worsening of symptoms and should be used with great caution in children who are acutely suicidal or actively using drugs or alcohol (Cohen, Berliner, et al., 2000; Cohen, Mannarino, et al., 2000).

Length of Treatment

This treatment approach has been used in 12-week treatment protocols. The length of treatment may be shortened if the traumatic impact appears to be less severe, and it may need to be lengthened if symptomatic resolution does not occur (Cohen, Berliner, et al., 2000; Cohen, Mannarino, et al., 2000).

Training and Prerequisites

The Center for Traumatic Stress in Children and Adolescents at Allegheny General Hospital in Pittsburgh provides a Child and Adolescent Psychiatry Residency Training Program (i.e., fellowships) and hosts trainees from graduate social work and clinical psychology programs. The standard 2-year program includes approximately 4 hours of didactic training, 3–5 hours of supervision, and 25–40 clinical practice hours per week) (Cohen, Berliner, et al., 2000; Cohen, Mannarino, et al., 2000).

Treatment Outcomes/Results

CBT interventions are efficacious in decreasing a variety of posttrauma and related symptoms in sexually abused children. The most rigorous of a number of studies include two randomized controlled trials (RCTs) on sexually abused children using the above treatment model: (1) 68 preschoolers (ages 3–7) and (2) 49 children and adolescents, (ages 8–14). In both studies, children were randomly assigned to either the trauma-focused CBT intervention or to nondirective supportive therapy (NST). Both studies included a therapist crossover design, rigorous adherence procedures, use of several methodologically sound instruments to measure symptomatology, and a 1-year follow-up design. The preschool study demonstrated that CBT was significantly superior to NST in decreasing PTSD symptoms (including sexualized behaviors), internalizing symptoms, and total behavior problems, and that these group × time differences were maintained during the 1-year follow-up (Cohen & Mannarino, 1996, 1997). The study of 8- to 14-year-olds demonstrated that the CBT intervention was significantly superior to NST in decreasing depressive symptoms and improving social competence (Cohen & Mannarino, 1997). Although no group × time effects were found with regard to sexualized behaviors, this may have been because these behaviors occurred less frequently in this cohort than in the preschoolers. Deblinger, Lippmann, and Steer (1996) conducted a RCT with the above CBT model, randomly assigning subjects to child-only, parent-only, child and parent, or standard community care (SCC) treatment cells. They found that the two treatment conditions in which the child received CBT experienced significantly greater improvement in PTSD symptoms, whereas the two treatment conditions in which the parent received CBT experienced significantly greater improvement in child's depressive symptoms and in parent's parenting skills. All three CBT conditions experienced greater symptomatic improvement than the SCC group.

Play Therapy

Play therapies help to reduce clinical symptoms and to remove impediments to continuing development. Terr (1983) suggests that a traumatized child needs to verbalize as well as to play. Methods of play therapy differ in their emphasis of play versus verbalization and in the amount of interpretation provided by the therapist (Webb, 1991). Traumatized children engage in play at older ages than do nontraumatized children (Terr, 1989). The method described below is an eclectic method in that it combines play with other methods, treats the child in context, emphasizes a strong therapeutic relationship, recognizes the child's successes, and reduces helplessness (Lehmann & Coady, 2000).

History and Precursors

Trauma/grief-focused therapy began as a semistructured research interview. The interview included a draw-a-picture/tell-a-story method and research questions developed at Cornell University by Drs. Ted Shapiro, Karen Gilmore, and Robert Pynoos (Eth & Pynoos, 1985; Nader, 1997). The initial specialized interview for traumatized children with innovations by Pynoos and Eth and additions by Nader was first published in detail in 1986 (Pynoos & Eth, 1986). It has continued to evolve in its clinical diagnostic and therapeutic use in response to the needs of traumatized children (Goenjian et al., 1997; Nader, 1994, 1997; Nader & Mello, 2000; Nader & Pynoos, 1991; Pynoos, 1993; Pynoos & Nader, 1993). As with all methods, there is some variation in the method among its primary users.

The techniques of this treatment cross psychotherapeutic boundaries and include principles found in a number of clinical theories. For example, directed and spontaneous symbolic or actual reenactments of traumatic episodes may find their precursors in the psychodrama of Gestalt therapy or the spontaneous play of play therapy (Amster, 1943; Axline, 1947); bringing subconscious traumatic impressions to clear consciousness as well as the assignment of new meaning is found in the cathartic abreactions of psychoanalytic treatment, the hypnotic elicitation and reframing of Milton Erikson's hypnotherapies (Erikson, 1985), and D. M. Levy's abreactive therapy (Levy, 1938); and emphasis of intense traumatic moments prior to redefinition are similar to the review, flooding, redefining, and sometimes desensitization of cognitive-behavioral therapies.

Methods

This method incorporates the use of play and drawings for children with an increase in discussion and role play or demonstration for adolescents. Toys or miniature replicas of the setting in which the trauma occurred are provided so that the child/adolescent can re-create and demonstrate the experience. The child reviews, on multiple occasions, the traumatic experience or its episodes, essentially rewinding the mental recording as needed within a single session to review and recapture details of the experience. This is accompanied by recognizing, verbalizing, and underscoring the child's traumatic impressions, emotions, desires for action (or inaction) in the situation (i.e., to intervene, flee, rescue or be rescued, prevent harm, self-protect, ward off, calm, etc.) and his or her successful actions (and inactions). This treatment method honors the intensity of traumatic impressions, identifications, emotions, and fantasies, facilitating their resolution (Nader, 1997; Nader & Mello, 2000; Pynoos & Eth, 1985; Pynoos & Nader, 1993). Symptoms may temporarily increase over the course of treatment as numbing and avoidance reduce. Abreactive processing in individual sessions is usually followed by a sense of relief, animation, increased expression, and resolution of related symptoms.

The initial session (Pynoos & Eth, 1985) examines the child's experience and worst moment. The focus of this and subsequent sessions are tailored to the child's timing and needs, and addresses personal symbolism and personal experience of the trauma. Drawings, verbalizations, behaviors, assessment measures and the reports of adults and friends give clues to areas of importance (Nader & Mello, 2000). Closure is achieved at the end of each session.

Family and group work provide important supplemental treatments (Nader & Mello, 2000). Child groups can be helpful in addressing issues such as injury or grief and in providing peer support and general coping strategies. For example, children who have previously resolved their own grief reactions are an asset to grief groups. Periodic meetings with parents and teachers are important to a child's progress. When a community has been affected, adult groups may assist parents to understand their children's responses, to adjust to regressions and other changes in the child, and to establish a rhythm with the child that enhances recovery. For example, severely traumatized or retraumatized children may need to reestablish a sense of trust, especially toward adults. Parents may benefit from support groups as well.

Population

Developmentally adapted for adolescent, school-age, or preschool children, this method has been used nationally and internationally (Goenjian et al., 1997; Nader, Pynoos, Fairbanks, Al-Ajeel, & Al-Asfour, 1993).

Length of Treatment

Children moderately-to-severely traumatized have benefited from 2 to 16 sessions. Moderately-to-severely traumatized children, especially those exposed to life threat and multiple bloody deaths or injuries, often require 1–2½ years of treatment to fully resolve their traumatic reactions. Child- and/or trauma-intrinsic factors may increase or decrease the length of treatment regardless of exposures. Additional sessions may be required in the course of the child's growth and development as a result of the interaction of trauma factors and life events or as traumatic impressions take on new meanings over time.

Training and Prerequisites

When provided by the present author (Nader), training in the use of this treatment method includes 24–40 hours of didactic training and additional supervision hours with opportunities for trainees to observe and, if desired, to be observed in sessions with children. Continued training over time addresses the progression of treatment and provides continued feedback regarding the progress of the children and of the clinicians in applying this treatment.

Treatment Outcomes/Results

A group of children traumatized by the 1988 Armenian earthquake were treated by clinicians using two to four sessions of this individual trauma/grief-focused therapy in combination with classroom discussions (Pynoos & Nader, 1988) and relaxation training (Goenjian et al., 1997). PTS and depressive reactions were measured pre- and postintervention (1½ and 3 years after the earthquake). PTS symptoms decreased among treated children and increased among nontreated children. Although depressive symptoms remained constant for the treatment group, they increased significantly in the nontreated group.

In 1989, a group of elementary school children in New York State were exposed to a tornado that collapsed a cafeteria wall, killing nine children and injuring others (Nader, 1997). A preliminary report was prepared for the school district 15 months after the event (Nader, 1991). Prior to the report, children were interviewed by clincians using the Childhood Post-Traumatic Stress Reaction Index (CPTS-RI; Frederick, Pynoos & Nader, 1992) 2 weeks, 11 months, and 15 months following the experience. Children with moderate and severe trauma levels were referred for treatment. After a period of initial training for the treatment team, between 3 and 14 months following the event, 111 children entered treatment. By 15 months after the event, 32 children remained on a waiting list and 17 had completed treatment. From 2 weeks to 11 months to 15 months following the tornado, the number of children with severe PTS levels had reduced from 39% to 22% to 7%, respectively. The number with doubtful-to-no PTS increased from 9% to 20% to 38%, respectively. The number of mild and moderate cases fluctuated as severely traumatized children began to recover (Nader, 1991). For this and other settings in which this treatment method was used, there were verbal reports over time from parents and children of recovery from trauma and improvement in the quality of life over pretrauma levels.

Therapies with a Physical Component

A few therapies include a physical component in their treatment methods. For example, Field, Seligman, Scafidi, and Schanberg (1996) were able to reduce anxiety, depression scores and cortisol levels using massage therapy. Another method, eye movement desensitization and reprocessing (EMDR), involves the movement of the eyes during traumatic reprocessing (Greenwald, 1999).

History and Precursors

In 1987, Francine Shapiro discovered that upsetting thoughts faded when the eyes moved spontaneously from side to side (Shapiro, 1989a, 1989b; Greenwald, 1998). EMDR has been adapted for children whose traumatic, loss, or stressful experiences have resulted in symptoms or problems (Pellicer, 1993; Greenwald, 1994, 1998).

In this approach, earlier trauma/loss is believed to potentially create vulnerability to subsequent stressors, especially those with the same theme or issue. Trauma and loss that do not meet DSM diagnosis and prerequisites are also treated with EMDR. An event does not have to qualify under criterion A of DSM-IV to be disturbing to the child or to cause symptoms. Any incompletely processed trauma/loss memory that seems to be contributing to a child/adolescent's problems or symptoms may become the focus of treatment (Greenwald, 1999).

Methods

EMDR procedures are complex and variable. Generally, a child is asked to focus intensely on a traumatic memory while moving the eyes rapidly from side to side by visually tracking the therapist's moving hand. This seems to render traumatic memories accessible to internal healing resources for work-through and integration. Treatment may include many "sets" of eye movements (10 seconds to a minute or more). The focus changes according to the child's status. Following a set of eye movements, the therapist "checks in" with the child to monitor progress and to refocus for the next set of eye movements. Subjective Units of Disturbance (SUDs) Scale ratings are taken at intervals. The child may experience imaginal reexperiencing, a progression of emotional responses, decreased distress, reduced vividness of images, physiological release (e.g., of tension), and the supplanting of negative self-statements and beliefs (Greenwald, 1994).

Some clinicians use a variety of adjunct treatments with EMDR (e.g., parent training, educational accommodations, behavior modification, and medication) to stabilize the environment and create conditions for healing and increased successful functioning. EMDR's purpose is to bring past trauma/loss memories to resolution. The preferred approach is to identify all possibly relevant memories (which may have contributed to the problem) and proceed in chronological order from earliest to latest. Although resolution of earlier trauma/loss memories may render the later memories less important, they are nevertheless addressed (Greenwald, 1999).

Population

EMDR has been used with all ages of children and for all kinds of loss and trauma (Greenwald, 1999). For younger children (e.g., toddlers exposed to accident or abuse, or who have witnessed violence), procedures are simplified and parent(s) may be more actively involved.

Length of Treatment

The more damaged (e.g., from chronic trauma) the child is, the more support (i.e., environmental; therapeutic relationship) the child is likely to require before facing traumatic memories and the more slowly the procedure may proceed (Greenwald, 1999).

Training and Prerequisites

Appropriate clinical competence in a specific area of practice (e.g., with traumatized children) is prerequisite. EMDR may be a very effective intervention when used appropriately, but it does not replace clinical judgment and skill, and should only be used within the context of an overall treatment plan. Licensed mental health professionals will need specialized training and supervised practice in EMDR methods. Many models of training are currently available. According to the EMDR International Association, the minimum standard for certification is approximately 40 hours of class, including a number of supervised small-group practice sessions. The 40 hours are staggered over at least 2 months to allow for practice with the basic approach before more complex aspects are learned. Following this phase, an additional 20 hours of supervision/consultation address EMDR in clinical practice (Greenwald, 1999).

Treatment Outcomes/Results

EMDR has been reported to dramatically increase efficiency in the treatment of traumatic memories for adults (Chemtob, Nakashima, Hamada, & Carlson, in press; Chemtob, Tolin, van der Kolk, & Pitman, 2000). Recent studies have demonstrated its successful use with children (Greenwald, in press; Puffer, Greenwald, & Elrod, 1998; Shapiro, 1989a; Soberman, Greenwald, & Rule, in press). In a case study of five children (ages 4–11) diagnosed with PTSD following exposure to Hurricane Andrew, one or two treatments of EMDR were administered. SUDs ratings were used to rate emotional reactivity during the procedure. Mother's ratings of children's symptoms/complaints on the Problem Rating Scale (PRS) of the SUDs showed score reductions in response to treatment. Follow-up 4 weeks later showed a return of all subjects to their pretrauma levels of functioning (Greenwald, 1994).

GROUP TREATMENT METHODS

Group methods have been used as important adjunct treatments for traumatized children (e.g., for parents; injured or grieving children or parents; support). A few group methods provide primary treatment for trauma (Yule & Williams, 1990). Glodich and Allen (1998) and Terr (1989) have detailed the advantages of group treatment. For example, children learn that there are others in their situation who have experienced similar emotions; groups help to overcome any "conspiracy of silence"; a larger number can be treated; children/adolescents may accept from peers what they will ignore from adults; members benefit from the work of others; and there are opportunities for listening without participating. Terr (1989), however, suggests that group treatment should be used in combination with other treatments for the following reasons: (1) development of new symptoms after hearing new types of horrors from others, (2) loss of credibility as courtroom witnesses because of group influence, and (3) the need for examination of internal mental processes stimulated by trauma. The significant influence of peer expectations can be both an advantage and a disadvantage of group treatment.

Cognitive-Behavioral Group Therapy

Trauma-focused coping (TFC) is a cognitive-behavioral group therapy treatment for children traumatized by single-incident traumas. TFC includes psychoeducation, cognitive therapy, exposure-based behavior therapy, generalization training, and relapse prevention. The direct antecedent of TFC, multimodality trauma treatment (MMTT), was developed by Drs. John March and Lisa Amaya-Jackson at Duke University and Dr. Edna B. Foa at the University of Pennsylvania. The following description of this method has been derived from materials provided by Dr. March (March, Amaya-Jackson, Foa, & Treadwell, 1999; March, Amaya-Jackson, Terry, & Costanzo, 1997; March, Amaya-Jackson, Murry, & Schulte, 1998).

History and Precursors

Derived from literature on evidence-based treatment for adult and pediatric posttraumatic reactions, TFC follows both cognitive (restructuring) and behavioral (exposure) principles. Treatment progress is reflected in an increasingly coherent narrative of the trauma that can be more readily integrated with the victim's existing schemas. Once a memory is so processed, the victim is able to conceive of the trauma as a distinct event rather than as a global representation, and thus, to discriminate between danger and safety. The self is then viewed as competent (March et al., 1999; also J. March, E-mail communication, August 25, 1999).

Theoretically, knowledge acquired throughout life is represented in memory in the form of abstract generic knowledge structures, or "schemas" (Bartlett, 1932; Neisser, 1976). Within an information processing framework, PTSD is conceptualized as founded in dysfunctional schemas in which the world is conceived as indiscriminately dangerous and the self is conceived as totally incompetent to cope with stress. These schemas are thought to have emerged through "overaccommodation" of pretrauma assumptions that the world is a safe place and the individual is competent (e.g., Foa, Steketee, & Rothbaum, 1989; Janoff-Bulman, 1989; McCann & Pearlman, 1990; Perloff, 1993; Resick & Schnicke, 1993). A few studies in children have found that an internal locus of control (a construct related to self-competence) was associated with chronic PTSD symptoms and may serve as a mediator in the maintenance of PTSD (Joseph et al., 1991; March, Amaya-Jackson, et al., 1997).

Recounting the traumatic memory decreases associated anxiety, thus allowing its reorganization (Foa & Rothbaum, 1997). When viewed through classical conditioning theory, the stressor, or traumatic event, is thought to act as an unconditioned stimulus that elicits an unconditioned (reflexive) response characterized by extreme fear and the cognitive perception of helplessness and terror. Cognitive, affective, physiological, and environmental cues accompanying the event (traumatic reminders) are conditioned stimuli. In turn, traumatic reminders become capable of eliciting a conditioned response (anxiety) which should decrease (habituate) with prolonged, repeated exposure in the absence of real threat. Through instrumental conditioning the child learns to reduce PTSD distress through cognitive and behavioral avoidance and sometimes anxiety-dampening rituals, such as checking or reassurance seeking. These anxiety-reducing behaviors preclude the extinction of trauma-relevant anxiety (March et al., 1999). The CBT therapist targets the distorted stimulus–stimulus and stimulus–response associations as well as dysfunctional evaluations and beliefs (Foa, 1997; Foa & Rothbaum, 1997; March, 1998). Treatment progress is reflected in an increasingly coherent narrative of the trauma that can be more readily integrated with the victim's existing schemas (March et al., 1999).

Methods

TFC involves 14 weekly sessions (see Table 12.3). The first few sessions build rapport, enlist the child's cooperation in the treatment process, and lay the groundwork for the child to think differently about PTSD. While the model is one of graded exposure, it is important for both children and adolescents to be informed early on about the treatment process, which begins with psychoeducation and cognitive therapy before moving to more exposure-based interventions.

Each session lasts approximately 50–60 minutes and includes a statement of goals; review of the preceding week; provision of new information; therapist-assisted practice; practice homework for the coming week; and monitoring procedures. The first 10 minutes of each session are spent checking in with each child and reviewing the previous week's homework. If a child was unable to complete homework, then this time is spent identifying what the obstacles were to completing it. The next 20 minutes are spent presenting and completing the goals for the current session. When session goals are completed, the final 10 minutes are spent helping each child choose the week's homework task and reviewing strategies that increase homework success. During the middle and end of treatment, 30–40 minutes of each session may be spent in therapist-assisted exposure tasks. After the child participates in the hard work of exposure, the end of a session may also be allocated to a social reward, such as playing a game or talking about something besides PTSD (March et al., 1999).

Even if indirectly related to PTSD, struggles with parents and peers, oppositional behavior, poor school performance, depression, and psychiatric symptoms (unless they constrain the treatment of PTSD) are not the focus of treatment. Secondary symptoms often remit once a child has some success in "bossing back" PTSD. While it is important to avoid getting sidetracked, each child is unique. When an intervention or exposure task is not working, revision is needed. The therapist peppers the group members with questions about

TABLE 12.3. Trauma-Focused Coping Therapy Sessions

Session 1: Overview of treatment process and group rules; information gathering; concept of "bossing back" PTSD

Session 2: Tripartite behavior regulation model; instruction in progressive, cue-controlled, differential muscle relaxation

Session 3: PTSD and traumatic reminders; fear thermometer; cognitive restructuring and positive self-talk

Session 4: The relationship of thoughts and feelings to behavior; behavioral coping skills to minimize avoidance

Session 5: Anger coping or grief work

Session 6: Videotape replay technique to develop an ideotypic stimulus hierarchy; systematic strategizing recall of the traumatic event in a moment-by-moment fashion (goals: input of corrective information and habituation of anxiety and increased cognitive mastery)

Session 7: Narrative exposure (briefly telling story to the group; summarizing stimulus hierarchy)

Sessions 8 and 9: Organizing a coherent trauma narrative toward habituation of trauma-based anxiety; imaginal exposure and, as homework, *in vivo* exposure; therapist and/or group members introduce corrective information regarding spatial/temporal distortions; global attributions reinforcing lack of personal efficacy; normalization; and positive coping

Session 10: Corrective information (cognitive restructuring) for PTSD-related schemas

Sessions 11 and 12: Cognitive/exposure-based interventions for the worst moment

Sessions 13 and 14: Practice, summary, review, reinforcement, and generalization of the techniques

Session 14: Graduation party (certificate for "becoming the boss of PTSD")

Source: Data from March et al. (1999).

their experiences "bossing" or being "bossed around" by PTSD. It is vital that the therapist remain on the side of the child, not of the PTSD (March et al., 1999). The therapist assists the child to "choose to be anxious." A consistently matter of fact stance models for the child that indeed, anxiety, though quite uncomfortable at times, can be tolerated and will eventually go away.

Adult Involvement in Treatment

To address limitations of generalization to the natural setting, parents receive an outline of skills to be covered in each session and are encouraged to cue their children when to use skills and to reinforce them for display of skills. Between sessions, children/parents know how to contact the group coleader and are given telephone numbers for a clinician who is on-call 24 hours/day, 7 days/week.

Population

TFC has been used effectively for children aged 8–18 years (March et al., 1998). It is designed to flexibly address the developmental level of children or adolescents in the treatment groups. Younger children use a storybook that includes drawing and role play; older children, a more discursive document and talking (March et al., 1999).

Training and Prerequisites

Before acting as a group leader, a clinician must be familiar with (1) the cognitive-behavioral treatment of pathological worry in youth, and (2) the treatment of PTSD in youth and must have supervision by experts in the application of CBT to pediatric PTSD. CBT requires a molecular understanding of specific symptoms, their triggers, the nature of PTSD, and how the patient copes successfully or unsuccessfully with PTSD symptoms.

Training is provided at the Program for Child and Adolescent Anxiety Disorders at Duke University, Durham, North Carolina, and includes 40 hours of training in the administration of CBT techniques under the supervision of Dr. John March, or at the Center for the Treatment and Study of Anxiety at the University of Pennsylvania, Philadelphia, by Dr. Edna B. Foa and Dr. Phil Kendall. Drs. March, Amaya-Jackson, Kendall, and Foa provide weekly supervision focused on the intervention (March et al., 1999).

Length of Treatment

TFC is 14 sessions and a booster session.

Treatment Outcomes/Results

Preliminary findings show that MMTT (TFC's precursor) decreased symptoms of PTSD and of anxiety, anger, depression, and disruptive behaviors in children and adolescents with a DSM-IV diagnosis of PTSD (March et al., 1998). Improvement continued after treatment termination. Of 14 youth participating in the TFC protocol, 12 no longer met criteria for PTSD at posttreatment. While results are not conclusive in the absence of a well-controlled outcome study, a study in progress aims to accomplish this.

In the fall of 1995, March and others screened 2,225 students from four schools—two elementary and two junior high—using the newly developed reliable and valid instrument for assessing pediatric PTSD, the Child and Adolescent Trauma Screen (CATS). They contacted approximately 20 students at each school with CATS T-scores above 65. From these students, the selection-to-treatment procedure eventually yielded from four to six consenting students per group with a DSM-IV diagnosis of PTSD. Treatment with the initial MMTT protocol was successful in reducing PTSD symptoms. Of 17 subjects, 14 completed treatment. Of these, 12 were PTSD negative on the CATS at posttreatment and remained so at 6-month follow-up. Repeated measures with analysis of variance (ANOVA) for the CATS demonstrated a clear treatment effect while confirming that the CATS is change sensitive. Problems with the initial version of the protocol generated the following changes: (1) reduction from 18 weeks to 14 weeks, plus a booster session; (2) separate developmentally sensitive manuals for children and adolescents; and (3) modification of the manual to make cognitive therapy and anxiety management training components more efficient. In year 2, children with disruptive behavior disorders on stable medications were included. While not as robust as the less comorbid sample, the results suggested clear benefits of the treatment. Samples across all 3 years reflected a variety of single-incident traumas, and the gender and racial composition reflected the population distribution (March et al., 1999).

Psychoeducational Groups

Psychoeducational groups have been used as important adjunct methods for traumatized children and their families. The following psychoeducational group for adolescents exposed to violence and abuse is described below by AnnMarie Glodich, PhD, & Jon G. Allen, PhD, of the Menninger Clinic Child and Family Center in Topeka, Kansas.

History and Precursors

In the 1980s, a psychoeducation model was used to treat schizophrenia and was subsequently used for treating depression, bipolar disorder, obsessive-compulsive disorder, chemical dependency, and medical illness (Holder & Anderson, 1990). It has been used with individual patients (e.g., borderline personality disorder) (Linehan, 1993; Siegmann & Long, 1995). Allen (1995), Benham (1995), and Lubin, Loris, Burt, and Johnson (1998) developed psychoeducational approaches for adults with trauma-related disorders. A number of authors have proposed their use be extended to children and adolescents with trauma-related disorders (AACAP Work Group on Quality Issues, 1998; Blechman, Dumas, & Prinz, 1994; Finkelhor & Strapko, 1992; Franklin & Streeter, 1992; Glodich & Allen, 1998; Glodich, 1999a, 1999b; Grusznski, Brink, & Edelson, 1988; Hazzard, 1993; Hazzard, Webb, Kleemeier, Angert, & Pohlin, 1991; Jones & Selder, 1996; Pescosolido, 1993; Rice, Herman, & Petersen, 1993; Schamess, 1993). Psychoeducational groups have provided helpful adjunct treatments for specific single-event traumas (Pynoos & Nader, 1988; Steinberg & Sunkenberg, 1994; Trolley, 1995). Wallen (1993) recommended psychoeducational groups that support self-esteem, promote a sense of competence, develop protection strategies for children exposed to ongoing neighborhood and/or family violence, and address the cumulative effects of repeated exposure to violence and abuse. Allen, Kelly, and Glodich (1997) and Glodich and Allen (1998) have articulated a psychoeducational approach tailored to children and adolescents exposed to ongoing violence and/or abuse. Reenactment and risk-taking behaviors are common among cumulatively traumatized children and adolescents. Glodich (1999a) seeks to fill the gap in the literature on the treatment of these behaviors in groups.

Methods

The Menninger Child and Family Center group protocol is specifically designed to provide education about the effects of trauma and violence and the connection of these effects to reenactment and risk-taking behaviors. Each session is structured with a specific focus and a task. Key topics are as follows: (1) prevalence of violence and trauma; (2) violence-related trauma and PTSD; (3) defenses; (4) avoiding further trauma and violence; (5) reexposure to trauma, reenactment, and diffusing violence to avoid further trauma; (6) combating helplessness, and the role of family in combating helplessness; and (7) review with a specific focus on reducing reenactment and risk-taking behaviors. Participants are encouraged to talk about as much of their experience as they wish, but they are not required to contribute their own personal experiences. Participants are not required to talk at all if they do not feel comfortable doing so. Each session begins and ends with antiviolence music (selected by the group leaders or participants). Two sessions feature role-play. This method has evolved over time; many sessions now include experiential exercises in addition to education.

The protocol is intended to increase knowledge of trauma and to decrease reenactment and risk-taking behaviors. Targeting these behaviors is critically important for averting traumatic reexposure and increased symptomatology. Description or detailed discussion of traumatic events is not elicited. Participants are provided factual information and possible coping strategies to help them develop a cognitive framework for processing events (Glodich, 1999a).

Population

This group intervention is suitable for violence-exposed adolescents aged 13–18 from various racial, ethnic, and socioeconomic groups. Potentially traumatic situations include the following: living in a high-crime area; being exposed to community violence; witnessing and/or participating in an attempted or actual drive-by shooting, other shooting, or stabbing; traumatic accidents; traumatic loss (traumatic death of parent, relative, or friend); rape; or family violence (physical, sexual, or emotional abuse witness/victim). The intervention is currently being adapted for younger children. All groups will be expanded and linked with violence prevention programs (Glodich, 1999a).

Training and Prerequisites

Allen and Glodich are currently preparing a Menninger Clinic training program in trauma treatment for therapists from all mental health disciplines (i.e., nurses, social workers, psychologists, and psychiatrists). Prerequisites are creativity, flexibility, ability to maintain group structure, and a comprehensive understanding of the impact of trauma and violence on children and adolescents. Therapists who have experience working with children exposed to violence and abuse may be best suited for this work. The method uses two coleaders (ideally male and female) (Glodich, 1999a).

Length of Treatment

Treatment has been expanded to 12 weekly sessions with pre- and post-assessments (Glodich, 1999, E-mail communication, April 16, 2001).

Adult Involvement in Treatment

To be maximally effective, the group demands close ongoing collaboration between those providing intervention, parents, and the school system (school and district administrators, counselors, social workers, and teachers) (Glodich, 1999a).

Treatment Outcomes/Results

Glodich (1999b) conducted a study of the efficacy of this psychoeducational intervention. Treatment group participants gained significantly in knowledge about trauma and its effects. Moreover, at posttest there was a statistically significant correlation between knowledge gained about trauma and more adaptive attitudes toward risk-taking behaviors. This study confirmed that psychoeducational groups have promise in decreasing trauma-exposed adolescents' propensities toward reenactment and perpetuation of the cycle of violence. The study generated additional features to strengthen the psychoeducational intervention, including lengthening groups, adding student mentors, including 2 police officers, and focusing more intensively on traumatic reminders. An additional study is in progress.

Family Therapy

Often an adjunct treatment, family therapy has been used as a major treatment component for sexually abused children (Gorham, 1997; Madanes,

1981, 1990; Sgroi, 1982, 1988). Described below by Mary Jo Barrett, director of the Center for Contextual Change in Skokie, Illinois, is a method based on a family treatment approach (Barrett, 1999).

History and Precursors

The multiple systems model is a systematic framework that divides the therapeutic process into stages and gives the clinician clear guidance in the face of the client's anxiety and overwhelming needs. The basis for the treatment is an organizational model (Trepper & Barrett, 1986) that calls for the treatment of abuse victims, nonoffending parents, nonabused siblings, and perpetrators. When a child is traumatized, the trauma happens in a context—the entire family is affected and disrupted by the traumatic event and its discovery. Consequently, the entire context must receive treatment whenever possible. The type of intervention—individual, family, or group—and the frequency of the sessions is determined by both client needs and clinician assessment. To assess the impact of the trauma, clinicians determine the nature of the event, the context of the abuse, and the meaning given to the event(s) by the client. This model has been used for the past 15 years in more than 75 programs throughout the United States, Europe, and Asia (Trepper & Barrett, 1986, 1989).

Methods

The most desirable treatment for victims of childhood abuse is a meta-model integrated into a clinician's own personal style and therapeutic interventions (Maddock & Larson, 1995). The multiple systems model is organized into three stages; although the treatment does not proceed linearly, the flow tends to occur within the boundaries of these three stages (Barrett, 1999).

The Therapeutic Team Approach. The clinician continually strives to build a team with the family, including the child, and all professionals involved (social service, judicial, and legal). The goal is to help clients rebuild a sense of power and control in their lives. Team relationships illustrate the value of all community members; interactions must represent healthy and meaningful relationships (i.e., respectful and articulate communication and appropriate problem-solving skills). As a part of this team, the family learns that positive, nonabusive relationships can and do exist.

Stage I: Creating a context for change. Stage I creates safety for the family and victim within the context of treatment. The clinician assesses safety inside and outside of treatment. Fluid assessment of individual and familial interactions and of individual strengths and difficulties takes place over time. Measurement tools and interviews are utilized. An ongoing treatment plan and goals are then designed and agreed upon with the entire community team (see below) and the family.

Stage II: Challenging patterns and expanding realities. During this stage, the team helps both individuals and families explore the patterns that created and maintained the sexual abuse, helping them create alternative behaviors, thoughts, and feelings. A combination of individual, family, play, and group therapy are utilized with both children and adults.

Stage III: Consolidation. In this relapse prevention stage, the family and the team review what they have learned and changed. Together they predict future difficulties and, based on current strengths, design a plan to assist with these difficulties and with the prevention of relapse.

Goals for Treatment. In follow-up interviews, both adults and children are asked to identify the most significant elements of the therapeutic process. Their answers become generic goals for treatment. Treatment plans and specific interventions can be designed with these ends in mind.

Recognition of Patterns. It is important for the family and child to recognize repetitious patterns of behavior, thoughts, and feelings that contribute to and maintain symptoms. For example, families should be aware of the patterns surrounding a victim's or perpetrator's sexually acting-out episode. Recognition of these predictable patterns can be discussed during Stage I (assessment), and interventions are designed and implemented in Stage II (Barrett, 1999).

Recognition of Strengths. It is important to help the family members recognize that they possess inherent strengths that can help them alter problematic behaviors (Wolin & Wolin, 1992). The emphasis on strengths helps to enhance empowerment and maintain hopefulness.

Boundaries and Safety. When working with traumatized individuals, it is imperative to focus sessions on building safety and to help them understand and design appropriate boundaries. Most traumas are boundary violations creating shifts in the person's sense of safety. The therapeutic process must help reestablish a personal sense of safety and boundaries that will keep children safe without hurting anyone else. Clinicians must also be continually aware of their own boundaries (Barrett, 1999).

Creating and Maintaining Hope. The process of discovery of and recovery from trauma is painful, frustrating, complicated, and often confusing for both client and clinician. Universally in follow-up interviews, clients comment that it was the hope of the team members that helped them through the maze of trauma recovery. Open communication between team members is imperative, as is ongoing supervision and consultation for clinicians that will allow them to maintain an ethical, well informed, and hopeful perspective on each and every case (Barrett, 1999).

Training and Prerequisites

Family therapists must integrate trauma and attachment theory into their body of knowledge. Understanding of Finkelhor's (1987) four-factor model of the traumagenic dynamics of childhood and Perry's (1993) theories on the physiological components of trauma are prerequisites.

The Center for Contextual Change, Skokie, Illinois, offers ongoing training to the community and to programs in other communities that base their work on this method. Trainees receive 30 hours of didactic training throughout the year, 1–2 hours weekly of individual supervision, and 2–3 hours weekly of team supervision, live supervision and consultation (Barrett, 1999).

Length of Treatment

Treatment for childhood trauma is complex. A multiple systems model can provide a clear therapeutic structure that will help a family successfully rebuild itself after a devastating trauma. The average length of treatment in this program is 2 years (Barrett, 1999).

Treatment Outcomes/Results

Clinical examples demonstrate the effectiveness of using family therapy with abuse victims. Treatment of a boy using Madanes's (1990) 16-step family therapy model decreased symptoms beginning after the first step (Gorham, 1997). A combination of individual, group, and family therapy has been successful in reducing symptoms of abused children (see the case of Andy in Roesler, Savin, & Grosz, 1993). Case examples show similar successes for a combination of play and family therapy (Sgroi, 1982, 1988).

Outcome of the multiple systems model is measured by follow-up and exit interviews. The most common childhood symptoms treated by this method are aggressive (sexual and general) behavior, inappropriate masturbation, dissociation, depression, developmentally delayed social skills, anxiety, learning disruptions, sleep difficulties, separation anxiety, eating disorders, and attachment disorders. Interviews have been conducted 6 months, 1 year, 5 years, and a few 10 years after consolidation of treatment. Results show that 78% of the families and individuals interviewed have reported that their families have remained abuse free and that symptoms have subsided.

TREATMENTS FOR SPECIAL POPULATIONS

For some traumatized children, issues other than PTSD are included among the priorities for treatment. Treatments for two special populations of traumatized children are described below.

Treatment for Dissociative Disorders

Models of dissociative identity disorder (DID) suggest a four-factor etiology: (1) biological capability for dissociation, (2) severe or overwhelming childhood traumatic events, (3) lack of a protective safe haven (an environment unable to absorb the distress or comfort the child), and (4) maintenance factors reinforcing dissociative adaptation (Peterson, 1996; Siegel, 1996). A main treatment philosophy includes some or all of the following: establishing safety, developing a working relationship with the alternate personalities ("alters"), hearing their stories, contracting, developing communication between the alters, working toward resolution and integration of personalities, and developing new coping skills (Kluft, 1986, 1990; Peterson, 1996; Putnam, 1989a; Siegel, 1996). A primary goal is shifting traumatic memories from implicit, nondeclarative memory into explicit, declarative memory, thus modulating the experience and putting it into the perspective of other life experiences (Peterson, 1996; Siegel, 1996). In contrast, the method described below by Joyanna L. Silberg (1999) minimizes focus on traumatic memories and emphasizes the child's recognizing and taking responsibility for the emotions and actions of each part of the self (alter).

History and Precursors

Although severe presenting dissociative symptoms occur without identifiable traumatic precursors (Malenbaum & Russell, 1987; Silberg, 1998a; Coons, 1996), severe dissociative disorders in children and adolescents are generally attributed to severe stressors such as chronic physical and sexual abuse (Silberg, 1998b) or, in some cases, to chronic medical problems requiring repeated surgical procedures (Dell & Eisenhower, 1990). A recent case history describes depersonalization disorder following HIV infection in an adolescent boy (Allers, White, & Mullis, 1997). In some cases, imitation of family dissociative disorders may be a contributing factor. Techniques have evolved from a synthesis of adult therapy for DID, play therapy, and family therapy techniques.

Methods

Silberg's treatment method is based on a multilevel intervention strategy where the child's emerging self-theories, the family system, and the child–therapist interaction system are intervention targets. Reconceptualizing the child's theory about him- or herself and avoiding rigid compartmentalization of self includes shaping perceptions of parts of the mind seen as separate. The goal is for the child to see the parts of mind as flexible skills, affects, or needs that the child simply has to learn to access at needed times. Dissociative children have learned to turn off affective states that serve as warning signals that will help to avoid difficulties. Analyzing the competing impulses that keep children stuck and encourage withdrawal into dissociative states is essential. Clinicians evaluate opposing feelings or alternate ideas and encourage resolution. It is often because of the fear of facing what seems to be an unresolvable emotional conflict that dissociative states result. Children who may have learned automatic coping strategies for facing conflicting feelings learn that no dilemma is unresolvable. These dilemmas have often resulted from a child being repeatedly in situations where there is no way out or viable choice to make, such as situations of trauma or abuse inflicted by attachment objects (Silberg, 1999).

A family treatment component targets interaction patterns that promote dissociative coping by teaching parents to validate children's feelings and promoting more open communication. These children are believed to expertly read covert family messages and act them out; openly revealing these hidden messages can liberate the child from double binds created by contradictory overt and metacommunications.

Therapist–child interaction system interventions emphasize the child's responsibility in decision making and avoid iatrogenesis when "alternate identities" are presented (Silberg, 1998a). The therapist is careful not to reinforce or encourage a fragmented view of self. For example, the well-known vocabulary of dissociative disorders (e.g., "switching" and "alters") conveys a reality to these experiences that they may not merit. Silberg recommends using the language of the child, or helping children find language to describe their experiences, with words that suggest similarities to normal phenomena. For example, the therapist might name the function and emphasize that it is indeed only a part of the self by saying, "That part of you that you call Doug, that helps you with getting angry." Over time, the therapist can omit the name and refer only to "the part of you that gets angry." Thus, the therapist's language approximates the normal experience of shifting self-states. Similarly, normalizing language to describe a switch into an active, self-protective state may include, for example, "You're going into action mode"— highlighting the logical function of that affect or mode of behavior in that situation. This way, the child continually learns to make the connections between his/her feeling states and actions, a primary deficit in dissociative children (Silberg, 1998a).

It might be necessary to ask the child to use language that feels incorrect or uncomfortable. For example, Jack, a 13-year-old boy, wanted to say, "Joey did this and is sorry," but was encouraged to say, "I broke the alarm clock because I felt mad about the way you woke me up, and I am sorry." Although Jack did not perceive this to be himself, Silberg asked him to go along with this way of apologizing. Technically it was his "body" that hurt the alarm clock, and of course everything in his mind really does belong to him. Language can also subtly shape experiences toward wholeness and unity through words suggesting choice, responsibility, and control. For example, when the therapist presumes that the child has responsibility and ownership of experiences, it influences the child to view himself as being an agent who makes informed choices (e.g., "When you decided to let Joey break the alarm clock, you must have been feeling pretty mad, I guess." Despite the child's resistance, the therapist's belief may encourage the child to examine more carefully underlying feelings and motivations leading to choices not as yet acknowledged (Silberg, 1998a).

Subtle environmental forces (e.g., parents, teachers, and siblings) may encourage dissociation by undue interest or fascination. For example, for their own entertainment, one family made a game of encouraging different parts to emerge. In the therapy session, the child is taught that information about his or her perceived parts of self is very personal and private. Nevertheless, the therapist does not relate directly to or develop separate relationships with the parts of self. It is preferable for the child to access other parts of self with internal communication—a more normal experience of self or mind. The clinician must react consistently and acceptingly with all self-states—no matter what part of the child presents—so that divergent reactions do not become a stimulus for shaping divergence rather than unity. If the child claims ignorance of things shared in a different state, the child is encouraged to find or discover it; the therapist assumes it can be readily discovered. Sometimes, parents are first to be confronted with separate personality states. Parents are encouraged not to develop private relationships or to vary their behaviors in response to each part. This may be difficult for parents; therefore, it is best, if possible, that parents' knowledge of the separate parts be minimal. When not possible, parents must be assisted to interact toward unity and responsibility (Silberg, 1998a).

Education about the ultimate goals of treatment helps to counterbalance unwitting shaping toward multiplicity. Every opportunity is used to point out gently how nice it will be when wholeness is achieved—the opportunities and increased trust the child will earn. Families can reinforce these messages gently and encouragingly, for example, with promises of a driver's license or privileges to be home alone as continuity of consciousness develops (Silberg, 1998a).

The focus of treatment is determined by a careful assessment of how much of the dissociative behavior is maintained by internal conflict, perceptions of ongoing threat, family patterns, secondary gains, and idiosyncratic self-theories. Following analysis, treatment addresses all of the factors that maintain the dissociative behavior and self-conception at the expense of adaptive coping. Traumatic memories are dealt with only on an "as needed" basis. If the reason a child continues to regress into a childlike state is discovered to be related to a stimulus cue that reminds a child of a traumatic memory, it is important to evaluate that memory, detoxify it, and sever any cues that automatically elicit reexperiencing of that event. Sometimes this best occurs with supportive, nurturing parents in the therapy room, who can listen to a child's account of a past trauma, provide reassurance that this will not reoccur, and provide the soothing that the child may have missed earlier. Processing these traumatic moments within the context of a safe and loving relationship is seen as the best way to detoxify their conditioned effects (Silberg, 1999).

Population

This method is appropriate for children with dissociative symptoms or DID.

Training and Prerequisites

This complex method takes great sensitivity to the many levels of systems that maintain dissociative behavior. Treatment must be tailored to each child. A high degree of professional knowledge and experience is required (Silberg, 1999).

Length of Treatment

Length will vary depending on the degree of severity of the dissociative symptoms, how entrenched the family is in their way of functioning, and the child's readiness to change. One study suggests that a moderate treatment length, under 2 years, was associated with the most favorable outcomes (Silberg & Waters, 1998).

Treatment Outcomes/Results

An outcome study by Silberg and Waters (1998) using a method less broad based than the one described here resulted in favorable outcomes for the majority of children with whom it was used. Successes with individual cases using Silberg's method include a 12- to 14-year-old with severe dissociative symptoms (Silberg, in press). Key therapeutic elements included using the therapeutic relationship to instill hope and attachment, the child's natural fantasy skills to help develop positive resources in the imagination, family work to extricate the patient from conflicting messages, and cognitive-behavioral skills to identify precursors to dissociative "shutdown" states. The child initially presented with a childlike alternate state for whose behavior she claimed to have no memory. In therapy, she learned to understand her dissociated feelings and her conflicting identifications and learned to express these feelings more directly to her parents. The patient was encouraged to take responsibility for her behavior even while in this childlike state. Her memory for her behavior quickly returned. After 2 years of treatment, no more dissociative problems were apparent, and today the youngster is reengaged in a productive life. Continued problems in the area of affect regulation are apparent and are the current focus of treatment.

Treatment of Inner-City Children and Adolescents

Although dramatic incidents of violence like the Columbine school shootings have occurred far too often over the past few years, small-scale massacres occur with a higher frequency in the inner city. Ethnicity, culture, and race operate interactively in multiply violence-traumatized inner-city children. They determine the nature of the assessment process and the therapeutic relationship, expectations of treatment outcome, problem definition, and the specific treatment process (Parson, 2000). Parson describes his method, posttraumatic child therapy (PTCT) below (Parson, 2000).

History and Precursors

Parson (1994) proposed the term urban violence traumatic stress syndrome (UVTS) to capture the damage to the inner-city child's self-structure. UVTS features five major dimensions: (1) *Damaged sense of self and confused self-identities* (e.g., viewing self as both victim and perpetrator)—perpetual sense of powerlessness to stop the violence or change the environment; persistent psychological distress; and vendetta rage (Garbarino et al., 1991, p. 379), hyperaggressivity and instrumental use of violence to cope with self-damage, death obsession, a sense of betrayal, and personal defilement. (2) *Severed attachment bonds*—UVTS interrupts vital attachment bonds and creates distrust of family, friends, neighbors, and society. (3) *Cognitive stress response*—"dematuring" is characterized by loss of conservation skills; loss of language skills; misalignment of emotion, time, and reality; disturbance in object constancy; and regressive use of primitive memory and functioning. (4) *Emotional stress response*—a profound intolerance for strong affect, despite ongoing sadness, grief, guilt, depression, shame, anxiety, anger, belligerence, revulsion, despair, poor impulse control, persistent fear states including anticipatory fear of being overwhelmed by strong affects, violent impulses, and/or terror. (5) *Moral stress response and distortion of ethnocultural values*—rupturing of values and morals and of ethnic mental structures.

PTCT is a multiphasic trauma treatment model (Brown, Scheflin, & Hammond, 1998, p. 454; Brown & Fromm, 1986; Burgess & Holstrom, 1974; Courtois, 1988; Herman, 1992; Parson, 1984, 1994, 1996a, 1996b, 1997) based on the early works of Pierre Janet (1889) and Sigmund Freud (see Breuer & Freud, 1893–1895/1955). Janet advanced a three-phase treatment approach: stabilization, containment, and symptom reduction; modification of traumatic memories; and personality integration and rehabilitation (van der Hart, Brown, & van der Kolk, 1989a, 1989b). In addition, PTCT recognizes the problem of arrested development in children after trauma (Parson, 1994, 1997). The PTCT model strives to increase memory management, related affect processing, and relational security and competence. Family and other adjunctant therapies assist this process.

Methods

The PTCT model emphasizes child and family education, expression of affects, deconditioning of negative affects, symptom management, coping augmentation, reversing cognitive distortions while facilitating self-identity and relational development (Brown et al., 1998; Parson, 1996a, 1996b, 1997). Each phase has specific goals for processing violence/trauma memories.

Memory functions in UVTS are organized in two basic systems: behavioral memory (trauma memories stored in impulsive actional forms) and autobiographical memory (Pillemer & White, 1989; Share, 1994). Treatment addresses fragmented, incomplete and often distorted memories. PTCT features four phases (see Table 12.4), but remains cognizant that each child and family are different. Successful treatment increases control and a better sense of self and reduces fragmentation and helplessness. The child learns to trust,

TABLE 12.4. Phases of Parson's Posttrauma Child Therapy Method

Phase 1: Pretherapy—includes modeling, role-play, relevant videotape programs, and other psychoeducational techniques; establishment of goals, benefits, focus, and methods.

Phase 2: Stabilization—involves cognitive-behavioral stress management including stress management/relaxation training, deconditioning of negative affects, biofeedback, systematic restructuring of assumptions, and (when indicated) psychopharmacology and/or residential treatment. Self-instructional training (Meichenbaum, 1986) is used in three steps: (1) negative thinking is explored; (2) the child learns how to generate incompatible thinking, facilitated by overt, positive self-statements later repeated subvocally; (3)behavioral rehearsal ensures the steady development of coping and mastery skills.

Phase 3: Return to scene—when sufficient trust has been developed in the therapeutic relationship and the child has mastered a relaxation procedure, EMDR techniques are used. The child is taken back to the actual scene of the occurrence and processes through cognitive and dynamic procedures (e.g., flooding).

Phase 4: Completion and integration of self—individual and play modalities, as dictated by the child's developmental needs; psychodynamic approaches (e.g., transference, dream interpretation) to facilitate the child's capacity to tolerate and integrate powerful trauma emotions.

Source: Data from Parson (2000).

to increase coping; to take responsibility for personal emotions and actions, and achieves integration and growth (including repaired attachments).

Population

Treatment is adapted for age and developmental level and is designed for inner-city children of African American, Latino, and Caucasian heritages. Children with schizophrenic, organic, and severe developmental anomalies may not do well with this method. Children with early sociopathic behavioral patterns will benefit from the PTCT approach. The proposed method is sufficiently broad to include traumatized children with a variety of personality and pathologic behavioral traits and patterns.

Training and Prerequisites

Knowledge of trauma and children and experience and training for physiological regulation of children are essential. Above all, trauma treatment with these children should be nurturing, corrective, engaging, child-sensitive, supportive, and fun. For violent, acting-out, impulse-driven African American and Latino boys Parson recommends a well-trained male therapist of African American or Latino cultural background when possible. Trauma treatment requires unconditional acceptance and caring. Those with revulsion and conscious or unconscious hostility toward them should not treat inner-city children. The absence of tolerance for difference disqualifies any therapist, regardless of race.

Length of Treatment

Estimated length of treatment is 12–18 months. For some children the time may be longer. The greater the family, community, and general social support available to the child—as adjunctive, facilitating elements—the faster and more successful the treatment is likely to be.

Treatment Outcomes/Results

Positive outcomes from using this method of treatment have included the following: (1) a greater sense of inner calm/peacefulness and self-soothing; (2) control over emotions, impulses, and negative behavioral expression; (3) less fear of emotional closeness; (4) increase in hopefulness and in positive possibilities for a violence-free future; (5) ability to internally process and then channel narcissistic, angry feelings into constructive action; (6) general enhanced coping; and (7) general enhanced ability to engage in moral reasoning, attitudes, and behaviors.

CONCLUSIONS

Used effectively, the innovative treatment methods described in this chapter have reduced symptoms of PTSD, reduced or prevented the escalation of depression and/or other trauma-associated symptoms, and enhanced or helped to recover the child's confidence, competence, and control. They provide an ally in the therapist and a sense that the child is not alone. Nevertheless, we know far less than we need to know about the effectiveness of our treatment methods. For example, we do not yet know whether different treatment methods may be most effective when used by clinicians with specific styles and attitudes, and when used in treatment of children with specific qualities and/or specific traumas.

Outcome studies that follow children into adulthood are needed to assess the long-term results of interventions. Children's reporting varies over time. Their reports may be influenced by perceived expectations, maturity levels, self-knowledge, and treatment. Moreover, measures of PTSD and associated symptoms do not investigate the translation of symptoms into patterns of thought and/or behavior or into vulnerabilities that develop over time. The link between these patterns/vulnerabilities and the trauma may not be evident. Some symptoms or vulnerabilities may become dormant until unleashed by the right set of triggers.

New measures and methods are needed to identify specific aspects of the child, the experience, and additional variables that influence the long-term consequences of trauma and treatment. We need to know more about the interplay of the child's history (e.g., attachments; family and school life), trauma symptoms (e.g., increased reactivity; changed attitudes), aspects of the specific event or ongoing exposures (e.g., intense traumatic impressions; the personal or impersonal nature of the assault whether by nature, person, or nation), characteristics of the child (e.g., temperament or personality style), and other variables. When we can identify and assess over time these additional variables, we will have clearer and more thorough information about the results of interventions and the needs of traumatized children.

ACKNOWLEDGMENTS

I am grateful to Dr. John P. Wilson, Dr. Fred Lerner, Dr. Sam Nader, Dr. Linda V. Berens, Dr. Christine Mello, Liz Hahn, Jackie George, Marilee Conant, Allison Spencer, Sheena Staff, and Chelsea Oldroyd for their kind assistance in gathering materials and information, typing, reading, and editing. I sincerely thank Dr. Joyanna L. Silberg, Dr. Judith A. Cohen, Dr. John March, Dr. Erwin R. Parson, Dr. AnnMarie Glodich, Dr. Rick Greenwald, and Dr. Mary Jo Barrett for their valuable contributions to this chapter.

REFERENCES

AACAP Work Group on Quality Issues (1998). Practice parameters for the assessment and treatment of children and adolescents with posttraumatic stress disorder (J. A. Cohen, principal author). *Journal of the American Academy of Child and Adolescent Psychiatry Supplement, 37*(10), 4S–26S.

Ainsworth, M. D. S. (1973). The development of infant–mother attachment. In B. M. Caldwell & H. Ricciuti (Eds.), *Review of child development research* (Vol. 3, pp. 1–94). Chicago: University of Chicago Press.

Allen, J. G. (1995). *Coping with trauma.* Washington, DC: American Psychiatric Press.

Allen, J. G., Kelly, K. A., & Glodich, A. M. (1997). A psychoeducational program for patients with trauma-related disorders. *Bulletin of the Menninger Clinic, 61,* 222–239.

Allers, C. T., White, J. F., & Mullis, F. (1997). The treatment of dissociation in an HIV-infected sexually abused adolescent male. *Psychotherapy, 34*(2), 201–206.

Alexander, P. C., Anderson, C. L., Brand, B., Schaeffer, C. M., Grelling, B. Z., & Kretz, L. (1998). Adult attachment and longterm effects in survivors of incest. *Child Abuse and Neglect, 22*(1), 45–61.

Amster, F. (1943). Differential use of play in treatment of young children. *American Journal of Orthopsychiatry, 13,* 62–68.

Axline, V. (1947). *Play therapy.* Boston: Houghton Mifflin.

Barrett, M. J. (1999, July 20). *Multiple systems model for the treatment of trauma.* E-mail communication.

Bartlett, F. C. (1932). *Remembering: A study in experimental and social psychology.* New York: Macmillan.

Benham, E. (1995). Coping strategies: A psychoeducational approach to posttraumatic symptomatology. *Journal of Psychosocial Nursing, 33*(6), 30–35.

Berens, L. V. (1985). *Comparison of Jungian function theory and Keirseyan temperament theory in the use of the Myers–Briggs Type Indicator.* Unpublished partial doctoral dissertation, United States International University, San Diego, CA.

Berens, L. V. (1998). *Understanding yourself and others: An introduction to temperament.* Huntington Beach, CA: Telos Publications.

Berens, L. V., & Nardi, D. (1999). *The 16 sixteen personality types: Descriptions for self-discovery.* Huntington Beach, CA: Telos Publications.

Blechman, E., Dumas, J., & Prinz, R. (1994). Prosocial coping by youth exposed to violence. *Journal of Child and Adolescent Group Therapy, 4,* 208–227.

Bloch, D., Silber, E., & Perry, S. (1956). Some factors in the emotional reaction of children to disaster. *American Journal of Psychiatry, 113,* 416–422.

Bowlby, J. (1969). *Attachment and loss: Vol. 1: Attachment.* New York: Basic Books.

Bowlby, J. (1973). *Attachment and loss: Vol 2: Separation.* New York: Basic Books.

Bretherton, I. (1990). Open communication and internal working models: Their role in the development of attachment relationships. In R. A. Thompson (Ed.), *Nebraska Symposium on Motivation: Vol. 36. Socioemotional development* (pp. 57–113). Lincoln: University of Nebraska Press.

Breuer, J., & Freud, S. (1955). Studies in hysteria. In J. Strachey (Ed. & Trans.), *The standard edition of the complete works of Sigmund Freud* (Vol. 2, pp. 1–311). London: Hogarth Press. (Original work published 1893–1895)

Briere, J. (1992). *Child abuse trauma: Theory and treatment of the lasting effects.* Newbury Park, CA: Sage.

Briere, J. (1995). *Trauma Symptom Checklist for Children Manual.* Odessa, FL: Psychological Assessment Resources.

Brodzinsky, D. M., Gormly, A. V., & Ambron, S. R. (1986). *Lifespan human development* (3rd ed., pp. 111–120). New York: Holt, Rinehart & Winston.

Brown, D., & Fromm, E. (1986). *Hypnotherapy and hypnoanalysis.* Hillsdale, NJ: Erlbaum.

Brown, D., Scheflin, A., & Hammond, C. (1998). *Memory, trauma treatment and the law: An essential reference on memory for clinicians, researchers, attorneys, and judges.* New York: Norton.

Burgess, A., & Holstrom, L. (1974). Rape trauma syndrome. *American Journal of Psychiatry, 131,* 981–986.

Carey-Trefzer, C. (1949). The results of a clinical study of war-damaged children who attended the Child Guidance Clinic, the Hospital for Sick Children, Great Ormond Street, London. *Journal of Mental Science, 95,* 535–559.

Carlson, E. B. (1997). *Trauma assessments.* New York: Guilford Press.

Chemtob, C. M., Nakashima, J., Hamada, R., & Carlson, J. (in press). Brief treatment for elementary school children with disaster-related PTSD: A field study. *Journal of Clinical Psychology.*

Chemtob, C. M., Tolin, D. F., van der Kolk, B. A., & Pitman, R. K. (2000). Eye movement desensitization and reprocessing. In E. B. Foa, T. M. Keane, & M. J. Friedman (Eds.), *Effective treatments for PTSD: Practice guidelines from the International Society for Traumatic Stress Studies* (pp. 139–154). New York: Guilford Press.

Chess, S., & Thomas, A. (1991). Temperament. In M. Lewis (Ed.), *Child and adolescent psychiatry: A comprehensive textbook* (pp. 145–159). Baltimore: Williams & Wilkins.

Cohen, J. A. (1999). *Treatment of traumatized children* (Trauma Therapy Audio Series). Thousand Oaks, CA: Sage.

Cohen, J. A., Berliner, L., & Mannarino, A. P. (2000). Treatment of traumatized children: A review and synthesis. *Journal of Trauma, Violence and Abuse, 1*(1), 29–46.

Cohen J. A., Deblinger, E, & Mannarino, A. P. (1997). *Treatment of PTSD in sexually abused children.* Funded grant application, National Institute of Mental Health, Bethesda, MD (No. 1R10 MH55963).

Cohen J. A., & Mannarino, A. P. (1993). A treatment model for sexually abused preschoolers. *Journal of Interpersonal Violence, 8*(1), 115–131.

Cohen, J. A., & Mannarino, A. P. (1996). A treatment outcome study for sexually abused preschool children: Initial findings. *Journal of the American Academy of Child and Adolescent Psychiatry, 35*(1), 42–50.

Cohen, J. A., & Mannarino, A. P. (1997). A treatment study for sexually abused preschool children: Outcome during a one year follow-up. *Journal of the American Academy of Child and Adolescent Psychiatry, 36*(9), 1228–1235.

Cohen, J. A., Mannarino, A. P., Berliner, L., & Deblinger, E. (2000). Trauma-focused cognitive behavioral therapy: An empirical update. *Journal of Interpersonal Violence, 15*(11), 1203–1223.

Combrinck-Graham, L. (1991). Development of school-age children. In M. Lewis (Ed.), *Child and adolescent psychiatry: A comprehensive textbook* (pp. 157–265). Baltimore: Williams & Wilkins.

Coons, P. M. (1996). Clinical phenomenology of 25 children and adolescents with dissociative disorders. *Child and Adolescent Psychiatric Clinics of North America, 5*, 361–374.

Courtois, C. (1988). *Healing the incest wound: Adult survivors in therapy.* New York: Norton.

Culbertson, J. L., & Willis, D. J. (1998). Interventions with young children who have been multiply abused. *Journal of Aggression, Maltreatment and Trauma, 2*(1), 207–232.

Danieli, Y. (Ed.). (1998). *International handbook of multigenerational legacies of trauma.* New York: Plenum Press.

Deblinger, E., & Heflin, A. H. (1996). *Treating sexually abused children and their nonoffending parents: A cognitive behavioral approach.* Thousand Oaks, CA: Sage.

Deblinger, E., Lippmann, J., & Steer, R. (1996). Sexually abused children suffering posttraumatic stress symptoms: Initial treatment outcome findings. *Child Maltreatment, 1*(4), 310–321.

Deblinger, E., McLeer, S. V., Atkins, M., Ralph, D., & Foa, E. (1989). Posttraumatic stress in sexually abused children, physically abused children and non-abused children. *Child Abuse and Neglect, 13*, 403–408.

Dell, D. F., & Eisenhower, J. W. (1990). Adolescent multiple personality disorder: A preliminary study of eleven cases. *Journal of the American Academy of Child and Adolescent Psychiatry, 29*(3), 359–366.

Delunas, E. (1992). *Survival games personalities play.* Carmel, CA: Sunflower Ink.

Dodge, K. A., Bates, J. E., Pettit, G. S., & Valente, E. (1995). Social information-processing patterns partially mediate the effect of early physical abuse on later conduct problems. *Journal of Abnormal Psychology, 104*(4), 632–643.

Erikson, M., Rossi, E. L., & Ryan, M. O. (1985). *Life reframing in hypnosis: Seminars, workshops, and lectures of Milton Erikson* (Vol. 2). New York: Irvington

Eth, S., & Pynoos, R. (1985). Psychiatric interventions with children traumatized by violence. In D. H. Schetky & E. P. Benedik (Eds.), *Emerging issues in child psychiatry and the law* (pp. 285–309). New York: Brunner/Mazel.

Fantuzzo, J. W. (1990). Behavioral treatment of the victims of child abuse and neglect. *Behavior Modification, 14*(3), 316–339.

Field, T., Seligman, S., Scafidi, F., & Schanberg, S. (1996). Alleviating posttraumatic stress in children following Hurricane Andrew. *Journal of Applied Developmental Psychology, 17*, 37–50.

Finkelhor, D. (1987). The trauma of child sexual abuse: Two models. *Journal of Interpersonal Violence, 2*(4), 348–366.

Finkelhor, D., & Strapko, N. (1992). Sexual abuse prevention education: A review of evaluation studies. In D. Willis, E. W. Holden, & M. Rosenberg (Eds.), *Prevention of child maltreatment: Developmental and ecological perspectives* (pp. 150–167). New York: Wiley.

Foa, E. B. (1997). Psychological processes related to recovery from a trauma and an effective treatment for PTSD. *Annals of the New York Academy of Sciences, 821*, 410–424.

Foa, E. B., & Rothbaum, B. O. (1997). Behavioural psychotherapy for post-traumatic stress disorder. *International Review of Psychiatry, 1*, 219–226.

Foa, E. B., Steketee, G., & Rothbaum, B. O. (1989). Behavioral/cognitive conceptualization of PTSD. *Behavior Therapy, 20*, 155–176.

Foulkes, D. (1990). Dreaming and consciousness. *European Journal of Cognitive Psychology, 2*(1), 39–55.

Foulkes, D., Hollifield, M., Sullivan, B., Bradley, L., & Terry, R. (1990). REM dreaming and cognitive skills at ages 5–8: A cross-sectional study. *International Journal of Behavioral Development, 13*(4), 447–465.

Franklin, C., & Streeter, C. (1992). Social support and psychoeducational interventions with middle class dropout youth. *Child and Adolescent Social Work Journal, 9*(2), 131–153.

Frederick, C., Pynoos, R., & Nader, K. (1992). *Childhood Post-Traumatic Stress Reaction Index* (CPTS-RI), a copyrighted semistructured interview for children with traumatic exposure. Available from Frederick or Pynoos at UCLA or from Nader (Knader@twosuns.org).

Freud, A. (1965). *Normality and pathology in childhood.* New York: International Universities Press.

Freud, A., & Burlingham, D. (1943). *War and children.* New York: Medical War Books.

Friedrich, W. N., Grambsch, P., Damon, L., Hewitt, S. K., Koverola, C., Lang, R., Wolf, V., & Broughton, D. (1992). The Child Sexual Behavior Inventory: Normative and clinical comparisons. *Psychological Assessment, 4,* 303–311.

Friedrich, W. N., Luecke, W. J., Beilke, R. L., & Place, V. (1992). Psychotherapy outcome of sexually abused boys: An agency study. *Journal of Interpersonal Violence, 7,* 396–409.

Garbarino, J. (1999). *Lost boys: Why our sons turn violent and how we can save them* (pp. 120–145). New York: Free Press.

Garbarino, J., Kostelny, K., & Dubrow, N. (1991). What children can tell us about living in danger. *American Psychologist, 46,* 376–383.

Glodich, A. M. (1999a, June 30). *Psychoeducational groups for adolescents exposed to violence and abuse.* An E-mail communication. (geothomps@cjnetworks.com)

Glodich, A. M. (1999b). *Psychoeducational groups for adolescents exposed to violence and abuse: Assessing the effectiveness of increasing knowledge of trauma to avert reenactment and risk-taking behaviors.* Unpublished doctoral dissertation, Smith College School for Social Work, Northampton, MA.

Glodich, A. M., & Allen, J. G. (1998). Adolescents exposed to violence and abuse: A review of the group therapy literature with an emphasis on preventing trauma reenactment. *Journal of Child and Adolescent Group Therapy, 8*(3), 135–155.

Goenjian, A. K., Karayan, I., Pynoos, R. S., Minassian, D., Najarian, L. M., Steinberg, A. M., & Fairbanks, L. A. (1997). Outcome of psychotherapy among early adolescents after trauma. *American Journal of Psychiatry, 154,* 536–542.

Goleman, D. (1992, July 21). Childhood trauma: Memory or invention? *New York Times,* p. B5.

Goodman, G. S., & Quas, J. A. (1996). Trauma and memory: Individual differences in children's recounting of a stressful experience. In N. Stein, P. A. Ornstein, B. Tversky, & C. J. Brainerd (Eds.), *Memory for everyday and emotional events* (pp. 267–294). Hillsdale, NJ: Erlbaum.

Gorham, E. L. (1997). Sixteen-step strategic family therapy for the treatment of child sexual abuse: A treatment adaptation and case example. *Psychotherapy in Private Practice, 16*(1), 21–37.

Greenwald, R. (1994). Applying eye movement desensitization and reprocessing (EMDR) to the treatment of traumatized children: Five case studies. *Anxiety Disorders Practice Journal, 1,* 83–97.

Greenwald, R. (1998). EMDR: New hope for children suffering from trauma and loss. *Clinical Child Psychology and Psychiatry, 3*(2), 279–287.

Greenwald, R. (1999, April 18). *EMDR for traumatized children*. An E-mail communication. (rg@childtrauma.com)

Greenwald, R. (in press). Motivation–Adaptive Skills–Trauma Resolution (MASTR) therapy for adolescents with conduct problems: An open trial. *Journal of Aggression, Maltreatment, and Trauma*.

Grusznski, R., Brink, J., & Edleson, J. (1988). Support and education groups for children of battered women. *Child Welfare, 67*(5), 431–443.

Gunnar, M. R., Brodersen, L., Krueger, K., & Rigatuso, J. (1996). Dampening of adrenocortical responses during infancy: Normative changes and individual differences. *Child Development, 67*, 877–889.

Hazzard, A. (1993). Psychoeducational groups to teach children sexual abuse prevention skills. *Journal of Child and Adolescent Group Psychotherapy, 3*(1), 13–23.

Hazzard, A., Webb, C., Kleemeier, C., Angert, L., & Pohl, J. (1991). Child sexual abuse prevention: Evaluation and one-year follow-up. *Child Abuse and Neglect, 15*, 123–138.

Heras, P. (1992). Cultural considerations in the assessment and treatment of child sexual abuse. *Journal of Child Sexual Abuse, 1*(3), 119–132.

Herman, J. (1992). *Trauma and recovery*. New York: Basic Books.

Herman, J. L., Perry, J. C., & van der Kolk, B. A. (1989). Childhood trauma in borderline personality disorder. *American Journal of Psychiatry, 146*, 490–495.

Holden, D., & Anderson, C. (1990). Psychoeducational family intervention for depressed patients and their families. In G. I. Keitner (Ed.), *Depression and families: Impact and treatment* (pp. 159–184). Washington, DC: American Psychiatric Press.

Howe, M. L. (1997). Children's memory for traumatic experiences. *Learning and Individual Differences, 9*(2), 153–174.

Howe, M. L., Courage, M. L., & Peterson, C. (1995). Intrusions in preschoolers' recall of traumatic childhood events. *Psychonomic Bulletin and Review, 2*(1), 130–134.

International Society for Traumatic Stress Studies [ISTSS]. (1998). *Childhood trauma remembered: A report on the current scientific knowledge base and its applications*. Chicago: Author.

James, B. (1994). *Handbook for treatment of attachment-trauma problems in children*. Lexington, MA: Lexington Books.

Janet, P. (1889). *L'automatisme psychologuque [Psychological automatisms]: essai ute psychologie experimentale sur les formes inferieures de l'activite humaine*. Paris: Feliz Alcan.

Janoff-Bulman, R. (1989). Assumptive worlds and the stress of traumatic events: Applications of the schema construct. *Social Cognition, 7*(2), 113–136.

Johnson, M. K., & Foley, M. A. (1984). Differentiating fact from fantasy: The reliability of children's memory. *Journal of Social Issues, 40*, 33–50.

Jones, F., & Selder, F. (1996). Psychoeducational groups to promote effective coping in school age children living in violent communities. *Issues in Mental Health Nursing, 17*(6), 559–571.

Joseph, S. A., Brewin, C. R., Yule, W., & Williams, R. (1991). Causal attributions and psychiatric symptoms in survivors of the Herald of Free Enterprise disaster. *British Journal of Psychiatry, 159*(542), 542–546.

Joseph, S. A., Brewin, C. R., Yule, W., & Williams, R. (1993). Causal attributions and post-traumatic stress in adolescents. *Journal of Child Psychology and Psychiatry, 34*(2), 247–253.

Jung, C. (1971). Psychological types. In *The collected works of C. G. Jung* (Vol. 6). Princeton: Princeton, NJ: University Press.

Keirsey, D. (1987). *Portraits of temperament*. Del Mar, CA: Prometheus Nemesis.

Keirsey, D., & Bates, M. (1978). *Please understand me*. Del Mar, CA: Prometheus Nemesis.

Kluft, R. P. (1986). Treating children who have multiple personality disorder. In B. G. Braun (Ed.), *Treatment of multiple personality disorder* (pp. 79–105). Washington, DC: American Psychiatric Press.

Kluft, R. P. (1990). *Incest-related syndromes of adult psychopathology*. Washington, DC: American Psychiatric Press.

Koss, M., Figueredo, A. J., Bell, I., Tharan, M., & Tromp, S. (1996). Traumatic memory characteristics: A cross-validated mediational model of response to rape among employed women. *Journal of Abnormal Psychology, 105,* 421–432.

Kostelny, K., & Garbarino, J. (1994). Coping with the consequences of living in danger: The case of Palestinian children and youth. *International Journal of Behavioral Development, 17*(4), 595–611.

Lacey, G. N. (1972). Observations on Aberfan. *Journal of Psychosomatic Research, 16,* 257–260.

Lehmann, P., & Coady, N. F. (Eds.). (2000). *Theoretical perspectives for direct social work practice: A generalist-eclectic approach*. New York: Springer.

Levy, D. M. (1938). Release therapy in young children. *Psychiatry, 1,* 387–390.

Levy, D. M. (1945). Psychic trauma of operations in children. *American Journal of Diseases of Children, 69,* 7–25.

Lewis, M. (1991). Normal growth and development: An overview. In J. M. Wiener (Ed.), *Textbook of child and adolescent psychiatry* (pp. 25–39). Washington, DC: American Psychiatric Press.

Lewis, M. (1995). Memory and psychoanalysis: A new look at infantile amnesia and transference. *Journal of the American Academy of Child and Adolescent Psychiatry, 34*(4), 405–417.

Lindsay, D. S., & Read, J. D. (1995). Memory work and recovered memories of childhood sexual abuse: Scientific evidence and public, professional, and personal issues. *Psychology, Public Policy, and Law, 1,* 846–908.

Linehan, M. M. (1993). *Cognitive-behavioral treatment of borderline personality disorder*. New York: Guilford Press.

Lubin, H., Loris, M., Burt, J., & Johnson, D. (1998). Efficacy of psychoeducational group therapy in reducing symptoms of posttraumatic stress disorder among multiply traumatized women. *American Journal of Psychiatry, 155,* 1172–1177.

Macksoud, M. S., Dyregrov, A., & Raundalen, M. (1993). Traumatic war experiences and their effects on children. In J. P. Wilson & B. Raphael (Eds.), *International handbook of traumatic stress syndromes* (pp. 625–632). New York: Plenum Press.

Madanes, C. (1981). *Strategic family therapy*. San Francisco: Jossey-Bass.

Madanes, C. (1990). *Sex, love and violence*. New York: Norton.

Maddock, J. W., & Larson, N. R. (1995). *Incestuous families: An ecological approach to understanding and treatment*. New York: Norton.

Main, M., Kaplan, N., & Cassidy, J. (1985). Security of infancy, childhood, and adulthood: A move to the level of representation. In I. Bretherton & E. Waters (Eds.), *Growing points of attachment theory and research* (pp. 66–106). Chicago: University of Chicago Press.

Malenbaum, R., & Russell, A. T. (1987). Multiple personality disorder in an eleven-year-old boy and his mother. *Journal of the American Academy of Child and Adolescent Psychiatry, 26*(3), 436–439.

Mannarino, A. P., & Cohen, J. A. (1996). Abuse related attributions and perceptions, general attributions, and locus of control in sexually abused girls. *Journal of Interpersonal Violence, 11*(2), 162–180.

Mannarino, A. P., Cohen, J. A., & Berman, S. R. (1994). Children's Attribution and Perception Scale: A new measure of sexual abuse-related factors. *Journal of Clinical and Child Psychology, 23*, 204–211.

Mannarino, A. P., Cohen, J. A., & Gregor, M. (1989). Emotional and behavioral difficulties in sexually abused girls. *Journal of Interpersonal Violence, 4*(4), 437–451.

March, J. (1998). *Manual for the Multidimensional Anxiety Scale for Children (MASC)*. Toronto, Canada: MultiHealth Systems.

March, J. (1999, August 25). E-mail communication.

March, J., Amaya-Jackson, L., Foa, E., & Treadwell, K. (1999). *Trauma-focused coping treatment of pediatric posttraumatic stress disorder after single-incident trauma (Version 1. 0)*. An unpublished protocol.

March, J., Amaya-Jackson, L., Murray, M., & Schulte, A. (1998). Cognitive-behavioral psychotherapy for children and adolescents with post-traumatic stress disorder following a single-incident stressor. *Journal of the American Academy of Child and Adolescent Psychiatry, 37*(6), 585–593.

March, J., Amaya-Jackson, L., Terry, R., & Costanzo, P. (1997). Post-traumatic stress in children and adolescents after an industrial fire. *Journal of the American Academy of Child and Adolescent Psychiatry, 36*(8), 1080–1088.

March, J., Frances, A., Kahn, D., & Carpenter, D. (1997). Expert consensus guidelines: Treatment of obsessive–compulsive disorder. *Journal of Clinical Psychiatry, 58*(Suppl. 4), 1–72.

Marsella, A. J., Friedman, M. J., Gerrity, E. T., & Scurfield, R. M. (Eds.). (1996). *Ethnocultural aspects of posttraumatic stress disorder: Issues, research, and clinical applications*. Washington, DC: American Psychological Association.

McCann, L., & Pearlman, L. (1990). *Psychological trauma and the adult survivor: Theory, therapy, and transformation*. New York: Brunner/Mazel.

McEwen, B. S. (1982). Glucocorticoids and hippocampus: Receptors in search of a function. In D. Ganen & D. Pfaff (Eds.), *Adrenal actions on the brain* (pp. 1–22). New York: Springer-Verlag.

Meichenbaum, D. (1986). *Stress inoculation training*. New York: Pergamon Press.

Meichenbaum, D. (1994). *A clinical handbook/practical therapist manual for assessing and treating adults with posttraumatic stress disorder (PTSD)*. Waterloo, Ontario, Canada: Institute Press.

Murray, C. C., & Son, L. (1998). The effect of multiple victimization on children's cognition: Variations in response. *Journal of Aggression, Maltreatment and Trauma, 2*(1), 131–146.

Myers, I. (1980). *Gifts differing*. Palo Alto, CA: Consulting Psychologists Press.

Myers, I., & McCaulley, M. (1985). *Manual: A guide to the use of the Myers–Briggs Type Indicator*. Palo Alto, CA: Consulting Psychologists Press.

Nachmias, M., Gunnar, M., Mangelsdorf, S., Parritz, R. H., & Buss, K. (1996). Behavioral inhibition and stress reactivity: The moderating role of attachment security. *Child Development, 67*, 508–522.

Nader, K. (1991, February 28). *Posttraumatic stress assessment: East Coldenham Elementary School.* Unpublished report.

Nader, K. (1994). Countertransference in treating trauma and victimization in childhood. In J. Wilson & J. Lindy (Eds.), *Countertransference in the treatment of PTSD* (pp. 179–205). New York: Guilford Press.

Nader, K. (1996a). Assessing traumatic experiences in children. In J. Wilson & T. Keane (Eds.), *Assessing psychological trauma and PTSD* (pp. 291–348). New York: Guilford Press.

Nader, K. (1996b). Children's traumatic dreams. In D. Barrett (Ed.), *Trauma and dreams* (pp. 9–24). Cambridge, MA: Harvard University Press.

Nader, K. (1997). Treating traumatic grief in systems. In C. R. Figley, B. E. Bride, & N. Mazza (Eds.), *Death and trauma: The traumatology of grieving* (pp. 159–192). London: Taylor & Francis.

Nader, K. (1998). Violence: Effects of a parents' previous trauma on currently traumatized children. In Y. Danieli (Ed.), *An international handbook of multigenerational legacies of trauma* (pp. 571–583). New York: Plenum Press.

Nader, K., Blake, D., & Kriegler, J. (1994). *Instruction Manual, Clinician-Administered PTSD Scale for Children and Adolescents CAPS-CA.* White River Junction, VT: National Center for PTSD.

Nader, K., Dubrow, N., & Stamm, B. (Eds.). (1999). *Honoring differences: Cultural issues in the treatment of traumatic stress.* Philadelphia: Taylor & Francis.

Nader, K., & Fairbanks, L. (1994). The suppression of reexperiencing: Impulse control and somatic symptoms in children following traumatic exposure. *Anxiety, Stress and Coping: An International Journal, 7,* 229–239.

Nader, K., Kriegler, J., Blake, D., & Pynoos, R. *Clinician-Administered PTSD Scale for children and adolescents (CAPS-C) (1994), a semi-structured interview for children with traumatic exposure.* White River Junction, VT: National Center for PTSD.

Nader, K., & Mello, C. (2000). Interactive trauma/grief-focused therapy. In P. Lehmann & N. F. Coady (Eds.), *Theoretical perspectives for direct social work practice: A generalist–eclectic approach* (pp. 382–401). New York: Springer.

Nader, K., & Pynoos, R. (1991). Play and drawing as tools for interviewing traumatized children. In C. Schaeffer, K. Gitlan, & A. Sandgrund (Eds.), *Play, diagnosis and assessment* (pp. 375–389). New York: Wiley.

Nader, K., & Pynoos, R. (1993). School disaster: Planning and initial interventions. *Journal of Social Behavior and Personality, 8*(5), 299–320.

Nader, K., Pynoos, R., Fairbanks, L., Al-Ajeel, M., & Al-Asfour, A. (1993). A preliminary study of PTSD and grief among the children of Kuwait following the Gulf crisis. *British Journal of Clinical Psychology, 32,* 407–416.

Neisser, U. (1976). *Cognition and reality: Principles and implications of cognitive psychology.* San Francisco: Freeman.

Odom, S. L., & Strain, P. S. (1984). Peer-mediated approach to promoting children's social interactions: A review. *American Journal of Orthopsychiatry, 54,* 545–557.

Parson, E. R. (1984). The reparation of the self: Clinical and theoretical dimensions in the treatment of Vietnam combat veterans. *Journal of Contemporary Psychotherapy, 14,* 14–56.

Parson, E. R. (1994). Post-traumatic ethnotherapy (P-TET): Processes in assessment and intervention in aspects of global psychic trauma. In M. B. Williams & J. F. Sommer (Eds.), *Handbook of post-traumatic therapy* (pp. 221–239). Westport, CT: Greenwood Press.

Parson, E. R. (1996a). It takes a village to heal a child: Necessary spectrum of expertise and benevolence by therapists, non-governmental organizations, and the United Nations in managing warzone stress in children traumatized by political violence. *Journal of Contemporary Psychotherapy, 26,* 251–286.

Parson, E. R. (1996b). Child trauma therapy and the effects of trauma, loss, and dissociation: A multisystems approach to helping children exposed to lethal urban community violence. *Journal of Contemporary Psychotherapy, 26,* 117–162.

Parson, E. R. (1997). Post-traumatic child therapy (P-TCT): Assessment and treatment factors in clinic work with inner-city children exposed to catastrophic community violence. *Journal of Interpersonal Violence, 12,* 172–194.

Parson, E. R. (2000). *Post-traumatic child therapy (P-TCT) with inner-city children and adolescents.* An E-mail communication. (BAIERP@aol.com)

Pellicer, X. (1993). Eye movement desensitization treatment of a child's nightmares: A case report. *Journal of Behavior Therapy and Experimental Psychiatry, 24,* 73–75.

Perloff, R. M. (1993). *The dynamics of persuasion.* Hillsdale, NJ: L. Erlbaum.

Perry, B. D. (1993). Medicine and psychotherapy: Neurodevelopment and the neurophysiology of trauma. *The Advisor, 6,* 1–18.

Pescosolido, R. (1993). Clinical considerations related to victimization dynamics and posttraumatic stress in the group treatment of sexually abused boys. *Journal of Child and Adolescent Group Therapy, 3*(1), 49–73.

Peterson, G. (1996). Treatment of early onset. In J. L. Spira & I. D. Yalom (Eds.), *Treating dissociative identity disorder* (pp. 135–181), San Francisco. Jossey Bass.

Piaget, J. (1952a). *The child's conception of number.* New York: Humanities Press International.

Piaget, J. (1952b). *The origins of intelligence in children.* New York: International Universities Press.

Piaget, J (1962), *Play, dreams and imitation in childhood.* New York: Norton.

Pillemer, D., & White, S. (1989). Childhood events recalled by children and adults. *Advances in Child Development and Behavior, 21,* 297–340.

Puffer, M. K., Greenwald, R., & Elrod, D. E. (1998). A single session EMDR study with twenty traumatized children and adolescents. *Traumatology, 3*(2). Available Internet: http://www.fsu.edu/~trauma/v3i2art6.html.

Putnam, F. W. (1989a). *Diagnosis and treatment of multiple personality disorder.* New York: Guilford Press.

Putnam, F. W. (1989b). Pierre Janet and modern views of dissociation. *Journal of Traumatic Stress, 2,* 413–429.

Pynoos, R., Frederick, C., Nader, K., Arroyo, W., Eth, S., Nunez, W., Steinberg, A., & Fairbanks, L. (1987). Life threat and posttraumatic stress in school age children. *Archives of General Psychiatry, 44,* 1057–1063.

Pynoos, R. S. (1993). Traumatic stress and developmental psychopathology in children and adolescents. In J. M. Oldham, M. B. Riba, & A. Tasman (Eds.), *American psychiatric press review of psychiatry* (Vol. 12, pp. 205–238). Washington, DC: American Psychiatric Press.

Pynoos, R. S., & Eth, S. (1985). Children traumatized by witnessing acts of personal violence: Homicide, rape, or suicide behavior. In S. Eth & R. S. Pynoos (Eds.), *Post-traumatic stress disorder in children* (pp. 17–43). Washington, DC: American Psychiatric Press.

Pynoos, R. S., & Eth, S. (1986). Witness to violence: The child interview. *Journal of the American Academy of Child Psychiatry, 25*(3), 306–319.

Pynoos, R. S., & Nader, K. (1988). Psychological first aid and treatment approach to children exposed to community violence: Research implications. *Journal of Traumatic Stress, 1*(4), 445–473.

Pynoos, R. S., & Nader, K. (1989). Children's memory and proximity to violence. *Journal of the American Academy of Child and Adolescent Psychiatry, 28*(2), 236–241.

Pynoos, R. S., & Nader, K. (1993). Issues in the treatment of post-traumatic stress disorder in children and adolescents. In J. P. Wilson & B. Raphael (Eds.), *The international handbook of traumatic stress syndromes* (pp. 535–539). New York: Plenum Press.

Pynoos, R. S., Nader, K., & March, J. (1991). Post-traumatic stress disorder in children and adolescents. In J. Weiner (Ed.), *Comprehensive textbook of child and adolescent psychiatry* (pp. 339–348). Washington, DC: American Psychiatric Press.

Rice, K., Herman, M., & Petersen, A. (1993). Coping with challenge in adolescence: A conceptual model and psycho-educational intervention. *Journal of Adolescence, 16,* 235–251.

Resick, P. A., & Schnicke, M. K. (1993). *Cognitive processing therapy for rape victims: A treatment manual.* Newbury Park, CA: Sage.

Roche, D. N., Runtz, M. G., & Hunter, M. A. (1999). Adult attachment: A mediator between child sexual abuse and later psychological adjustment. *Journal of Interpersonal Violence, 14*(2), 184–207.

Roesler, T. A., Savin, D., & Grosz, C. (1993). Case study: Family therapy of extrafamilial sexual abuse. *Journal of the American Academy of Child and Adolescent Psychiatry, 32*(5), 967–970.

Rossman, B., Bingham, R. D., & Emde, R. N. (1997). Symptomatology and adaptive functioning for children exposed to normative stressors, dog attack, and parental violence. *Journal of the American Academy of Child and Adolescent Psychiatry, 36*(8), 1089–1097.

Saigh, P. A. (1992). The behavioral treatment of child and adolescent posttraumatic stress disorder. *Advances in Behavior Research and Therapy, 14,* 247–275.

Schamess, G. (1993). Group psychotherapy with children. In H. Kaplan & B. Sadock (Eds.), *Comprehensive group psychotherapy* (pp. 560–577). Baltimore: Williams & Wilkins.

Scheeringa, M. S., & Zeanah, C. H. (1995). Symptom expression and trauma variables in children under 48 months of age. *Infant Mental Health Journal, 16*(4), 259–270.

Sgroi, S. M., (1982). Family treatment. In S. M. Sgroi (Ed.), *Handbook of clinical intervention in child sexual abuse* (pp. 241–267). Lexington, MA: Lexington Books.

Sgroi, S. M. (Ed.). (1988). *Vulnerable populations: Evaluation and treatment of sexually abused children and adult survivors.* Lexington, MA: Lexington Books.

Shannon, M. P., Lonigan, C. J., Finch, A. J., & Taylor, C. M. (1994). Children exposed to disaster. I. epidemiology of posttraumatic symptoms and symptom profiles. *Journal of the American Academy of Child and Adolescent Psychiatry, 33,* 80–93.

Shapiro, F. (1989a). Efficacy of the eye movement desensitization procedure in the treatment of traumatic memories. *Journal of Traumatic Stress, 2,* 199–223.

Shapiro, F. (1989b). Eye movement desensitization: A new treatment for posttraumatic stress disorder. *Journal of Behavior Therapy and Experimental Psychiatry, 20,* 211–217.

Share, L. (1994). *If someone speaks, it gets lighter: Dreams and the reconstruction of infant trauma.* Hillsdale, NJ: Analytic Press.

Siegel, D. J. (1996). Cognition, memory and dissociation. *Child and Adolescent Psychiatric Clinics of North America, 5*(2), 509–536.

Siegmann, R. M., & Long, G. M. (1995). Psychoeducational group therapy changes the face of managed care. *Journal of Practical Psychiatric and Behavioral Health, 1,* 29–36.

Silberg, J. L. (1998a). Afterword. In J. L. Silberg (Ed.), *The dissociative child: Diagnosis, treatment, and management* (2nd ed.). Lutherville, MD: Sidran Press.

Silberg, J. L. (Ed.). (1998b). *The dissociative child: Diagnosis, treatment, and management.* Lutherville, MD: Sidran Press.

Silberg, J. L. (1999, May 4). *Treatment for children's dissociative disorders.* E-mail communication. (JLSIlberg@aol.com)

Silberg, J. L. (2001). Treating a young teenage girl with maladaptive dissociation. In H. Orvaschel, J. Faust, & M. Herson (Eds.), *Handbook of conceptualization and treatment of child psychopathology* (pp. 449–474). Oxford, UK: Elsevier Science.

Silberg, J. L., & Waters, F. W. (1998). Factors associated with positive therapeutic outcome. In J. L. Silberg (Ed.), *The dissociative child: Diagnosis, treatment, and management* (2nd ed., pp. 105–112). Lutherville, MD: Sidran Press.

Soberman, G. S., Greenwald, R., & Rule, D. L. (in press). A controlled study of eye movement desensitization and reprocessing (EMDR) for boys with conduct problems. *Journal of Aggression, Maltreatment, and Trauma.*

Solomon, A., Moshe, K., & Mikulincer, M. (1988). Combat-related posttraumatic stress disorder among second-generation Holocaust survivors: Preliminary findings. *American Journal of Psychiatry, 145*(7), 865–868.

Stamm, B. H. (Ed.). (1996). *Measurement of stress, trauma and adaptation.* Lutherville, MD: Sidran Press.

Stein, N., Wade, E., & Liwag, M. D. (1996). A theoretical approach to understanding and remembering harmful events. In M. Stein, P. A. Ornstein, B. Tversky, & C. J. Brainerd (Eds.), *Memory for everyday and emotional events.* Hillsdale, NJ: Erlbaum.

Steinberg, R., & Sunkenberg, M. (1994). A group intervention model for sexual abuse: Treatment and education in an inpatient child psychiatric setting. *Journal of Child and Adolescent Group Therapy, 4*(1), 61–73.

Stillwell, B. M., Galvin, M., & Kopta, S. M. (1991). Conceptualization of conscience in normal children and adolescents, ages 5 to 17. *Journal of the American Academy of Child and Adolescent Psychiatry, 30*(1), 16–21.

Styron, T., & Janoff-Bulman, R. (1997). Childhood attachment and abuse: Long-term effects on adult attachment, depression, and conflict resolution. *Child Abuse and Neglect, 21*(10), 1015–1023.

Suomi, S. J. (1995, February 17). *Genetic and experiential factors influencing bio-behavioral reactions to stress in primates.* Paper presented at the first annual meeting of the Trauma, Loss and Dissociation Conference, Alexandria, VA.

Suomi, S. J., & Levine, S. (1998). Psychobiology of intergenerational effects of trauma. In Y. Danieli (Ed.), *International handbook of multigenerational legacies of trauma* (pp. 623–637). New York: Plenum Press.

Terr, L. C. (1979). Children of Chowchilla: Study of psychic trauma. *Psychoanalytic Study of the Child, 34,* 547–623.

Terr, L. C. (1983). Chowchilla revisited: The effects of psychic trauma four years after a school-bus kidnapping. *American Journal of Psychiatry, 140,* 1542–1550.

Terr, L. C. (1985). Remembered images and trauma: A psychology of the supernatural. *Psychoanalytic Study of the Child, 40,* 493–533.

Terr, L. C. (1989). Treating psychic trauma in children: A preliminary discussion. *Journal of Traumatic Stress, 2*(1), 3–20.

Terr, L. C. (1991). Childhood traumas: An outline and overview. *American Journal of Psychiatry, 148*(1), 10–20.

Terr, L. C. (1994). *Unchained memories: True stories of traumatic memories, lost and found.* New York: Basic Books.

Thomas, A., & Chess, S. (1977). *Temperament and development.* New York: Bruner/Mazel.

Thompson, R. A. (1991). Attachment theory and research. In M. Lewis (Ed.), *Child and adolescent psychiatry: A comprehensive textbook* (pp. 100–108). Baltimore: Williams & Wilkins.

Trepper, T. S., & Barrett, M. J. (1986). Vulnerability to incest: A framework for Assessment. In T. S. Trepper & M. J. Barrett (Eds.), *Treating incest: A multiple systems perspective* (pp. 13–25). New York: Haworth Press.

Trepper, T. S., & Barrett, M. J. (1989). *Systemic treating of incest: A therapeutic handbook.* New York: Brunner/Mazel.

Trolley, B. (1995). Group issues and activities for female teen survivors of sexual abuse. *Child and Adolescent Social Work Journal, 12*(2), 101–118.

van der Hart, O., Brown, P., & van der Kolk, B. A. (1989a). La traitement psychologique du stress posttraumatique de Pierre Janet [Pierre Janet's psychological treatment of posttraumatic stress]. *Annales Medico-Psychologiques, 147*(9), 976–982.

van der Hart, O., Brown, P., & van der Kolk, B. (1989b). Pierre Janet's treatment of post-traumatic stress. *Journal of Traumatic Stress, 2,* 379–395.

van der Kolk, B. A. (Ed.). (1987). *Psychological trauma.* Washington, DC: American Psychiatric Press.

van der Kolk, B. A., & Sapporta, J. (1991). The biological response to psychic trauma: Mechanisms and treatment of intrusion and numbing. *Anxiety Research, 4,* 199–212.

Wallen, J. (1993). Protecting the mental health of children in dangerous neighborhoods. *Children Today, 22*(3), 24–28.

Webb, N. B. (1991). *Play therapy with children in crisis: A casebook for practitioners.* New York: Guilford Press.

Westerlundh, B., & Johnson, C. (1989). DMT defences and the experience of dreaming in children 12 to 13 years old. *Psychological Research Bulletin, 29*(6), 1–23.

Wolff, S. (1991). Moral development. In M. Lewis (Ed.), *Child and adolescent psychiatry: A comprehensive textbook* (pp. 187–194). Baltimore: Williams & Wilkins.

Wolin, S. J., & Wolin, S. (1992). *The resilient self: How survivors of troubled families rise above adversity.* New York: Villard Books.

Wozencroft, T., Wagner, W., & Pellegrin, A. (1991). Depression and suicidal ideation in sexually abused children. *Child Abuse and Neglect, 15,* 505–511.

Yates, T. (1991). Theories of cognitive development. In M. Lewis (Ed.), *Child and adolescent psychiatry: A comprehensive textbook* (pp. 109–128). Baltimore: Williams & Wilkins.

Yule, W., & Williams, R. M. (1990). Post-traumatic stress reactions in children. *Journal of Traumatic Stress, 3,* 279–295.

Zeanah, C. H., & Zeanah, P. D. (1989). Intergenerational transmission of maltreatment: Insights from attachment theory and research. *Psychiatry, 52,* 177–196.

13

Treatment of PTSD
in Families and Couples

LAURIE HARKNESS and NOKA ZADOR

An essential feature of the traumatic experience and its aftermath is the crushing and indelible sense of one's aloneness and disconnection from others. By its very nature, posttraumatic stress disorder (PTSD) can damage one's capacity for making and sustaining relationships. It is therefore not surprising that PTSD can lead to interpersonal difficulties, which in turn can exert a profoundly disruptive influence on the victim's significant relationships. What is surprising is that relatively little has been written about the significant role that the family can play in either helping or impeding the traumatized individual's recovery process, as well as the complex and dysfunctional patterns of interactions that can result when the impact of trauma goes unrecognized. In addition, little empirical research has been done to validate clinical observations on the efficacy of couples and family treatments.

This chapter examines the nature of the impact of trauma on family life and the implications this has for treatment. We first review how the disturbances in the traumatized individual's interactions with others reflects different facets of the symptoms of PTSD and its associated features. We then examine how these individual patterns effect and become woven into the family system and highlight common dysfunctional patterns of family interaction. We also examine how the dialectical nature of the individual's struggle to come to terms with his or her traumatic experience can be enacted in the family life. Finally, we review some of the core issues that need to be addressed in the clinical work with these individuals and their families. Clinical vignettes are shared which demonstrate key clinical issues. In addition, we emphasize the effects of chronic severe PTSD rather than acute traumatic stress reactions on family interactions, with the focus primarily on individuals suffering from combat-related and prolonged exposure traumas.

IMPACT OF PTSD ON HOW THE SURVIVOR RELATES TO OTHERS

In examining the ways in which the symptoms of PTSD can effect the quality of the survivor's relationship to others, the three general clusters of PTSD symptoms serve as a framework. First, the reexperiencing cluster (i.e., the disturbances in memory) affects the survivor's ability to be present in the present. Second, the numbing and avoidance symptoms interfere with the individual's capacity to identify, modulate, and express feelings. Third, the hyper-arousal symptoms impact on the survivor's sense of safety and capacity to trust. All affect one's capacity for interpersonal relatedness. In addition, several associated features of PTSD seem to contribute to relationship difficulties and make it difficult for the survivor to tolerate the feelings of vulnerability inherent in the process of forming and maintaining attachments. These include (1) unresolved grief feelings and the fear of reexperiencing devastating losses, (2) the demoralizing effect of the trauma and PTSD, (3) unresolved guilt feelings, and (4) self-hate, low self-esteem, and shame.

Trauma survivors' interpersonal difficulties tend to fall into two broad categories: problems with aggression and problems with a pervasive sense of emotional detachment. These problems with aggression and connection are often multidetermined, and their underlying causes can be traced to at least one, and more often to a combination, of the PTSD symptoms and associated features. There is also clearly a dynamic interplay between these disturbed modes of relating (which we explore later). Let us now look at each of these interpersonal problem areas separately.

Aggression

Many individuals with severe chronic PTSD have tremendous difficulty in the modulation and appropriate expression of anger. Traumatized individuals fear losing control and getting angry, and yet it may take little to light their fuse. The high rate of domestic and emotional abuse has been well documented in the literature. The fear of hurting others may lead to withdrawal and isolation as a form of protection.

All three clusters of PTSD symptoms can potentially contribute to problems with aggression and anger. The reexperiencing symptoms, especially when they have violent content, evoke a sense of being threatened and humiliated. The hyperarousal symptoms foster chronic irritability and outbursts of rage, a pervasive sense of mistrust and danger, and low frustration tolerance. Hypervigilance can lead to the tendency to misinterpret and overreact to environmental cues as being threatening. And the avoidance symptoms can lead to the stressful buildup of unresolved problems. Unrealistic self-expectations, self-hate, and guilt may be externalized, projected into others, and become a common source of aggressive behavior.

Emotional Detachment

The most obvious sources of emotional detachment are the avoidance symptoms. Within the avoidance cluster, it has been found that emotional numbing is the main source of emotional and social constriction (Riggs, Byrue, Weathers, & Litz, 1998). Other sources of detachment include the self-absorption stemming from a preoccupation with traumatic memories and unresolved feelings of guilt and grief. The vulnerability that comes from a fear of loss and a foreshortened sense of the future is another salient contributing factor to detachment. Detachment can also be a way to protect oneself from being overstimulated. Finally, problems with trust, shame, and feelings of worthlessness and inadequacy can all contribute to the wish to avoid interpersonal interactions.

Of course, there is also a dynamic relationship between these two sets of problems. Emotional detachment can be a means by which the survivor tries to protect others from his or her anger and its destructive consequences. Not surprisingly, this effort to protect others often backfires as the avoidance of interaction with others leads to festering conflicts, unmet needs, and a pervasive sense of aloneness.

IMPACT OF PTSD ON THE FAMILY SYSTEM AS A WHOLE

Traumatized individuals develop and have many different kinds of family units. In our experience, a common thread in all these different familial patterns is a pronounced and pervasive sense of emotional estrangement, even among those who have been able to sustain long-term relationships. The following is a review of commonly described constellations of problems and dilemmas that family members experience and confront every day. Obviously, not all families struggle with all of these issues.

"It's Like Living with the Iceman"

Living with someone who has become emotionally unavailable or detached can feel like, as one wife put it, "constantly dealing with the presence of an absence and the absence of a presence." Rosenheck and Thomson (1986) described that one of the most serious problems posed by PTSD for family life is the emotional emptiness that results from the veteran's self-absorption, isolation, and irritability. The lack of emotional responsiveness and involvement in family life may take on many forms and degrees of severity, including "spacing out," not really paying attention, spending hours in front of the television set, to being physically absent, isolating in the "bunker" or leaving home for days at a time. Family members, especially children, may fill in this void with a sense of responsibility and guilt.

Family members may also become acutely sensitive to the veteran's vulnerability to being overwhelmed by social encounters, and try to organize their lives around "not disturbing" the veteran. Among the more serious consequences of this pattern on family members is a pervasive sense of alienation, rejection, abandonment, and resentment.

"He's on the Outside Looking In"

A pernicious consequence of the veteran's estrangement from the family is the "serious, functional loss of the husband/father from stage-specific tasks and routines of family life" (Rosenheck & Thomson, 1986, p. 562) He/she is no longer an actively participating member of family life, often missing out on the family events, ceremonies, and rites of passage that are critical to the development of a sense of family belonging and identity. This is also one of the factors that leads to the "lopsided relationships" often cited in the PTSD literature, in which the wife is overfunctioning and "running the show," with the veteran passive and on the sidelines.

Although married for 25 years and a loyal husband and father, George, a Vietnam veteran with PTSD, suffered from profound emotional numbing and detachment. Married before he went to Vietnam, he was described by his wife as "vibrant and affectionate." In his job in grave registration, he dealt day after day with the dead bodies of fellow soldiers, many of whom were his own age. Initially he felt this job to be most sacred as he prepared the bodies for return home; gradually, however, he found himself physically unable to bear the sense of sorrow and disgust that this endless stream of corpses evoked in him. He felt that something inside of him died: "my heart iced over." Returning home to his wife and a 1-year-old child he had never met, the only feeling he recalled experiencing was guilt over not having any feelings about reuniting with his family. He tried hard to provide and be with his family, but as the years went on he found himself isolating, spending more time alone in his room than with his wife and children, disappearing for days and sometimes for months at a time. As he missed out on more and more of his children's important social and school events, his wife stated she became the "mother, father, caretaker of the entire family." The children quickly learned not to knock on the door of their father's office—even when he spent days at a time locked in that room.

"It's Like Living with Dr. Jekyll and Mr. Hyde"

Problems with anger can lead to volatile outbursts or impulsive, violent, destructive behavior, but these eruptions are often followed by periods of withdrawal and relative calm. In more severe cases, this can lead to violent acting out or physical abuse. It is not unusual for relatively high-functioning individuals with PTSD to experience intermittent episodes of volatile outbursts. One wife stated, "He's like a hot and cold water faucet. He can be fine and nice one minute and a raging lunatic the next minute."

Some of the obvious consequences have to do with problems connected to any family in which anger is inappropriately and/or destructively expressed. The family is fearful, hurt, and angry. The unpredictable nature of the outbursts contributes to a family atmosphere pervaded by tension, anxiety, a kind of hypervigilance, a feeling of "walking on eggshells," and a need to keep feelings bottled up. This in turn can lead to depression, somatic complaints, or destructive acting out in family members.

"It's Like Living with Ghosts"

Individuals who suffer from chronic PTSD are emotionally and psychologically haunted; so are their families. Through the reexperiencing symptoms and subsequent reenactment of trauma-related issues, the family often finds itself responding to past events as if they were occurring in the present. This often occurs with little or no awareness that this is happening. For example, one father reported his struggle to feel close to his son, whom he dearly loved but could not hold, as being caught in a conflict that if he held his son he would have to let go of his buddy who died in his arms. Another father described how he had become avoidant of his 13-year-old daughter, with whom he had had a very close relationship. Through treatment, the father was able to voice his guilt at having killed a 13-year-old girl in self-defense and then realized the avoidance of his own daughter was connected to these unresolved feelings. Meanwhile, the daughter had begun to feel that there was something bad inside of her that was scaring the father away. Although not able to disclose to his daughter the real truth, once the father realized what was occurring he reassured her his distancing had nothing to do with her and that he loved her. He made an effort to be with her and to deal with the feelings she evoked within the treatment setting.

One 4-year-old girl was referred for evaluation after she began exhibiting the following symptoms: oppositional behavior, frequent tantrums, intense separation anxiety, and frequent nightmares. Both parents and nursery school teachers found this behavior extremely difficult to manage. These symptoms had emerged relatively abruptly in what had been a healthy, well-functioning child. After numerous individual and family sessions, the little girl described her fantasy that she needed to go to Vietnam and find her father's eye, which in fact he had lost in a grenade attack. Although he had never discussed with her his own obsession with this injury, the little girl sensed that his pain, sleep difficulties, and other symptoms were associated with his lost eye. In addition, it was learned that the father himself was experiencing an anniversary reaction. Through drawings and talking, the therapist taught her about the Vietnam War and some of the terrifying things that happened in that war, especially focusing on how the war affected her father. All this was done in a language that she could grasp and relate to. In addition, family meetings were held where the father acknowledged his pain about the injury but also emphasized that he was getting the help he needed and learning to take better care of himself. When she was reassured that her perceptions were valid and that he could be a whole, giving father, even without his eye, the girl was both relieved and able to feel safe once again.

"It's Like Living in Two Different Time Zones"

As one colleague stated, "trauma nails you to the floor of time." The individual is often psychologically stuck in the past while the family is concerned with the present and the future. The individual and family find themselves leading separate, parallel lives, often with different sets of values and sources of meaning. The reexperiencing symptoms can make events that happened decades ago seem more vivid and real than what's happening in the present. Furthermore, if the individual experiences the present as an incessant, endless source of demands and expectations he or she can't live up to, the trauma experiences can, in fact, be a source of comfort and "soothing." For Vietnam veterans, their combat experiences can end up representing the most exciting, meaningful time in their lives, when they were most heroic, alive, valued, competent, and when friendships were most intense and profound. Vietnam can become an impossible act to follow.

When a family is polarized in this fashion, for example, it can become stuck in mutually invalidating patterns of interaction. The partner and/or children feel that their day-to-day concerns and struggles are minimized, and that the interests and issues that matter to them are not appreciated or even recognized. Family members may feel that their own experiences are, in fact, trivial when compared to the veteran's, leading to a tendency to romanticize or glorify the veteran's experiences and to devalue their own. However, the family can also become impatient with and angry at the veteran's preoccupation, wishing he would "get over it" and move on with his life, frustrated by the tenacity of the past's hold over him. The veteran often feels that the power and uniqueness of his experiences are not appreciated or even under-

stood by his family. The wife feels her work, needs, and interests are minimized, children feel devalued, and the veteran feels 'they' can never understand what it's like to be haunted daily by the image of having his buddy die
in his arms.

This issue is connected to one of the essential features of the trauma experience: it is unspeakable, incomprehensible, cannot be released, and cannot be absorbed. Judith Herman (1992) talks about this as the dialectical dynamic between the wish to forget and the need to make sense of and
integrate the experience. The polarized family seems to represent a failure to
live with the tension of this paradox posed by the trauma: the need to find a
way to live with the past, without being its prisoner, and the need to remember and move on. As this is a critical issue in understanding PTSD and the
family, it will be explored in greater depth later in the treatment section.

"It's Like He Can't Live with Us, He Can't Live without Us"

These relationships are often marked by intense ambivalence. The sources of
this ambivalence center around the struggle between the compulsion to isolate and the fear of losing others that one cares about and/or is dependent
on. Traumatized individuals often feel tremendous guilt and shame toward
their family for not being able to give enough, for being a burden, and/or for
hurting them. Yet, this guilt also keeps them from leaving; they do not want
to abandon, disappoint, and hurt their loved ones anymore. Most often, they
genuinely love and care about their family. Many veterans will state that their
spouse and/or child is their sole reason for existing and responsible for keeping them alive. This can be very confusing to the family and can create a
sense of insecurity and instability as well as burden them with a sense of responsibility to keep the veteran alive and happy.

COMMON PATTERNS OF INTERACTION

Several authors have identified and described patterns of family interaction
that can develop in response to dealing with the traumatized individual.
Danieli (1981), in describing her observations of families of Holocaust survivors, identified salient "adaptational styles" (families of fighters, the numb
family and the families of those who made it) in which unresolved issues or
themes of the survivor's life permeates and shapes the family dynamics.
Harkness (1993; see also Harkness & Giller, 1995) identified three dysfunctional interactional styles found in families of Vietnam veterans with PTSD.
She used key concepts of Minuchin (1974) to examine disturbances in the
roles and boundaries of family members and subsystems. Families with disengaged relationships are marked by alienation from and lack of involvement

with each other; enmeshed families are characterized by undifferentiated role boundaries with a kind of "us against them" way of perceiving their relationship with the world. Families in which the veteran is prone to violence tend to be chaotic and crisis driven. In all three cases, the most profound impact of PTSD on family life centers around the emotional inaccessibility of the father.

Both Daneli (1987) and Harkness (1993) developed their categorizations of styles based on their own clinical observations; further research to study or even verify the existence of certain family styles or types has yet to be done. However, over and over again in the literature on families, writers have noted patterns similar to the ones described by Harkness, with the common denominator being the veteran's alienation from the family. Vietnam veterans are often described as living on the periphery of family life, and—even when involved—his or her role is usually that of the "soldier/protector," a role which has little to do with emotional closeness and availability. Another common structural pattern that results is the tendency for the boundaries between the mother and children to be diffuse and the boundaries between this subsystem and the veteran to be rigid and impermeable. Consequently, the mother and children sometimes form cross-generational alliances, as wives tend to form dysfunctional alliances with their children in reaction to the father's remoteness and unpredictability. This can undermine the parental subsystem and the appropriate differentiation of roles and authority.

IMPACT OF PTSD ON FAMILY SUBSYSTEMS AND INDIVIDUAL FAMILY MEMBERS

Family of Origin

The impact of chronic PTSD on one's family of origin has received little attention. Perhaps this is because teasing out the influence of premorbid functioning from the ramifications of the trauma itself, and looking at how these two forces interact, is a rather formidable challenge. From clinical observations, we have been struck by the existence of certain enduring static patterns of estrangement and misconceptions. For many families, the dramatic changes in personality and behavior are bewildering and inexplicable.

For example, John grew up in the South in an intact, close-knit working-class family. He reported no history of any abuse. As the youngest of four children, at times he felt pampered and overprotected, but also very special. He was described by his family as affectionate, sensitive, and connected to both friends and family. He excelled in school. John enlisted in the U.S. Army for patriotic reasons as well as to get a scholarship for school. He completed one tour of duty in Vietnam, during which he was exposed to a great deal of combat. He witnessed atrocities and the horrific death of his best friend.

Upon returning from Vietnam, the family noticed that John was "not the same boy he was when he left." He was irritable, began to drink heavily, and would disappear for days at a time. The family's attempts to help him were invariably rebuffed. Eventually, contact with John was so painful and at times frightening that they stopped trying to interact with him. John spent most of his time alone in the woods. His father, himself a World War II combat veteran, avoided asking John about his war experiences and did not share his own, as they too were painful. He did not understand why his son couldn't get on with his life as he had.

Years later, during a family session with the 76-year-old mother (the father was deceased), John's mother cried as she spoke of being overwhelmed with feelings of helplessness and guilt in the face of her son's self-destructiveness. The mother believed she was responsible for her son's condition: "If I had been the mother I should have been, I would have found some way to reach him. I could do that when he was a boy, but after the war, no matter what I did, it wasn't enough. I failed him." His sisters were less guilt ridden but expressed a profound sense of loss: "What we saw was his ghost."

No family members were aware of the impact John's behavior had on each of them, and the sisters were "shocked" to discover that their mother felt so responsible for his problems. During one family session, she recalled an incident where he had barricaded himself in his room and was threatening to shoot anyone who tried to get in. He was calling out names she had never heard. His mother contacted the police, who brought him to a hospital. He felt betrayed by his family and did not return home. During the meeting, she revealed that, to this day, she questions whether she did the right thing.

The chasm created by John's traumatic experiences could not be bridged by his family, despite intensive efforts on their part to help him maintain a connection. Furthermore, for years his family experienced tremendous conflict about how and when to push John to get him more involved with family life, and frustration and helplessness because no matter what they did John did not get better and drifted further away. However, even in families where the veteran is able to maintain more consistent contact, there is often a pervasive sense of the "before and after" picture of the brother or son who "came back from the war a different person." Without treatment or education, questions about why the veteran "couldn't get over it" persists, often feeding the veteran's own sense of being a failure and misunderstood.

Marital/Couple Relationships

Much of the literature on PTSD and the family has focused on the impact of PTSD on the marital/couple relationships. As we have already discussed, disturbances in the survivor's capacity to trust, to feel, and to tune into the present wreak havoc on his or her capacity for intimacy. Frequently, the spouses assume most of the emotional, practical, and financial responsibilities of family life. Z. Solomon (1998) describes this as the "redistribution of roles and redivision of labor." Rabin and Nardi (1991) describe this overfunctioning as a way to avoid conflict by decreasing the demands that the partner makes on the traumatized individual. This can lead to a vicious cycle: overfunctioning may eventually reinforce underfunctioning, which increases the demands on the partner. Scaturo and Hayman (1992), in their paper on the impact of combat trauma across the life cycle, point out that "massive amounts of psychic energy, a portion of which might otherwise be directed toward career development, have been diverted toward keeping traumatic recollections and PTSD symptoms under control." They continue: "These veterans may find themselves at mid-life working at jobs which do not sufficiently challenge them or are below their vocational potential" (p. 281). Some veterans become completely disabled by their symptoms. Many experience a profound sense of failure and emasculation from this experience, and by midlife this may seriously effect their hierarchical position within the family. Rather than the husband and wife functioning as coequals in the family hierarchy, the traumatized individual's ability to function within the marriage is perceived as "inadequate" while the spouse's is seen as "overadequate." Overfunctioning and being a full-time caretaker for the entire family can create feelings of resentment and of being overburdened and lead to increased levels of stress, vulnerability to depression, and loss of identity.

Connected to these feelings of being overburdened and responsible for the family's well-being, is the tendency for the spouse, in most cases the wife, to oscillate between feeling that she is to blame for the veteran's marital problems, on the one hand, and resenting and blaming the veteran for the situation, on the other. Like many parents of veterans, wives seem to believe they should be able to heal them through love, although this attitude could change over time with the wife attributing all the problems in the marriage to the veteran's problems. Z. Solomon (1998) writes about the "compassion trap" the wife is caught in: she has little control over his PTSD, yet feels responsible for his well-being. Women in one family group were all in agreement when one of the women summed up the conundrum they face this way: "If I pay attention to his problems and needs, I stop paying attention to myself, and I'm afraid I end up enabling him. However, if I try to take better care of myself, I feel like I'm abandoning him—or at the very least, being a neglectful wife!" Many spouses also use the Al-Anon concept of the 3 C's to describe their tendency to feel that they cause, can control, and should be able to cure their spouse's problems.

Researchers have repeatedly found that, in couples and families of Vietnam veterans with PTSD, there are increased marital and family difficulties. The divorce rate is quoted as being twice that of their peer group, with common findings including a higher incidence of domestic violence, communication problems, poor problem-solving skills, and sexual problems. The impact of poor communication and problem-solving skills on these couples' ability to deal with or resolve problems within the family often leads to the buildup of emotional distress and anger, which can then lead to guilt, withdrawal, passivity, as well as aggression.

TREATMENT ISSUES: MOVING ON IS NOT A BETRAYAL OF THE PAST

In this chapter, we do not attempt to offer a single model for working with couples and families where one of the adult members suffers from PTSD. Models for working with these families have been reviewed elsewhere and include the whole continuum of treatments available, from classical systems-oriented family treatment to psychoeducational to cognitive behavioral to the more traditional modes of treatments, which include group, individual, and family/couple therapies. Obviously, what models, styles and/or techniques are used will reflect the clinician's theoretical orientation and be responsive to the family's strengths, needs, and issues. No one theory or treatment modality has been found to be more effective than others; what is necessary is a comprehensive understanding of PTSD and its impact on relationship issues. As with any kind of family treatment, a comprehensive clinical assessment is the tool that identifies family strengths, as well as the pathogenic agent or agents responsible for the relationship problems seen in the family. This assessment includes issues related to the families of origin of both adults, premorbid functioning, present stressors, as well as the nature of the trauma and the individual and family's stage of recovery. All these factors, and the complicated interaction between them, are usually involved in the genesis and perpetuation of family patterns and dysfunction. The PTSD-specific treatment interventions on which this chapter focuses can be integrated into any treatment modality.

There are three essential treatment components to any successful PTSD family/couple treatment. Although each is reviewed separately below, in the treatment process they are overlapping and interconnected. To what degree one component is emphasized over another will be determined by the family's needs and stage of recovery. The components are as follows: (1) *psychoeducational,* which facilitates an understanding of the impact of trauma and PTSD; (2) *disclosure of traumatic material,* which builds on this understanding and identifies the myths, reenactments, and distorted worldviews that are common consequences of living with PTSD; and (3) *addressing the dialectical nature of living with PTSD,* which enables the clinician to help the family live with the tension of the compelling past while still appreciating the day-to-day demands of the present. The following subsections elaborate on these three key components.

First, a cautionary note: A precondition for any PTSD treatment is the need to establish a sense of safety for all members. It is well documented that people who have been traumatized can act out in ways that are destructive to self and to others. Any family assessment should begin with identifying the presence of domestic violence, sexual abuse, the existence of guns, and the occurrence of suicidal behavior and threats that can hold the family hostage. Clinicians must also screen for substance abuse. The need for these issues/problems to be addressed and alleviated is a priority in any family treatment just as it is in any individual treatment.

Psychoeducation

The psychoeducational process is indispensable to any couple/family work with this population. This process includes teaching family members about the PTSD symptoms and issues related to the traumatic event. The focus of this process includes how these symptoms affect the individual and his or her functioning, perception of the world, and—most importantly—relationships with others. This gives the family a chance to understand how they have reacted and adapted to the traumatized individual and the PTSD symptoms; often family members become aware for the first time of the behaviors to which they have been reacting. Framing the behavior as a common reaction to a traumatic experience that others also struggle with provides the individual and family with the opportunity to change their perception of the behavior from one of blaming or fixing self or other to an ongoing collaborative and problem-solving process that can involve the entire family.

There are many different ways that information about PTSD and trauma can be disseminated, including literature, videos, and lectures. Ideally, this should occur within a therapeutic and/or supportive setting. Any psychoeducational process will focus on two broad categories: (1) the symptoms themselves and (2) the context in which the trauma occurred. Even though a rape victim and a PTSD combat veteran may share similar PTSD symptoms, the impact on interpersonal and family issues may be very different. The rape victim may be dealing more with issues of sexual intimacy, and the veteran more with issues related to aggression management. Understanding the context in which the trauma occurred may help facilitate empathy as well as demystify otherwise bewildering behaviors. One 13-year-girl's bullying behavior toward her classmates was a source of consternation and confusion to her parents and teachers until she was able to reveal in her individual therapy that she found weakness in others intolerable as it reminded her of her vulnerability, which she detested. She had been sexually abused for years and despised herself for what she perceived to be her weakness and inability to fight back. Through giving her family and teachers information about the effects of sexual abuse on a developing adolescent's sense of identity and self-esteem, their reactivity, anger, and frustration gave way to understanding and patience.

The psychoeducational approach frequently reduces blame, shame, and stigmatization. This in turn decreases the defensive responses that prevent family members from engaging in a constructive dialogue with each other. Decreasing blame can enhance the family's ability to assume responsibility for the treatment process itself and to improve family functioning. The family and survivor need to know that the survivor is not responsible for the trauma or for the PTSD that he or she developed as a result of the traumatic experience. Information and knowledge allows survivors and their families to develop more appropriate and realistic role and behavior expectations. This psychoeducational approach shifts the spotlight from focusing on the survivor as the source of the family difficulties as "identified patient" to a new focus on the "trauma and its wake." By engaging every member of the family in an objective inquiry into the impact of PTSD, commitment to changing behavior becomes based on understanding rather than guilt and shame. Helping family members understand the PTSD sequelae and their effects on the family, while exploring alternatives and compromises that meet the needs of the family, becomes crucial. One wife complained about her husband's constant unwillingness to go out to dinner and do anything "special" with her. She believed he did not want to do anything with her because he "did not care." Although their 8-year relationship was stable, she was growing increasingly frustrated and resentful of this behavior. In the couple's work, she learned for the first time about the severity of her husband's hyperarousal symptoms and was surprised to discover that her husband felt extremely guilty about his inability to give her more. He had not been able to share these feelings with her because he felt ashamed of the fearfulness that kept him from going out in public. The couple's learning about how symptoms of avoidance and hyperarousal lead to isolative behavior enabled the wife to feel empathy and the husband to feel less guilty. This in turn made it possible for the couple actively to seek compromises that allowed both of their needs to be met. With the therapist's help, they came up with the idea of having picnics in the backyard and candlelight dinners at home.

Even in the early stages of treatment where clinicians are obtaining important clinical information to formulate a couple/family assessment, the sharing of information and reframing of behavior can create surprisingly profound changes in the couple's understanding of the problems and the ways that they deal with them. In a group for partners of veterans with PTSD, a new member realized for the first time that her husband's angry outbursts were not about her but a manifestation of his own very severe hyperarousal symptoms. She also realized that her tendency to reassure and appease him during these outbursts was not helpful and set her up to be blamed. In the group she realized, "It is not all me," and learned not to personalize his behavior. Other wives in the group not only agreed with her but also supported her in finding new ways to deal with this.

A common concern of family members is that understanding can be used as an excuse for unacceptable behavior. The husband of the wife in the example above had severe problems with anger management. Couple work included teaching them that even though he might not be able to stop his emotional reactions (anger), he needed to learn alternative, nondestructive ways of expressing his anger.

Disclosure

In many of these couples/families, at the heart of the disconnection is the reality of the traumatic experience itself, which can be terrifying and overwhelming to all who encounter it. In fact, the difficulty in addressing traumatic material is what makes working with these families different than working with other dysfunctional couples/families. An important aspect of the psychoeducational process is that it helps to "detoxify" the traumatic material so that it can be approached by the family and trauma survivor in a manner that makes it possible to be integrated into the family history. Without some form of disclosure, the family is often caught up in the previously described dysfunctional patterns of interactions that are based on reenactments of certain aspects of the trauma or on distorted worldviews. This also inevitably leads to a certain kind of alienation and misunderstanding that will permeate the family atmosphere.

Before clinicians can effectively help the family deal with other issues that all families struggle with, like communication and difficulties in intimacy, the reality of the trauma must be addressed. Rosenheck and Thomson (1986) write about reducing a mysterious event into approachable knowledge. Disclosure includes two parts: what and when. How much to disclose, what aspects to reveal versus what aspects to conceal, and the timing of the disclosure will vary depending on the individual's and family's need, ability, and willingness to share. Not all details need to be shared all the time. The goal is to transform an event that is unspeakable and elusive into knowledge that is approachable and meaningful.

Disclosure can be on the general or personal level and range from just needing to acknowledge having been a victim of rape or a soldier in Vietnam to a much more detailed personal description of the experiences that the person had. Whether or not to reveal the more personal-level experiences, especially if the traumatic content contains violence or unresolved feelings of guilt and shame, depends on the survivor's level of acceptance and the family's ability to hear and adaptively process the data. In general, it is the survivors themselves that must initially come to some level of tolerance for these feelings; otherwise, they will be looking to their families for forgiveness or to resolve issues that need to be dealt with from within themselves. When and how much to reveal is an ongoing process. Certainly, as discussed above, the veteran father of the 13-year-old girl did not need to share the trigger of his withdrawal from his daughter. What he did need to do in his individual treatment, however, was identify the trigger and work through this as he struggled to be closer to his daughter. He also needed to share with his daughter enough about his trauma so that both were aware that what they were struggling with was related to the trauma and not to her.

As clinicians help survivors and family members acknowledge the traumatic experience, timing is of course very important. The age of children, psychological stability, the family's level of functioning, and the level of commitment of the various family members to the treatment process and to each other—all are important factors in determining the timing of disclosure. The couple and family need to be prepared for the disclosure process, and generally this takes time. Prematurely addressing these issues can have disastrous consequences, as it may overwhelm family members and precipitate the family into fleeing treatment. Disclosure can be a lifelong process, and complete disclosure should not be held up as some ultimate ideal goal for all to attain. This is a delicate process in which the complicated trade-offs involved in the pros and cons of knowing must be weighed against the survivor's and family's ability to make sense of this material without being overwhelmed by it.

Dialectical Dilemma

Just as one of the central challenges of a survivor's life is to learn how to live with, rather than be a prisoner of, his or her past, the family also faces an ongoing conundrum: they must find ways to acknowledge the unique and profound nature of the survivor's experience without allowing it to overshadow and diminish all other experiences. The ways in which family members deal with their loved one's struggles is fraught with difficulties stemming from the paradoxical nature of the psychological consequences of trauma. Both the family and survivor are caught up in the struggle to find a manageable way to express the impact of the trauma without being overwhelmed by it. Some families become paralyzed by the double-binding "go away closer" signals embedded in the PTSD symptoms themselves. The family's response often parallels the individual's conflictual wish/fear around confronting and finding expression for the trauma versus forgetting and defending against it. Within this "dialectic of psychological trauma" (Herman, 1992) and the way it gets played out in the family, lies the family's potential for both paralysis and growth. If the family can find ways to hold and contain (as opposed to resolve) the tension inherent in this dialectical dilemma, then reframing the experience is possible so that it becomes a source of meaning and vitality.

As previously described, some families become polarized and live parallel lives: both the family and the survivor feel alone, misunderstood, and unsupported. This polarization is a consequence of the inability to understand, integrate, appreciate, and move beyond this dialectical dilemma. The family needs help in recognizing the poignancy of the struggle they are caught in;

most family members genuinely want to understand the survivor's experience, and survivors often long to become an active participating member of the family. The ability to recognize this is the key to transforming mutually invalidating patterns of interaction to mutually supportive ones. During their second couple session, one wife, married for more than 15 years to a Vietnam veteran with severe PTSD, described how often she felt as though they were roommates leading separate lives that rarely overlapped. Even though he never talked about it, she knew that during his many hours in the basement he was mulling over Vietnam memories because he would listen to music from the 1960s and look through his photographs from Vietnam. When she asked him to talk to her about Vietnam he would become irritable and taciturn, often saying "It's not important." At the same time, when she would discuss problems at her work he would repeatedly compare it to "being on a mission," which made her feel that these experiences which he said were too insignificant to be discussed were, in fact, the measuring stick by which all life events were judged. She also at times felt he was selfish and self-indulgent. Her impatience with him made him feel both criticized and ashamed. Both withdrew even further from each other. When she was educated about the compelling nature of the reexperiencing symptoms, she became thoughtful and stated, "I just did not realize that what he had been through so long ago could still have control over how he thinks and feels about things."

In this session for the first time the veteran began talking about the trauma of losing his best friend and stated that part of the depression and withdrawal he was experiencing was connected to the anniversary of this death. The wife cried and said, "How horrible for you." For the first time the veteran felt understood rather than judged for his withdrawal. Her reaction also allowed him to begin to share how guilty he felt about his lack of involvement with her. This surprised the wife: "I always thought he just got fed up with me." As she became more interested and respectful of his experiences, he began to feel more motivated to find ways to not let his reexperiencing symptoms consume him. Through this interaction they experienced a shift which allowed them to become more active participants in each other's lives.

The family can play an integral and crucial role in helping the survivor move from vulnerability to resiliency and from constriction to more expansive ways of experiencing the world. Once the indelible imprint that trauma leaves can be validated, then the individual and the family can begin to address the crucial issues that affect day-to-day life. However, it is important to remember that moving on is not the same as forgetting and that letting go is not the same as betraying the significance of what happened. Survivors are living witnesses to a profound "historical truth." Weaving the impact of this history into present goals helps give meaning and purpose to the present which both the survivor and the family can share. One veteran, whose worst combat experiences occurred during Christmas, would withdraw into his "bunker" rather than be with his family during the holidays. Following several months of individual and family treatment, it was recommended that one way of honoring this experience would be for the family to do something that was of service, especially if other veterans were involved. The family decided to volunteer at a local soup kitchen during the holiday season. For the first time, the veteran was able to tolerate being with his family and they all valued being together as they honored the significance of the past and the significance of the family.

It is really the therapist's task to reframe traumatic experiences so that they can be seen as sources of wisdom and guidance. With one couple struggling with the survivor's belief that he did not deserve an intimate and close relationship, the therapist asked, "How would your best friend [who died in combat] advise you now?" "Life is precious . . . enjoy what you have and the people in your life," was his response. Associated with his struggle of being close was the fear of yet another devastating loss: the loss of his wife. His imagining his friend's advice allowed him to shift from a preoccupation with the fear of loss and the precariousness of life to an appreciation of the preciousness of the moment with his loved one.

Another example of constructively reframing the meaning of the past involves a 9-year-old boy who was beating up children at school. He said to his father, "I want to be a soldier like you." The boy's behavior can be seen as an attempt to identify and appease the father and/or defend against the father's guilt over his aggressive behavior in Vietnam. With the therapist present the father explained to his son that what he learned from being a soldier in Vietnam was that it hurt to hurt people and that, for him, he was struggling to do things that would not hurt others. As a result the boy stopped being such a bully and was finally able to make friends. For the veteran father, this experience facilitated the process of transforming painful guilt inducing memories into a moral lesson that he could pass on to his son.

These three clinical components—psychoeducation, disclosure, and the dialectical struggle—enable the family to hear, appreciate, and validate the survivor's issues. As this occurs, more energy is freed up within the family system to effectively address here-and-now needs and concerns. Dealing with a child's school problems or with a spouse's need for greater intimacy is no longer seen as trivial, as long as these issues are not seen as disavowing the survivor's past. The past and present need not cancel each other out, and the family does not need to be caught up in an either/or struggle. Shortly after a Vietnam veterans' wives group began, they all asked the therapist, "How do we help our husbands get better?" The therapist responded, "Help them get better?" When the therapist wondered aloud where their needs fit into the picture of their lives, the group, after some discussion, identified the following dilemma: "If I attend to his needs am I enabling him and neglecting myself? Or if I take care of myself, am I abandoning him?" After two years of both supportive and psychoeducational treatment in this group, these wives were able to acknowledge the legitimacy of their needs without invalidating their husband's needs.

As the family addresses the treatment components identified above, the family's expectation of involvement of all members in the day-to-day life of the family can be seen as facilitating healing. One veteran stated that when his son called him "Daddy," he was not responding to the veteran part of him but to one of his other identities—in this case, that of being a father. Helping family members develop realistic family and role expectations now becomes the therapeutic work at hand. Helping parents function as parents and children fulfill their roles as children now can be addressed.

In conclusion, by utilizing an understanding of the complex relationship between the traumatic material and the dynamics of the family, and the clinical components identified in this chapter, the family can learn to live with—rather than be controlled by—derivatives of traumatic experiences. These experiences can become a source of meaning and strength. If healing from trauma is about finding positive ways to integrate the past into the ongoing narrative of one's life, then family life provides the setting in which this can be most successfully accomplished.

REFERENCES

Danieli, Y. (1981, Sept./Oct.). Differing adaptational styles in families of survivors of the Nazi Holocaust. *Children Today*.

Harkness, L., & Giller, E. L. (1995). Families of Vietnam veterans with post-traumatic stress disorder syndrome: Child social competence and behavior. In D. Rhodes, M. Leaveck, & J. Hudson (Eds.), *The legacy of Vietnam veterans and their families*. Agent Orange Class Assistance Program, Washington, DC.

Harkness, L. (1993). Trangenerational transmission of war-related trauma. In J. P. Wilson & B. Raphael (Eds.), *International handbook of traumatic stress syndromes* (pp. 635–643). New York: Plenum Press.

Herman, J. L. (1992). *Trauma and recovery*. New York: Basic Books.

Minuchin, S. (1974). *Families and family therapy*. Cambridge, MA: Harvard University Press.

Rabin, C., & Nardi, C. (1991). Treating post-traumatic stress disorder couples: A psychoeducational program. *Community Mental Health Journal, 27*(3), 209–223.

Riggs, D. S., Byrne, C. A., Weathers, F. W., & Litz, B. T. (1998). The quality of intimate relationships of male Vietnam veterans: Problems associated with post-traumatic stress disorder. *Journal of Traumatic Stress, 11*(1), 87–101.

Rosenheck, R., & Fontana, A. (1998). Warrior fathers and warrior sons: Intergenerational aspects of trauma. In Y. Danieli (Ed.), *International handbook of multigenerational legacies of trauma* (pp. 225–241). New York: Plenum Press.

Rosenheck, R., & Thomson, J. (1986). "Detoxification" of Vietnam War trauma: A combined family–individual approach. *Family Process, 25,* 559–570.

Scaturo, D. J., & Hayman, P. M. (1992). The impact of combat trauma across the family life cycle: Clinical considerations. *Journal of Traumatic Stress, 5,* 272–288.

Solomon, Z. (1998). The effect of combat-related post-traumatic stress disorder on the family. *Psychiatry, 51,* 323–329.

14

Treatment of PTSD in Persons with Severe Mental Illness

KIM T. MUESER and STANLEY D. ROSENBERG

Over the past two decades there has been a tremendous growth in recognition of the high rate of psychological trauma in the general population. One result of this heightened awareness has been increased research on the most common psychiatric consequence of trauma: posttraumatic stress disorder (PTSD). More recently, especially over the past decade, a similar awareness has been emerging regarding the prominence of trauma in the lives of persons with severe and persistent mental illness. Findings to date suggest that this is a crucial area of study because rates of trauma exposure appear to be extremely high in this group, its effects may be amplified, and clients and clinicians are expressing an immediate need for effective treatments for these posttraumatic disorders.

However, only limited research has evaluated the prevalence and impact of PTSD in these patients, and even less work has focused on the treatment of comorbid PTSD in the severely mentally ill population. Therefore, the extant knowledge about PTSD in people with severe mental illness (SMI), including prevalence, impact, phenomenology, and treatment, is quite limited. At the same time, some of the conceptual and pragmatic complexities of studying PTSD in people with SMI are becoming manifest. To pose but a few of the difficult questions confronting clinicians and researchers. (1) Is the accurate diagnosis of PTSD technically feasible in people with disorders characterized by hallucinations, delusions, memory, and other cognitive impairments, as well as with symptoms which overlap those of PTSD (e.g., flattening of affect, social withdrawal)? (2) To what extent can PTSD itself represent a chronic disorder, presenting in some individuals as a SMI (or misdiagnosed as such)? (3) Are the best practices for treatment and community support for people with SMI compatible with the most efficacious treatments for PTSD, or will the latter require significant modifications for more vulnerable populations?

These questions are indicative of how early we are in the process of developing knowledge that can guide the treatment of people with primary psychotic illness and comorbid PTSD. In general, the field now has only a small but growing body of clinical lore on the treatment (particularly of women) with both SMI and PTSD. Published accounts of programs providing such interventions for the SMI, like those developed for combat veterans with chronic PTSD (e.g., Seidel et al., 1994; Frueh et al., 1996), generally emphasize their complex, multifaceted, and long-term nature. However, no published accounts exist of a "model" program which has been replicated at a second site.

Because of our limited understanding of the interface between PTSD and SMI, the scope of this chapter is necessarily broad and to some extent speculative. We begin the chapter with a review of the high prevalence of trauma in patients with severe mental illness, followed by a discussion of the correlates of trauma in this population. We next review research on the prevalence of PTSD in severe mental illness. We summarize a model we have recently developed which posits that PTSD mediates the effects of trauma on the course and outcome of SMI, and we consider both the theoretical and clinical implications of this model for assessment and treatment in this population. Following the explication of this model, we consider the range of different treatments that have been developed for trauma or PTSD in persons with SMI and propose a taxonomy for classifying these interventions. We conclude with suggestions for clinical intervention and future research in this area.

TRAUMA IN SEVERE MENTAL ILLNESS

Definitions

In this chapter we refer to *trauma* as the experience of an uncontrollable event that the person perceives to threaten his or her psychological or physical integrity (Herman, 1992; Horowitz, 1986; van der Kolk, 1987). In our discussion of PTSD, we employ the more narrow definition of a traumatic event provided by DSM-IV (American Psychiatric Association, 1994), which includes events involving direct threat of bodily or psychological harm that the person finds at the time of the event to be intensely distressing. Common examples of traumatic events include childhood sexual abuse, rape, experiencing or witnessing physical assault, direct threat with a weapon, combat exposure, being the victim of an accident or natural disaster, and learning of the sudden and unexpected death of a loved one.

Severe mental illness (SMI) is a general term frequently used to describe individuals with psychiatric disorders that have a profound impact on functioning in a wide range of range of domains, such as the ability to work, to care for oneself and live independently in the community, and to maintain rewarding interpersonal relationships (Schinnar et al., 1990). Psychotic symptoms such as hallucinations or delusions are common but not universal in this population. Due to their difficulties working and living independently in the community, patients with SMI frequently receive disability income, such as Social Security Disability Income (SSDI) or Social Security Supplemental Income (SSSI). The most common diagnoses typically include schizophrenia, schizoaffective disorder, bipolar disorder, or severe cases of major depression. Many states include people with severe personality disorders (e.g., borderline personality) as well as chronic PTSD in the SMI category, but we will limit the current discussion to the four primary disorders listed above.

PREVALENCE OF TRAUMA

Before addressing the rates of exposure to traumatic events in persons with SMI, it is helpful to review the epidemiology of trauma in the general population. In the National Comorbidity Survey, lifetime rate of exposure to any trauma, defined according to DSM-III-R (American Psychiatric Association, 1987), was 56% (Kessler et al., 1995). In a study of the epidemiology of trauma in 1007 young subjects (aged 21–30) living in southeastern Michigan, 39% reported at least one lifetime trauma; when these subjects were prospectively followed up 3 years later, 19% had been subsequently exposed to a traumatic event (Breslau et al., 1991, 1995). In general, men are more likely to have experienced or witnessed physical assault, whereas women are more likely to have been sexually victimized (Breslau et al., 1995; Kessler et al., 1995).

The high rate of sexual assault in women is further supported by numerous surveys indicating that between 15% and 33% of females are sexually abused as children (Finkelhor et al., 1990; Russell, 1986; Saunders et al., 1992; Wyatt, 1985). In addition, between 14% and 25% of women are raped during adulthood (Burt, 1979; Kilpatrick et al., 1987; Koss, 1993; National Victims Center, 1992; Russell, 1986; Searles & Berger, 1987; Sorenson et al., 1987; Wyatt, 1992). These high rates of trauma are of special concern when we consider the bias toward underreporting traumatic events inherent in retrospective study designs (Kessler et al., 1995) and due to factors such as reluctance to discuss unpleasant memories (Dill et al., 1991), fear of responses of the person to whom the event is disclosed (Symonds, 1982), or desire to protect perpetrators of abuse with whom they may have ongoing relationships (Della Femina et al., 1990). Thus, trauma is fairly common in the general population.

A growing body of evidence indicates an even higher prevalence of trauma among persons with a SMI, as recently reviewed by Goodman et al. (1997). Between 34% and 53% of persons with SMI report childhood sexual or physical abuse (Greenfield et al., 1994; Jacobson & Herald, 1990; Mueser, Goodman, et al., 1998; Rose et al., 1991; Ross et al., 1994). Over the lifetime, estimates of exposure to interpersonal violence, either physical or sexual, in persons with SMI vary between 43% and 81% (Carmen et al., 1984; Hutchings & Dutton, 1993; Jacobson, 1989; Jacobson & Richardson, 1987; Lipschitz et al., 1996). In addition, significant rates of exposure to noninterpersonal trauma have also been found in the SMI population. For example, Mueser, Goodman, et al. (1998) stated that 43% of persons with SMI reported experiencing a car or work accident and 14% reported being victims of a natural or human-made disaster.

Furthermore, exposure to interpersonal violence over the past year is high for persons with SMI living with family members or significant others, as indicated by two recent studies reporting rates of 29% in the United States (Cascardi et al., 1996) and 38% in Sweden (Bergman & Ericsson, 1996). As recently summarized by Goodman et al. (1997), studies of the prevalence of interpersonal trauma in homeless women with SMI suggest that these patients are especially vulnerable to victimization. For example, one study of episodically homeless women with SMI indicated that 97% had been exposed to interpersonal violence (Goodman et al., 1995), and a second study found that 77% of homeless women with SMI had been sexually or physically abused as children (Davies-Netzley et al., 1996).

Thus, persons with SMI appear to be more likely to have experienced traumatic events than people in the general population, although to our knowledge no study has directly compared rates across these populations. This high rate of trauma is reported in a recently completed study by Mueser, Goodman, et al. (1998), who found that 98% of a sample of 275 patients with SMI had experienced at least one traumatic event in their lives. The apparently increased rate of trauma in persons with psychiatric illnesses is consistent with the results of Kessler et al. (1995), who reported that most people with PTSD also had other comorbid disorders. The high exposure of persons with SMI to traumatic events suggests that trauma should be regarded as normative experience in this population.

Clinical Correlates of Trauma

Exposure to trauma in childhood, especially sexual abuse, has been repeatedly linked to the later development of adult psychiatric disorders (Bagley & Ramsey, 1986; Browne & Finkelhor, 1986; Bushnell et al., 1992; Duncan et al., 1996; Polusny & Follette, 1995). In addition, trauma exposure is related to psychiatric symptoms in the SMI population. Specifically, sexual and physical abuse, in either childhood or adulthood, has been reported to be associated with greater severity across a wide range of different symptoms in persons with SMI, including hallucinations and delusions, depression, suicidality, anxiety, hostility, interpersonal sensitivity, somatization, and dissociation (Beck & van der Kolk, 1987; Briere et al., 1997; Bryer et al., 1987; Craine et al., 1988; Carmen et al., 1984; Davies-Netzley et al., 1996; Figueroa et al., 1997; Goff et al., 1991a, 1991b; Goodman et al., 1997; Greenfield et al., 1994; Muenzenmaier et al., 1993; Ross et al., 1994; Swett & Halpert, 1993).

In addition to more severe psychiatric symptoms, trauma in SMI patients has been found to be related to higher levels of substance abuse (Briere et al., 1997; Carmen et al., 1984; Craine et al., 1988; Goodman & Fallot, 1998; Rose et al., 1991). The more severe symptoms and substance abuse problems in these patients results in higher utilization of expensive health services, such as emergency room visits or inpatient hospitalizations (Briere et al., 1997; Carmen et al., 1984).

PTSD IN SEVERE MENTAL ILLNESS

Although exposure to interpersonal violence among SMI patients has been found to be related to more severe psychiatric symptoms in numerous studies, less research has examined either the prevalence of PTSD or its role in mediating the effects of trauma in this population. In this section we review research on the prevalence of PTSD in patients with SMI and consider the clinical implications of failing to diagnose this important comorbid disorder.

Prevalence of PTSD

Recent estimates of lifetime prevalence of PTSD in the general population range between 8% and 12% (Breslau et al., 1991; Kessler et al., 1995; Resnick et al., 1993). Only four studies have examined PTSD in patients with SMI, but each study suggests notably higher rates of PTSD. Craine et al. (1988), studying history of sexual abuse in 105 female state hospital patients, reported that 34% met criteria for PTSD, or 66% of the patients who had been abused. In a study of exposure to domestic violence over the past year in 69 acute psychiatric inpatients living with family or partners, Cascardi et al. (1996) found that 29% had PTSD, or 48% of patients who had been abused.

Both the Craine et al. (1988) and Cascardi et al. (1996) studies were limited with respect to the traumas assessed and the setting in which the assessment took place. Craine et al. evaluated only sexual abuse in women, whereas Cascardi et al. examined only recent domestic violence in patients living with family or partners. Both investigations were limited to psychiatric inpatients and were conducted in one setting. More recently, Mueser, Goodman, et al. (1998) examined the prevalence of PTSD based on a comprehensive survey of exposure to traumatic events over the lifetime in 275 patients with SMI. Both psychiatric inpatients and outpatients were assessed in public sector facilities in an urban and a rural setting. Exposure to the following different types of traumatic events were evaluated in both childhood and adulthood: sexual assault, physical assault without a weapon, physical assault with a weapon, witnessing, sudden unexpected death of a loved one, accident or human-made disaster, and natural disaster.

The results indicated that most patients had experienced at least one type of traumatic event (98%) and that 43% met DSM-IV criteria for current PTSD. As was found in studies of trauma in the general population (e.g., Breslau et al., 1991; Kessler et al., 1995), women were more likely to have been sexually assaulted and men were more likely to have been physically assaulted and to have witnessed violence to others. Also in line with research in the general population, the number of different types of trauma and sexual assault in childhood were the most significant unique predictors of PTSD (Astin et al., 1995; Kessler et al., 1995; King et al., 1996; Resnick & Kilpatrick, 1994). These findings have recently been replicated in a large sample of 181 urban outpatients, in which 40% (42% of those exposed to trauma) were diagnosed with PTSD (Switzer et al., 1999) Interestingly, in contrast to studies of PTSD in the general population which have found higher rates of PTSD in women than men (Kessler et al., 1995), neither Cascardi et al. (1996), Mueser, Goodman, et al. (1998), nor Switzer et al. (1999) found gender differences in PTSD in their patients with SMI. Moreover, the likelihood of developing PTSD, given exposure to a traumatic event, appears to be elevated in people with SMI.

Underdiagnosis of PTSD in Persons with Severe Mental Illness

A potentially important finding across all three studies of PTSD in patients with SMI was the absence of chart documentation of PTSD. Despite the high rates of PTSD, Craine et al. (1988) and Cascardi et al. (1996) reported that no patients had diagnoses of PTSD in their charts, and in Mueser, Goodman, et al. (1998) only 3 of 119 (2%) patients with PTSD had this as a chart diagnosis. There are several reasons why PTSD may be so frequently underdiagnosed in the SMI population. In general, clinicians working with SMI patients tend to neglect the assessment of interpersonal violence history. Almost universally, studies that assess trauma history in patients with SMI through direct interviews report that in only a fraction of the positive cases is the history documented in the patient's chart (Cascardi et al., 1996; Craine et al., 1988; Jacobson, 1989; Jacobson & Herald, 1990; Mitchell et al., 1996).

Furthermore, even when evaluation of trauma histories in SMI patients is mandated and duly recorded, clinicians neglect to follow up positive histories by examining PTSD symptoms (Eilenberg et al., 1996). Since one of the symptoms of PTSD is avoidance of stimuli that remind the person of the traumatic event(s), patients who are not directly queried about their traumatic experiences will often not spontaneously volunteer the information (Redner & Herder, 1992). Finally, clinicians may not pursue trauma histories and PTSD more vigorously in their patients with SMI because they do not know how to incorporate such information into treatment planning.

The failure to detect and treat PTSD in patients with SMI could have important implications for the course and outcome of their illnesses. The causal relationships between PTSD and SMI are likely complex and interacting. There is evidence both that early trauma predicts the later development of psychiatric illness and that persons with mental disorders are more vulnerable to develop PTSD after exposure to a traumatic event than are nonmentally ill persons (Blanchard et al., 1995; Breslau et al., 1995). Furthermore, persons with a SMI are more likely to be interpersonally victimized (Goodman et al., 1995), thereby increasing their vulnerability and chance of developing PTSD. In the next section, we summarize a model which posits that PTSD plays an important role in mediating the effects of trauma and retraumatization on the course of SMI.

A HEURISTIC MODEL OF TRAUMA, PTSD, AND THE COURSE OF SEVERE MENTAL ILLNESS

This model (Mueser, Rosenberg, et al., in press), an adaptation of the stress–vulnerability model (Falconer, 1965; Liberman et al., 1986), assumes that the severity of SMI has a biological basis determined early in life by genetic and early environmental factors. *Stress*, including discrete events such as traumas and exposure to ongoing conditions such as a hostile environment, can impinge on vulnerability, precipitating relapses and use of acute care services. Conversely, *coping* resources, such as adaptive skills or the ability to obtain support, can minimize the negative effects of stress on relapse and rehospitalization.

In our heuristic model, illustrated in Figure 14.1, we hypothesize that PTSD is mainly responsible for the relationships between trauma and more severe clinical presentation in patients with SMI. PTSD is given a central mediating role in this model because the symptoms which define PTSD, as well as its common clinical correlates, can be theoretically linked to a worse prognosis of SMI. PTSD is hypothesized to both directly and indirectly increase symptom severity and risk of relapse in patients with SMI. PTSD can directly affect SMI through increased avoidance behavior, distress related to reexperiencing the trauma, and physiological overarousal. Common corre-

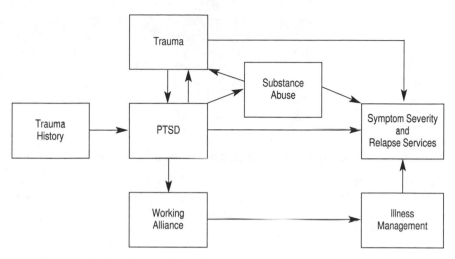

FIGURE 14.1. Heuristic model of trauma, PTSD, and severe mental illness (SMI). PTSD is hypothesized to worsen the severity and course of SMI through the direct effects of PTSD symptoms (e.g., reexperiencing the trauma, overarousal) and indirectly through the effects of PTSD on substance abuse, retraumatization, and a poor working alliance with clinicians, leading to receipt of fewer preventative illness management services.

lates of PTSD can also indirectly affect SMI, including retraumatization, a poor working alliance, and substance abuse. We provide more details about this model below.

Direct Effects of PTSD on Severe Mental Illness

We hypothesize that each of the three symptom clusters required to diagnose PTSD—*avoidance of stimuli* related to the trauma, distress related to *reexperiencing the trauma,* and *heightened physiological arousal*—affect SMI. As the most common traumas experienced are interpersonal in nature, avoidance of trauma-related stimuli (e.g., close relationships, sex) in PTSD often leads to social isolation (American Psychiatric Association, 1994). There is abundant evidence that lack of social contacts is a strong prospective predictor of symptom relapses and rehospitalizations in patients with SMI (Avison & Speechley, 1987; Harrison et al., 1996; Strauss & Carpenter, 1977). Social isolation may increase vulnerability to psychotic symptoms because of the lack opportunities for reality testing with others, the absence of meaningful stimulation such as work, or the failure to experience the buffering effects of a supportive social network (Bell et al., 1996; Cresswell et al., 1992). Thus, severe avoidance due to PTSD is expected to worsen symptom severity in patients with SMI.

Distress due to reexperiencing the trauma and heightened physiological arousal can be conceptualized as a chronic stress. Extensive research shows that both discrete stressors (e.g., life events) and exposure to chronic stress (e.g., a stressful environment) can worsen SMI (Butzlaff & Hooley, 1998). Similarly, increased physiological arousal, especially chronic overactivation, is associated with a poor prognosis in patients with SMI (Dawson & Nuechterlein, 1984; Straube & Öhman, 1990; Zahn, 1986).

Indirect Effects of PTSD on Severe Mental Illness

In addition to the direct effects, common clinical correlates of PTSD are hypothesized to indirectly influence SMI, including *retraumatization*, a *poor treatment alliance*, and *substance abuse*. We next discuss each of these indirect pathways in turn.

Retraumatization

Research on the sequelae of trauma has often noted a tendency for victimization to lead to retraumatization over the lifetime (Burnam et al., 1988; Polusny & Follette, 1995). Indeed, the high rate of multiple traumas experienced by patients with SMI has often been noted (Goodman et al., 1995; Lipschitz et al., 1996; Mueser, Goodman, et al., 1998; Muezenmaier et al., 1993). Furthermore, evidence indicates that the number of traumatic events experienced is a strong predictor of PTSD in the general population (Astin et al., 1995; King et al., 1996; Resnick & Kilpatrick, 1994) and among persons with SMI (Mueser, Goodman, et al., 1998).

Multiple traumatization may both contribute to the development of PTSD and be a by-product of PTSD as well. For example, a foreshortened sense of future may lead to retraumatization due to the inability or unwillingness to anticipate and prevent negative events. In addition, early trauma and onset of PTSD may interfere with the acquisition of social skills necessary to avert exposure to at least some interpersonal violence (Harris, 1996; Mueser & Taylor, 1997). Regardless of the precise pathways, PTSD is related to revictimization, and exposure to traumatic events and victimization in patients with SMI can worsen the course of illness (Bebbington & Kuipers, 1992; Lam & Rosenheck, 1998).

Treatment Alliance

PTSD and interpersonal dysfunction are closely linked (Escobar et al., 1983; Glover, 1984; Jordan et al., 1992). Problems related to hypervigilance, recurrent disturbing memories, efforts to avoid stimuli reminiscent of the trauma, anger, and mistrust have an impact on the person's ability to form and maintain close relationships with others (Browne & Finklehor, 1986; Roessler &

McKenzie, 1994). Efforts to keep secrets or avoid topics related to traumatic events can interfere with close relationships and ultimately exacerbate anxiety about the experiences themselves (Kelly & McKillop, 1996).

The difficulties that patients with PTSD experience confiding in others may also influence their ability to establish a treatment alliance with providers. Poor relationships with treatment providers can result in receiving fewer services necessary to manage the psychiatric illness (e.g., medication checks, case management), with increasing risk of symptom exacerbations. Several studies suggest that the quality of the alliance with the case manager in patients with SMI is related to symptom severity (Gehrs & Goering, 1994; Neale & Rosenheck, 1995; Priebe & Gruyters, 1993; P. Solomon et al., 1995), although this has not been examined in patients with SMI and PTSD.

Substance Abuse

Patients with PTSD often have comorbid alcohol and drug use disorders (Chilcoat & Breslau, 1998; Deering et al., 1996; Keane & Wolfe, 1990; Mc-Farlane, 1998; Rundell et al., 1989; Stewart, 1996; Stewart et al., 1998; Triffleman et al., 1995). There is also a high prevalence of substance use disorders in the SMI population (Cuffel, 1996; Mueser, Yarnold, et al., 1990, 1992; Regier et al., 1990). Prospective research has shown that substance abuse in persons with SMI contributes to a wide range of negative outcomes, including worse symptom severity (e.g., Drake et al., 1989, 1996; Kozaric-Kovacic et al., 1995; Linszen et al., 1994). PTSD, therefore, may increase vulnerability to substance abuse in patients with SMI, worsening the course of illness.

Clinical Implications of the Heuristic PTSD and Severe Mental Illness Model

Our model suggests that the failure to assess and treat PTSD in patients with SMI may have dire consequences, resulting in a more severe course of both illnesses. Intervention designed to ameliorate the symptoms of PTSD may improve the course of SMI by lessening its direct effects, such as lowering physiological overarousal and decreasing social isolation due to avoidance of trauma-related stimuli. Effective treatment may also influence indirect pathways by which PTSD impacts on the course of SMI, such as through reduction of substance abuse, decreasing vulnerability to retraumatization, and improving the working alliance with treatment providers. This model also suggests that to the extent substance abuse is maintained partly by efforts to decrease overarousal and distress due to recollections of traumatic events, targeting PTSD may be critical for improving substance abuse in patients with SMI. Furthermore, effective treatment of PTSD in these "triply" diagnosed patients (SMI, PTSD, substance abuse disorder) could reduce both substance abuse and vulnerability to subsequent retraumatization, as shown by evidence linking PTSD, substance abuse, and retraumatization in the general population (Kilpatrick et al., 1997).

CURRENT CLINICAL PRACTICES AND TREATMENT MODELS OF PTSD IN SEVERE MENTAL ILLNESS

Despite the apparent high prevalence and negative clinical impact of PTSD in the chronic population, assessment and treatment of PTSD have been largely ignored, or has been a low-priority issue, in most clinical settings serving the SMI. For example, only very recently and in only a few states have departments of mental health mandated and supported posttraumatic assessments and treatments for patients receiving public sector care for SMI (National Association of State Mental Health Program Directors [NASMHP], 1998).

We conducted a computerized search of the literature over the past 31 years on PTSD treatment for people with SMI using the search terms "trauma," "PTSD," "sexual abuse," "physical abuse," "mental illness," "severe mental illness," "serious mental illness," "schizophrenia," "bipolar," and "treatment." The search of PsychInfo yielded 130 publications of potential interest, and the PILOTS database yielded 105 such publications. We examined the identified publications for descriptions of programs offering any or all of the currently used techniques for treating PTSD in other (non-SMI) populations including psychoeducation, stress management/relaxation, cognitive restructuring, exposure-based treatments, supportive interventions, skills training, pharmacological treatment, and interpersonal psychotherapy (IPT) or psychodynamic psychotherapy. Both individual and group treatment modalities, as well as in- and outpatient programs, were included. This search narrowed the list of publications of interest to 17.

Reviewing even this modest literature is complicated by several facts: (1) Most of the interventions were directed at diverse diagnostic groups, not all of whom would meet the standard definition of SMI cited above (e.g., patients with borderline personality disorders or substance use disorders). (2) Interventions were often explicitly designed for women and did not include males with PTSD and SMI. (3) Several of the programs described in the literature seem to be directed not at treatment of PTSD per se but at a much broader spectrum of posttraumatic responses associated with childhood sexual abuse; indeed, focused PTSD treatments appeared to be excluded in some of these treatment programs (e.g., Scheidt, 1994; Talbot et al., 1998), since explicit discussion of trauma experiences may be avoided in the belief that patients are too clinically unstable to manage such discussions. (4) Conversely, patients with PTSD secondary to non-CSA traumas (e.g., nonsexual assaults, rape trauma in adulthood) seem not be included in these programs for SMI trauma survivors, limiting generalizability. (5) The interventions described tended to be multipronged (e.g., group psychoeducation combined with art therapy in the context of an inpatient treatment program). (6) It is often unclear as to which aspect of the complex treatments were directed at attempts to ameliorate symptoms/dysfunction resulting from SMI and/or SUD and which were directed at postabuse or PTSD symptoms.

Our search located no randomized clinical trials of PTSD interventions for people with possible SMI, four single-case studies, and six open trials (or descriptions of treatment programs). The open trials were generally reported without quantitative measures of change. None of the published reports met or even approached the "gold standard" criteria for outcomes studies of PTSD treatment outlined by Foa and Meadows (1997): clearly defined target symptoms; reliable outcome measures; manualized, replicable treatment programs; etc. It is also unclear to what degree the target population described in these reports are truly individuals with SMI and PTSD. That is, some of the patients described may well have been cases of chronic complex PTSD without an independent SMI (e.g., Nishith et al., 1995; Herder & Redner, 1991).

Nishith et al. (1995) and Mueser and Taylor (1997) reported single-case design studies of cognitive-behavioral treatment of PTSD provided to women with severe symptomatology (e.g., major depression, suicidality with delusions). Symptoms of PTSD, depression, and distress were assessed pretreatment, posttreatment, and at 3-month (Nishith et al., 1999) and 3-year (Mueser & Taylor, 1997) follow-ups. In both instances, improvement followed treatment which included standard hospital care, as well as exposure and broad-based cognitive-behavioral interventions directed at PTSD and trauma-related symptoms. Contrary to expressed concerns in the literature (Litz et al., 1990; S. D. Solomon, 1997), both patients were able to tolerate the exposure intervention and suffered no other symptom exacerbation or dysfunction as a treatment side effect. A cautionary note is, however, warranted. The case histories presented left ambiguity as to whether PTSD was the primary diagnosis for either or both of the patients treated, with the depressive symptoms being secondary. The difficulty distinguishing primary PTSD from PTSD that is comorbid with another Axis I diagnosis is further compounded when evidence is considered that psychotic symptoms can occur secondary to PTSD (Butler et al., 1996; Hamner, 1997; Mueser & Butler, 1987; Sautter et al., 1999). This could limit the generalizability of the reported case experience in regards to patients with a primary SMI, and the translation of these case studies for schizophrenia-spectrum disorders and bipolar disorder remains unexplored.

Although programmatic (i.e., multipronged) interventions explicitly directed at people with both SMI and posttraumatic symptoms have existed for at least 10 years, there appear to be virtually no scientific data on the effectiveness of these PTSD treatments. At least four reports have been published describing experimental treatment approaches, usually embedded in larger programs of comprehensive case management or acute inpatient treatment. These programs primarily target women with chronic and severe psychiatric disorders who also have suffered childhood sexual abuse and usually a variety of other interpersonal traumas. The interventions are directed at a full range of symptoms, including those associated with PTSD diagnoses and DESNOS (Disorders of Extreme Stress Not Otherwise Specified). No quantitative outcome data are provided in any of these reports.

These reports do reflect some consensus about useful program characteristics. PTSD treatments for SMI patients should include (or at least assume) comprehensive case management, housing supports, attention to safety issues, medication management, integration of the treatment team, and inclusion of a full range of posttraumatic services (e.g., psychoeducation, support, exposure, and cognitive restructuring), and should also take a long-term perspective with a recognition of stages of recovery and relapse in regards to both primary psychiatric disorder and PTSD symptoms. Program reports also convey some optimism that PTSD interventions can be useful in the SMI population. Case vignettes are provided in some reports, suggesting that these interventions can be beneficial across a broad spectrum of symptoms and disability (e.g., social withdrawal, substance abuse, and self-care).

At the very least, the clinical experiences described, which probably now include many hundreds of patients, provide support for the idea that trauma interventions are feasible, even in the context of acute and/or chronic psychotic illness and comorbid substance abuse disorders (Talbot et al., 1998; Harris, 1997; Stowe & Harris, 1997; Herder & Redner, 1991). As in the single-case reports, program experiences appear to challenge the common recommendations regarding treatment eligibility or treatment readiness (e.g., stable sobriety) generally found in the PTSD literature. The results of these experimental programs, based on clinician evaluation and nonstandardized patients' feedback, appear to provide support for the field to proceed to more systematic, controlled studies of PTSD interventions for people with SMI. Such interventions would likely share many characteristics of treatments designed for veterans with chronic combat-related PTSD in combination with other Axis I and Axis II disorders (e.g., Frueh, 1996; Seidel et al., 1994). These programs are multiphasic, contain both group and individual components, and address cognitive dimensions and coping skills in structured and supportive environments.

The studies and program descriptions reviewed also emphasize two types of treatment modifications: (1) modified treatments of the patient's psychotic disorder in light of trauma effects including PTSD, and (2) modifications of treatments for PTSD in light of the issues and limitations introduced by the presence of a chronic SMI. In the former category, such issues as the boundaries of case management or the use of inpatient hospitalization or restraints for patients' safety must be considered in the light of trauma reactions. In the latter category, the need for adjunctive supports for people with unstable housing or impoverished social networks must be considered in establishing the timing and context of PTSD treatments.

Case Example

Given the current state of programming in most mental health care systems, clinicians typically must cobble together these treatment elements when they encounter patients with both PTSD and SMI. Patients ordinarily would neither have been identified as trauma survivors nor diagnosed with PTSD when referred, and the issue of which disorder is primary may not be clear during the initial stages of treatment. The following case is illustrative of many of the issues outlined in this review:

Ms. SW, a divorced woman in her mid–30s, was transferred for treatment to a new clinician following a job switch by her former therapist. She had seen the previous therapist for about 6 months of outpatient treatment, which was initiated after she had taken a medical leave from her job as a primary grade teacher due to "emotional strain." She had become increasingly unable to function in the classroom after learning that one of her female students had been physically and sexually assaulted. SW's leave had not proved helpful, but rather she had become increasingly withdrawn, depressed, anxious, and intermittently suicidal. Although she liked the former therapist, the patient had done rather poorly during the treatment, spending increasing amounts of her time housebound, weepy, and unable to concentrate on even simple tasks. Along with weekly psychotherapy for depression (supportive and cognitive-behavioral emphases), SW was also advised to take an antidepressant, to which she reluctantly agreed. However, she soon stopped the medication, complaining of various side effects.

Although the precipitating events of SW's depressive episode raised the suspicion of posttrauma history, no direct information in this regard was forthcoming, and both diagnosis and treatment focused on affective problems. Fairly early in treatment, SW exhibited hypomanic symptoms, and a past history of suspected bipolar disorder contributed to a revised diagnosis. A trial of lithium was begun and then terminated at the patient's request, despite the fact that both the therapist and a consulting psychiatrist felt the medication to be necessary. The transfer to treatment with the new therapist was superficially smooth, but SW's symptoms remained largely unchanged and she was unable to return to her teaching position the following term, as had been originally planned. Indeed, it appeared that her level of functioning was continuing to deteriorate. Presentation in therapy was generally quite muted, with frequent moments of tense silence. Given the poor clinical course, the therapist began taking a more solution-focused, rehabilitative approach, encouraging SW to resume more leisure activities and hobbies that would involve social contact. The patient agreed that this would be helpful but appeared to experience even such small steps as difficult to achieve and as "too much pressure." Manic symptoms began to appear at this time, along with apparently delusional material about deceased family members attempting to harm her. Antipsychotic medication was then reluctantly agreed to by the patient and reintroduced, but her response was limited. Suicidal ideation became more prominent, as did social withdrawal. SW very reluctantly agreed to a brief inpatient stay, primarily because of safety concerns. During this hospitalization, she revealed to nursing staff (albeit in vague terms) that she had suffered both physical and sexual abuse as a child.

This disclosure allowed more direct discussion of posttraumatic symptoms in therapy and helped to clarify why treatment of SW's affective symptoms were ineffective. For example, self-isolation was not simply a depressive sign but also represented a phobic avoidance of situations where SW might have to interact with older males, contact with whom could cause reexperiencing symptoms. Her dislike of psychotropic medication was partially complicated by issues of obedience to and control by authorities of what entered her body, particularly her mouth. While aware of this symbolic and irrational component of her response to medication suggestions, SW reported that her feelings about doctors and medicines had always been skewed by suspicion, anger, and the need to "stand up for herself." In addition, her chronic sense of fatigue was partially due to frequent sleep disturbance associated with trauma-related nightmares.

The therapist, an older male, was also often perceived as a threatening presence, accounting for much of the silence and hesitancy encountered in therapy. SW was able to acknowledge that any rehabilitative suggestions made by the therapist were perceived by her as directive and controlling, thus evoking feelings of revictimization. Exploration of these issues made clear that treatment of her mood disorder would require modification based on her PTSD symptomatology. In addition, treatment of SW's posttraumatic difficulties required titration based on her vulnerability to both depression and manic symptomatology when under stress. It was made clear to the patient that the pace of PTSD treatment would be under her control, so that even the factual recounting of the earlier abuse experiences was achieved in small steps with frequent "time-outs." Support in daily activities, as well as some consistent interpersonal contact, appeared to be important during this phase of treatment, and SW was linked with a case manager who helped provide these resources. As SW became slightly less agoraphobic, she also began participating in a peer support program in the local community and began to learn more about other people who had learned to cope with both affective illness and posttraumatic disorders. This multipronged approach, which included psychopharmacological treatment, crisis intervention, environmental manipulation, case management, social supports, cognitive-behavioral, and interpersonal components, has led to considerable improvement. SW has now returned to work and is finding it easier to resume earlier activities. However, the continued use of external supports and further cognitive and interpersonal treatment appear to be useful in ensuring more stable recovery.

APPLICATION OF EMPIRICALLY SUPPORTED PTSD INTERVENTIONS TO SMI

Table 14.1 presents a taxonomy of PTSD interventions that have been attempted with severely and chronically disabled patients and which likely will constitute the backbone of effective treatments for this population. As can be seen, some of these interventions overlap with current best-practice treatments for SMI, creating possible efficiencies or synergies in the treatments of the two (or more) disorders typically suffered by this population. Conversely, some treatments may have negative interactions, requiring careful titration or modification.

The ability of community mental health programs to successfully implement evaluation and intervention strategies for SMI patients with PTSD

TABLE 14.1. Taxonomy of Interventions for PTSD, SMI, and Related Problems

| Intervention | Disorder | | | |
	PTSD	Childhood sexual abuse	SMI	Substance abuse disorder
Psychoeducation	R	R	R	N
Stress management/innoculation	E	R	R	N
Cognitive restructuring	E	R	E	R
Exposure	E	R	NA	NA
Skills training	F	R	E	E
Supportive psychotherapy	N	R	N	R
Interpersonal/psychodynamic therapy	F	R	T	R
Self-help groups	U	R	F	R
Psychopharmacology	F	U	E	E
Intensive case management	U	U	E	NA
Housing supports	U	U	R	U
Financial and employment supports	U	U	R	U
Family intervention	F	U	E	E

Note. E, efficacy demonstrated; R, recommended by clinical experience and/or open trial; F, known to be feasible, but effectiveness unknown; U, unknown effects; T, known to be toxic; C, believed by clinicians to be contraindicated; N, not effective; NA, not applicable hinges on two issues: (1) fears or ignorance among providers about dealing with posttraumatic issues, and (2) cost concerns at agency or systems levels.

As witnessed by the explosion of lawsuits, books in the popular press, media depictions, and self-help groups, the topic of trauma, and especially sexual abuse and "repressed memories," has become quite controversial in recent years (Brandon et al., 1998; Herman, 1992; Loftus & Ketcham, 1994; Pope & Hudson, 1995; Wakefield & Underwager, 1992). Many clinicians are understandably reluctant to enter into the fray by assessing trauma and its consequences in their patients with SMI, preferring to steer clear of the topic altogether. At the same time, most patients with trauma histories and PTSD are more than willing to oblige in avoiding discussion of traumatic experiences, as avoidance of trauma-related memories is a symptom of their PTSD. The problem of mutual avoidance is further exacerbated by the lack of clear guidelines for the treatment of patients with SMI and comorbid PTSD, resulting in an attitude among clinicians that exploring trauma and PTSD in their patients amounts to "opening Pandora's box."

Attitudes about the assessment and treatment of trauma-related syndromes in patients with SMI are likely to change slowly over time, with the accumulation of evidence documenting that valid assessments can be conducted and that well-defined interventions can produce reliable and substantial improvements in patient functioning. Clinicians' fears about addressing the sequelae of trauma in their patients are related to not only their ignorance of presentation and treatment of trauma-related syndromes in the SMI population but the more widely shared ignorance of the field in general. As the lack of knowledge about the potential importance of trauma is frequently supplanted by inaccurate information, stereotypes, and beliefs based on clinicians' personal experiences, clinical practices are likely to change only very gradually in response to reeducation efforts and, more critically, personal successes in treating PTSD in patients with SMI. Clinical research is needed in order to establish the assessment and treatment guidelines that will be the focus of training with clinicians. However, in the absence of empirically supported guidelines for working with SMI patients with traumatic experiences, simply mandating the assessment of trauma history will have a negligible effect on the ability of clinicians to address trauma syndromes in their patients.

Once treatments have been developed and established for patients with SMI and PTSD, how will health maintenance organizations (HMOs) and health insurance providers be persuaded to pay for these services? From a strictly fiscal perspective, the most convincing argument for paying for the treatment of trauma syndromes in patients with SMI would be evidence that such interventions are not only clinically beneficial but that they also result in lower utilization of high-cost services such as emergency room and inpatient treatment. Our heuristic model of PTSD and SMI suggests that untreated PTSD leads to a more severe course of psychiatric illness, including use of higher-cost services, as recently reported by Switzer et al. (1999). More evidence supporting both the impact of persistent PTSD on the course of psychiatric illness and the costs of treatment, as well as lower overall costs associated with successful treatment of PTSD, would provide a strong case for the coverage of PTSD in patients with SMI.

RECOMMENDATIONS AND FUTURE DIRECTIONS

Clearly, systematic empirical study is needed before we can specify best-practices treatments for people with both SMI and PTSD. Furthermore, there is a need for interventions to be developed that can be tailored to the specific interactions between trauma, PTSD, and the course of SMI unique to each patient. In our heuristic model, we suggest several direct and indirect mechanisms by which PTSD may be expected to worsen SMI and service utilization, but the specific pathways involved will differ from one patient to the next. Interventions need to be sufficiently flexible to allow clinicians to target the specific factors related to PTSD that most contribute to problems in community living and psychiatric severity. For example, substance abuse (due to efforts to mollify the effects of intrusive memories of traumatic events) and retraumatization (secondary to substance abuse) may be the most critical consequences of PTSD that need to be addressed in one patient, whereas physiological overarousal, avoidance of trauma-related stimuli, and a poor working alliance may be more important in another patient. Naturally, treatment for two such patients would be expected to differ in some respects (e.g., focus on addressing intrusive symptoms vs. avoidance of trauma-related stimuli), while overlapping in other ways (e.g., psychoeducation about PTSD).

Manualized treatments that are safe, feasible, and practical must be developed and systematically tested using reliable and valid outcome measures. The limited data currently available support the possibility of utilizing PTSD treatments which have been validated in the general population and adapting these for patients with SMI. More specifically, psychoeducation, cognitive-behavioral techniques (including exposure and cognitive restructuring), anxiety management (including stress inoculation), and social skills training have all shown efficacy in other PTSD populations and appear to be tolerated by patients with SMI if delivered in a context of comprehensive mental health care. Neither pharmacotherapy directed at PTSD symptoms nor group support modalities currently have the same degree of evidential support regarding efficacy, but clinicians working with SMI patients with PTSD often advocate use of these modalities as adjunctive or partial alternatives to the interventions listed above.

Combined PTSD treatments appear to be necessary for these patients for two reasons. First, their multiple disorders are interactive and cannot be successfully managed in isolation. Second, since no single intervention is likely to ameliorate all PTSD symptoms in all patients, exposure, anxiety management, and cognitive interventions will need to be used sequentially or conjointly to reduce the morbidity associated with PTSD in this population. While exposure treatments may be generally efficient in reducing intrusive symptoms, it is not yet clear whether—or under what circumstances (e.g., phase of illness, degree of social isolation)—such treatments will be well tolerated by people with SMI. Similarly, considering the cognitive deficits often present in persons with SMI, it is unclear how many will have the cognitive resources to participate in and benefit from cognitive restructuring. From a stage-of-treatment perspective, where engagement and trust building may well be necessary (and lengthy) prerequisites to active treatment, it may be crucial to prepare patients for PTSD treatment through psychoeducation and support. After patients are engaged and clinically stable, treatments can then progress to coping and skills-building modules, which could in turn prepare patients for the initiation of exposure and cognitive restructuring.

In addition, the interactions between PTSD symptoms, psychotic symptoms, and substance abuse disorder issues must be considered in the design and sequencing of services. How will patients be supported so that potentially stressful phases of treatment, like the initial sessions of exposure, do not lead to relapse of substance abuse as a means of avoidance of painful affect? Etiological and nosological questions will also require careful observation of patients, as well as clinicians with sophisticated knowledge of both (or all three) disorders. For example, not only do symptoms of reexperiencing represent acute stressors for patients with SMI, but such PTSD symptoms may well be confused for primary psychotic symptoms—such as hallucinations or delusions—if clinicians are not sensitive to posttraumatic presentations and symptom course (Jennings, 1994; Oruč & Bell, 1995; Waldfogel & Mueser, 1988).

Given the available state of knowledge in the field, as well as the degree of consensus that exists among experts, we would suggest a valuable approach for PTSD interventions may be found in the best-practices models for integrated dual diagnosis (i.e., SMI and substance use disorder) treatment (Drake et al., 1993; Minkoff, 1989; Mueser, Drake, & Noordsy, 1998). These models were also developed to adapt theoretically motivated treatment technologies from the general population to the SMI. After a decade of experimentation, they have demonstrated their ability to successfully address the multifaceted needs of the dual disorders population in a cost-effective manner (Drake et al., 1998). First, many—if not most—SMI patients with PTSD also suffer from substance abuse problems (Briere et al., 1997; Carmen et al., 1984; Craine et al., 1988; Rose et al., 1991). Second, the basic principles employed by dual-diagnosis programs (i.e., assertiveness, integration of providers, comprehensiveness of interventions, long-term perspective, stage-of-treatment focus to match intervention to the patient's motivational state, flexibility, and need for optimism) appear to fit well with the experience of clinicians working with SMI with PTSD.

Dual-diagnosis treatment programs have been forced to deal with issues of denial and secretiveness in SMI patients, who are often distrustful of the providers' motives and fearful of further stigmatization and legal entanglements. The same dynamics appear to be true for SMI patients with trauma histories and PTSD. All these factors point to the importance of psychoeducation as an initial step for PTSD treatment in the SMI. The field of mental health treatment has become much more aware of substance use disorder as a common and toxic factor in people with psychiatric illnesses. PTSD is much less widely recognized by providers (Cascardi et al., 1996; Mueser, Goodman, et al., 1998) and appears to be poorly understood by patients and their families. Given the high rates of trauma and PTSD in people with SMI, we would advocate universal education for providers and mental health consumers about trauma, PTSD, and their possible relationship to other psychiatric and medical conditions. Such psychoeducation can help to destigmatize abuse and to open a dialogue between consumers and providers on the issue of posttraumatic reactions and their treatment.

As with dual-diagnosis treatment models, a long-term perspective is required for durable change to occur. Like substance use disorder, PTSD can be a chronic, relapsing condition which is frequently misunderstood or denied (Friedman & Rosenheck, 1996; Kessler et al., 1995). Helping patients to recognize and acknowledge their PTSD, and then move through stages of change toward recovery, requires patience, understanding, and frustration tolerance on the part of the therapist. Clinicians must be ready to meet patients at their own level of illness recognition, both encourage and allow patients to move at their own pace, and provide hope when relapse occurs. Given the long-term sense of stigma, inferiority, and lack of efficacy reported by SMI patients with abuse histories, it will also be important for treatment programs to fully employ a collaborative ideology which allows for an optimization of patient participation and a sense of control over the treatment environment and program design. These same considerations would also suggest the inclusion of a range of treatment options, such as group versus individual treatment, as well as control by patients over the timing and ultimately the selection of modalities used in their own treatment.

Just as dual-diagnosis programs attend to the environments and life circumstances which lead SMI patients to substance abuse relapse, so will clinicians need to increase their recognition of the dangerousness of PTSD/SMI patients' typical environments. As the cited trauma surveys indicated, the lives of people with SMI tend to be filled with multiple and frequently overwhelming dangers. When these environments must be negotiated by people with already limited coping resources, and often limited cognitive resources as well, it becomes clear that the need to enhance patient safety and avoid retraumatization during treatment must be a core feature of PTSD interventions for this group.

Given the resource restrictions currently being placed on mental health providers, it will also be incumbent on the field to develop interventions which incorporate the key elements of PTSD treatment into supportable, cost-effective formats. Use of such efficiencies as time-limited or patient-run groups may make the difference between programs that are implemented in clinical practice and those which agency administrators refuse to support in the face of other pressures and priorities. Advocates for patient-operated programs point out that trauma and its consequences are frequently ignored by the mental health profession (Fisher, 1992; Jennings, 1994) and that psychiatric treatment itself often has iatrogenic traumatic (or retraumatizing) effects (Deegan, 1990; Fisher et al., 1996; Miller, 1990). Client-run education and support groups for trauma survivors may have the advantage of providing needed ongoing support to patients in a context free of the usual power hierarchies of the mental health system that have been argued to perpetuate and worsen the effects of earlier sexual and physical trauma (Beale & Lambric, 1995; Deegan, 1992).

Finally, we feel that it will be crucial to explore the tolerance of SMI patients with varying primary psychiatric disorders, as well as differing trauma backgrounds and other comorbidities, for PTSD interventions of different intensities and types. Once we can be assured that such treatments "do no harm," the utility of exposure-based and other cognitive-behavioral and psychosocial treatments for PTSD in people with SMI can be systematically evaluated. While experience to date suggests that such treatments are likely to be translatable for more vulnerable, multiproblem populations, they are also likely to require the use of adjunctive supports, treatment preparation, and attention to clinical indicators of readiness for PTSD treatment. The development of standardized yet flexible interventions for PTSD that can be provided in conjunction with comprehensive rehabilitation-based programs offers the best promise for improving the long-term outcome of patients with SMI, and thereby enabling these individuals to get on with their lives.

REFERENCES

American Psychiatric Association (1987). *Diagnostic and statistical manual of mental disorders*. (3rd ed., rev.). Washington, DC: Author.

American Psychiatric Association (1994). *Diagnostic and statistical manual of mental disorders*. (4th ed.) Washington, DC: Author.

Astin, M. C., Ogland-Hand, S. M., Coleman, E. M., & Foy, D. W. (1995). Posttraumatic stress disorder and childhood abuse in battered women: Comparisons with maritally distressed women. *Journal of Consulting and Clinical Psychology, 63*, 308–312.

Avison, W. R., & Speechley, K. N. (1987). The discharged psychiatric patient: A review of social, social–psychological, and psychiatric correlates of outcome. *American Journal of Psychiatry, 144,* 10–18.

Bagley, C., & Ramsey, R. (1986). Sexual abuse in childhood: Psychological outcomes and implications for social work practice. *Journal of Social Work and Human Sexuality, 4,* 33–47.

Beale, V., & Lambric, T. (1995). *The recovery concept: Implementation in the mental health system* (A report by the Community Support Program Advisory Committee). Columbus: Ohio Department of Mental Health, Office of Consumer Services.

Bebbington, P., & Kuipers, L. (1992). Life events and social factors. In D. J. Kavanaugh (Ed.), *Schizophrenia: An overview and practical handbook* (pp. 126–144). London: Chapman & Hall.

Beck, J. C., & van der Kolk, B. A. (1987). Reports of childhood incest and current behavior of chronically hospitalized psychotic women. *American Journal of Psychiatry, 144,* 1474–1476.

Bell, M. D., Lysaker, P. H., & Milstein, R. M. (1996). Clinical benefits of paid work activity in schizophrenia. *Schizophrenia Bulletin, 22,* 51–67.

Bergman, B., & Ericsson, E. (1996). Family violence among psychiatric inpatients as measured by the Conflict Tactics Scale (CTS). *Acta Psychiatrica Scandinavica, 94,* 168–174.

Blanchard, E. B., Hickling, E. J., Taylor, A. F., & Loos, W. (1995). Psychiatric morbidity associated with motor vehicle accidents. *Journal of Nervous and Mental Disease, 183,* 495–504.

Brandon, S., Boakes, J., Glaser, D., & Green, R. (1998). Recovered memories of childhood sexual abuse: Implications for clinical practice. *British Journal of Psychiatry, 172,* 296–307.

Breslau, N., Davis, G. C., & Andreski, P. (1995). Risk factors for PTSD-related traumatic events: A prospective analysis. *American Journal of Psychiatry, 152,* 529–535.

Breslau, N., Davis, G. C., Andreski, P., & Peterson, E. (1991). Traumatic events and posttraumatic stress disorder in an urban population of young adults. *Archives of General Psychiatry, 48,* 216–222.

Briere, J., Woo, R., McRae, B., Foltz, J., & Sitzman, R. (1997). Lifetime victimization history, demographics, and clinical status in female psychiatric emergency room patients. *Journal of Nervous and Mental Disease, 185,* 95–101.

Browne, A., & Finkelhor, D. (1986). Impact of child sexual abuse: A review of the research. *Psychological Bulletin, 99,* 66–77.

Bryer, J. B., Nelson, B. A., Miller, J. B., & Krol, P. A. (1987). Childhood sexual and physical abuse as factors in adult psychiatric illness. *American Journal of Psychiatry, 144,* 1426–1430.

Burnam, M. A., Stein, J. A., Golding, J. M., Siegel, J. M., Sorenson, S. B., Forsythe, A. B., & Telles, C. A. (1988). Sexual assault and mental disorders in a community population. *Journal of Consulting and Clinical Psychology, 56,* 843–850.

Burt, M. R. (1979). *Attitudes supportive of rape in American culture.* Rockville, MD: U. S. Department of Health & Human Services.

Bushnell, J. A., Wells, J. E., & Oakely-Browne, M. (1992). Long-term effects of intrafamilial sexual abuse in childhood. *Acta Psychiatrica Scandinavica, 85,* 136–142.

Butler, R. W., Mueser, K. T., Sprock, J., & Braff, D. L. (1996). Positive symptoms of psychosis in posttraumatic stress disorder. *Biological Psychiatry, 39,* 839–844.

Butzlaff, R. L., & Hooley, J. M. (1998). Expressed emotion and psychiatric relapse. *Archives of General Psychiatry, 55,* 547–552.

Carmen, E., Rieker, P. P., & Mills, T. (1984). Victims of violence and psychiatric illness. *American Journal of Psychiatry, 141,* 378–383.

Cascardi, M., Mueser, K. T., DeGirolomo, J., & Murrin, M. (1996). Physical aggression against psychiatric inpatients by family members and partners: A descriptive study. *Psychiatric Services, 47,* 531–533.

Chilcoat, H. D., & Breslau, N. (1998). Investigations of causal pathways between PTSD and drug use disorders. *Addictive Behaviors, 6,* 827–840.

Craine, L. S., Henson, C. E., Colliver, J. A., & MacLean, D. G. (1988). Prevalence of a history of sexual abuse among female psychiatric patients in a state hospital system. *Hospital and Community Psychiatry, 39,* 300–304.

Cresswell, C. M., Kuipers, L., & Power, M. J. (1992). Social networks and support in long-term psychiatric patients. *Psychological Medicine, 22,* 1019–1026.

Cuffel, B. J. (1996). Comorbid substance use disorder: Prevalence, patterns of use, and course. *New Directions for Mental Health Services, 70,* 93–105.

Davies-Netzley, S., Hurlburt, M. S., & Hough, R. (1996). Childhood abuse as a precurser to homelessness for homeless women with severe mental illness. *Violence and Victims, 11,* 129–142.

Dawson, M. E., & Nuechterlein, K. H. (1984). Psychophysiological dysfunctions in the developmental course of schizophrenic disorders. *Schizophrenia Bulletin, 10,* 204–232.

Deegan, P. E. (1990). Spirit breaking: When the helping professions hurt. *The Humanistic Psychologist, 18,* 301–313.

Deegan, P. E. (1992). The Independent Living Movement and people with psychiatric disabilities: Taking back control over our own lives. *Psychosocial Rehabilitation Journal, 15,* 3–19.

Deering, C. G., Glover, S. G., Ready, D., Eddleman, H. C., & Alarcon, R. D. (1996). Unique patterns of comorbidity in posttraumatic stress disorder from different sources of trauma. *Comprehensive Psychiatry, 37,* 336–346.

Della Femina, D., Yaeger, D., & Lewis, D. (1990). Child abuse: Adolescent records vs. adult recall. *Child Abuse and Neglect, 14,* 227–231.

Dill, D., Chu, J., & Grob, M. (1991). The reliability of abuse history reports: A comparison of two inquiry formats. *Comprehensive Psychiatry, 32,* 166–169.

Drake, R. E., McHugo, G., & Noordsy, D. L. (1993). Treatment of alcoholism among schizophrenic outpatients: Four-year outcomes. *American Journal of Psychiatry, 150,* 328–329.

Drake, R. E., Mercer-McFadden, C., Mueser, K. T., McHugo, G. J., & Bond, G. R. (1998). Review of integrated mental health and substance abuse treatment for patients with dual disorders. *Schizophrenia Bulletin, 24,* 589–608.

Drake, R. E., Mueser, K. T., Clark, R. E., & Wallach, M. A. (1996). The natural history of substance disorder in persons with severe mental illness. *American Journal of Orthopsychiatry, 66,* 42–51.

Drake, R. E., Osher, F. C., & Wallach, M. A. (1989). Alcohol use and abuse in schizophrenia: A prospective community study. *Journal of Nervous and Mental Disease, 177,* 408–414.

Duncan, R. D., Saunders, B. E., Kilpatrick, D. G., Hanson, R. F., & Resnick, H. S.

(1996). Childhood physical assault as a risk factor for PTSD, depression, and substance abuse: Findings for a national survey. *American Journal of Orthopsychiatry, 66*, 437–448.

Eilenberg, J., Fullilove, M. T., Goldman, R. G., & Mellman, L. (1996). Quality and use of trauma histories obtained from psychiatric outpatients through mandated inquiry. *Psychiatric Services, 47*, 165–169.

Escobar, J. I., Randolph, E. T., Puente, G., Spiwak, F., Asamen, J. K., Hill, M., & Hough, R. L. (1983). Post-traumatic stress disorder in Hispanic Vietnam veterans: Clinical phenomenology and sociocultural characteristics. *Journal of Nervous and Mental Disease, 171*, 585–596.

Falconer, D. S. (1965). The inheritance of liability to certain diseases estimated from the incidence among relatives. *Annuals of Human Genetics, 29*, 51–76.

Figueroa, E. F., Silk, K. R., Huth, A., & Lohr, N. E. (1997). History of childhood sexual abuse and general psychopathology. *Comprehensive Psychiatry, 38*, 23–30.

Finkelhor, D., Hotaling, G., Lewis, I. A., & Smith, C. (1990). Sexual abuse in a national survey of adult men and women: Prevalence, characteristics, and risk factors. *Child Abuse and Neglect, 14*, 19 28.

Fisher, D. B. (1992). Humanizing the recovery process. *Resources, 4*, 5–6.

Fisher, W. A., Penney, D. J., & Earle, K. (1996). Mental health services recipients: Their role in shaping organizational policy. *Administration and Policy in Mental Health, 23*, 547–553.

Foa E. B., & Meadows, E. A. (1997). Psychosocial treatments for posttraumatic stress disorder: A critical review. *Annual Review of Psychology, 48*, 449–480.

Friedman, M. J., & Rosenheck, R. A. (1996). PTSD as a persistent mental illness. In S. Soreff (Ed.), *The seriously and persistently mentally ill: The state-of-the-art treatment handbook* (pp. 369–389). Seattle, WA: Hogrefe & Huber.

Frueh, B. C., Turner, S. M., Beidel, D. C., Mirabella, R. F., & Jones, W. J. (1996). Trauma management therapy: A preliminary evaluation of a multicomponent behavioral treatment for chronic combat-related PTSD. *Behaviour and Research Therapy, 34*, 533–543.

Gehrs, M., & Goering, P. (1994). The relationship between the working alliance and rehabilitation outcomes of schizophrenia. *Psychosocial Rehabilitation Journal, 18*, 43 54.

Glover, H. (1984). Themes of mistrust and the posttraumatic stress disorder in Vietnam veterans. *American Journal of Psychotherapy, 37*, 445–452.

Goff, D. C., Brotman, A. W., Kindlon, D., Waites, M., & Amico, E. (1991a). Self-reports of childhood abuse in chronically psychotic patients. *Psychiatry Research, 37*, 73–80.

Goff, D. C., Brotman, A. W., Kindlon, D., Waites, M., & Amico, E. (1991b). The delusion of possession in chronically psychotic patients. *Journal of Nervous and Mental Disease, 179*, 567–571.

Goodman, L. A., Dutton, M. A., & Harris, M. (1995). Physical and sexual assault prevalence among episodically homeless women with serious mental illness. *American Journal of Orthopsychiatry, 65*, 468–478.

Goodman, L. A., & Fallot, R. (1998). HIV risk behaviors and poor urban women with severe mental disorders: Association with childhood physical and sexual abuse. *American Journal of Orthopsychiatry, 68*, 73–83.

Goodman, L. A., Rosenberg, S. D., Mueser, K. T., & Drake, R. E. (1997). Physical and sexual assault history in women with serious mental illness: Prevalence, impact, treatment, and future directions. *Schizophrenia Bulletin, 23,* 685–696.

Greenfield, S. F., Strakowski, S. M., Tohen, M., Batson, S. C., & Kolbrener, M. L. (1994). Childhood abuse in first-episode psychosis. *British Journal of Psychiatry, 164,* 831–834.

Hamner, M. B. (1997). Psychotic features and combat-associated PTSD. *Depression and Anxiety, 5,* 34–38.

Harris, M. (1996). Treating sexual abuse trauma with dually diagnosed women. *Community Mental Health Journal, 32,* 371–385.

Harris, M. (1997). Modifications in service delivery. In M. Harris & C. L. Landis (Eds.), *Sexual abuse in the lives of women diagnosed with serious mental illness* (pp. 3–20). Amsterdam: Harwood Academic Publishers.

Harrison, G., Croudace, T., Mason, P., Glazebrook, C., & Medley, I. (1996). Predicting the long-term outcome of schizophrenia. *Psychological Medicine, 26,* 697–705.

Herder, D. D., & Redner, L. (1991). The treatment of childhood sexual trauma in chronically mentally ill adults. *Health and Social Work, 16,* 50–57.

Herman, J. L. (1992). *Trauma and recovery.* New York: Basic Books.

Horowitz, M. J. (1986). *Stress response syndromes* (2nd ed.). New York: Aronson.

Hutchings, P. S., & Dutton, M. A. (1993). Sexual assault history in a community mental health center clinical population. *Community Mental Health Journal, 29,* 59–63.

Jacobson, A. (1989). Physical and sexual assault histories among psychiatric outpatients. *American Journal of Psychiatry, 146,* 755–758.

Jacobson, A., & Herald, C. (1990). The relevance of childhood sexual abuse to adult psychiatric inpatient care. *Hospital and Community Psychiatry, 41,* 154–158.

Jacobson, A., & Richardson, B. (1987). Assault experiences of 100 psychiatric inpatients: Evidence of the need for routine inquiry. *American Journal of Psychiatry, 144,* 508–513.

Jennings, A. (1994). Imposing stigma from within: Retraumatizing the victim. *Resources, 6,* 11–15.

Jordan, B. K., Marmar, C. R., Fairbank, J. A., Schlenger, W. E., Kulka, R. A., Hough, R. L., & Weiss, D. S. (1992). Problems in families of male Vietnam veterans with posttraumatic stress disorder. *Journal of Consulting and Clinical Psychology, 60,* 916–926.

Keane, T. M., & Wolfe, J. (1990). Comorbidity in post-traumatic stress disorder: An analysis of community and clinical studies. *Journal of Applied Social Psychology, 20,* 1776–1788.

Kelly, A. E., & McKillop, K. J. (1996). Consequences of revealing personal secrets. *Psychological Bulletin, 120,* 450–465.

Kessler, R. C., Sonnega, A., Bromet, E., Hughes, M., & Nelson, C. B. (1995). Posttraumatic stress disorder in the National Comorbidity Survey. *Archives of General Psychiatry, 52,* 1048–1060.

Kilpatrick, D. G., Acierno, R., Resnick, H. S., Saunders, B. E., & Best, C. L. (1997). A 2-year longitudinal analysis of the relationships between violent assault and substance use in women. *Journal of Consulting and Clinical Psychology, 65,* 834–847.

Kilpatrick, D. G., Saunders, B. E., Veronen, L. J., Best, C. L., & Von, J. M. (1987).

Criminal victimization: Lifetime prevalence, reporting to police, and psychological impact. *Crime and Delinquency, 33,* 479–489.

King, D. W., King, L. A., Foy, D. W., & Gudanowski, D. M. (1996). Prewar factors in combat-related posttraumatic stress disorder: Structural equation modeling with a national sample of female and male Vietnam veterans. *Journal of Consulting and Clinical Psychology, 64,* 520–531.

Koss, M. P. (1993). Rape: Scope, impact, interventions, and public policy responses. *American Psychologist, 48,* 1062–1069.

Kozarić-Kovačić, D., Folnegović-Šmalc, V., Folnegović, Z., & Marušić, A. (1995). Influence of alcoholism on the prognosis of schizophrenic patients. *Journal of Studies on Alcohol, 56,* 622–627.

Lam, J. A., & Rosenheck, R. (1998). The effect of victimization on clinical outcomes of homeless persons with serious mental illness. *Psychiatric Services, 49,* 678–683.

Liberman, R. P., Mueser, K. T., Wallace, C. J., Jacobs, H. E., Eckman, T., & Massel, H. K. (1986). Training skills in the psychiatrically disabled: Learning coping and competence. *Schizophrenia Bulletin, 12,* 631–647.

Linszen, D. H., Dingemans, P. M., & Lenior, M. E. (1994). Cannabis abuse and the course of recent-onset schizophrenic disorders. *Archives of General Psychiatry, 51,* 273–279.

Lipschitz, D. S., Kaplan, M. L., Sorkenn, J. B., Faedda, G. L., Chorney, P., & Asnis, G. M. (1996). Prevalence and characteristics of physical and sexual abuse among psychiatric outpatients. *Psychiatric Services, 47,* 189–191.

Litz, B. T., Blake, D. D., Gerardi, R. G., & Keane, T. M. (1990). Decision making guidelines for the use of direct therapeutic exposure in the treatment of posttraumatic stress disorder. *The Behavior Therapist, 13,* 91–93.

Loftus, E., & Ketcham, K. (1994). *The myth of repressed memory.* New York: St. Martin's Press.

McFarlane, A. C. (1998). Epidemiologic evidence about the relationship between PTSD and alcohol abuse: The nature of the association. *Addictive Behaviors, 6,* 813–825.

Miller, J. S. (1990). Mental illness and spiritual crisis: Implications for psychiatric rehabilitation. *Psychosocial Rehabilitation Journal, 14,* 29–45.

Minkoff, K. (1989). An integrated treatment model for dual diagnosis of psychosis and addiction. *Hospital and Community Psychiatry 40,* 1031–1036.

Mitchell, D. G., Laurenzano, C. G., & Laurenzano, C. (1996). Sexual abuse assessment on admission by nursing staff in general hospital psychiatric settings. *Psychiatric Services, 47,* 159–164.

Muenzenmaier, K., Meyer, I., Struening, E., & Ferber, J. (1993). Childhood abuse and neglect among women outpatients with chronic mental illness. *Hospital and Community Psychiatry, 44,* 666–670.

Mueser, K. T., & Butler, R. W. (1987). Auditory hallucinations in chronic combat-related posttraumatic stress disorder. *American Journal of Psychiatry, 144,* 299–302.

Mueser, K. T., Drake, R. E., & Noordsy, D. L. (1998). Integrated mental health and substance abuse treatment for severe psychiatric disorders. *Practical Psychiatry and Behavioral Health, 4,* 129–139.

Mueser, K. T., Goodman, L. B., Trumbetta, S. L., Rosenberg, S. D., Osher, F. C., Vidaver, R., Auciello, P., & Foy, D. W. (1998). Trauma and posttraumatic stress disorder in severe mental illness. *Journal of Consulting and Clinical Psychology, 66,* 493–499.

Mueser, K. T., Rosenberg, S. D., Goodman, L. B., & Trumbetta, S. L. (in press). Trauma, PTSD and course of severe mental illness: An interactive model. *Schizophrenia Research.*

Mueser, K. T., & Taylor, K. L. (1997). A cognitive-behavioral approach. In M. Harris & C. L. Landis (Eds.), *Sexual abuse in the lives of women diagnosed with severe mental illness* (pp. 67–90). Amsterdam: Harwood Academic Publishers.

Mueser, K. T., Yarnold, P. R., & Bellack, A. S. (1992). Diagnostic and demographic correlates of substance abuse in schizophrenia and major affective disorder. *Acta Psychiatrica Scandinavica, 85,* 48–55.

Mueser, K. T., Yarnold, P. R., Levinson, D. F., Singh, H., Bellack, A. S., Kee, K., Morrison, R. L., & Yadalam, K. G. (1990). Prevalence of substance abuse in schizophrenia: Demographic and clinical correlates. *Schizophrenia Bulletin, 16,* 31–56.

National Association of State Mental Health Program Directors [NASMHPD]. (1998, April 2–3). *Responding to the behavioral healthcare issues of persons with histories of physical and sexual abuse.* Paper presented at a national trauma experts meeting of the NASMHPD, Alexandria, VA.

National Victims Center (1992). *Rape in America: A report to the nation.* Arlington, VA: Author.

Neale, M. S., & Rosenheck, R. A. (1995). Therapeutic alliance and outcome in a VA intensive case management program. *Psychiatric Services, 46,* 719–721.

Nishith, P., Hearst, D. E., Mueser, K. T., & Foa, E. B. (1995). PTSD and major depression: Methodological and treatment considerations in a single case design. *Behavior Therapy, 26,* 319–335.

Oruč, L., & Bell, P. (1995). Multiple rape trauma followed by delusional parasitosis: A case report from the Bosnian war. *Schizophrenia Research, 16,* 173–174.

Polusny, M. A., & Follette, V. M. (1995). Long-term correlates of child sexual abuse: Theory and review of the empirical literature. *Applied and Preventive Psychology, 4,* 143–166.

Pope, H. G., Jr., & Hudson, J. I. (1995). Can memories of childhood sexual abuse be repressed? *Psychological Medicine, 25,* 121–126.

Priebe, S., & Gruyters, T. (1993). The role of the helping alliance in psychiatric community care: A prospective study. *Journal of Nervous and Mental Disease, 181,* 552–557.

Rapkin, A. J., Kames, L. D., Darke, L. L., Stampler, F. M., & Naliboff, B. D. (1990). History of physical and sexual abuse in women with chronic pelvic pain. *Obstetrics and Gynecology, 76,* 92–96.

Redner, L. L., & Herder, D. D. (1992). Case management's role in effecting appropriate treatment for persons with histories of childhood sexual trauma. *Psychosocial Rehabilitation Journal, 15*(3), 37–45.

Regier, D. A., Farmer, M. E., Rae, D. S., Locke, B. Z., Keith, S. J., Judd, L. J., & Goodwin, F. K. (1990). Comorbidity of mental disorders with alcohol and other drug abuse: Results from the Epidemiologic Catchment Area (ECA) study. *Journal of the American Medical Association, 264,* 2511–2518.

Resnick, H. S., & Kilpatrick, D. G. (1994). Crime-related PTSD: Emphasis on adult general population samples. *PTSD Research Quarterly, 5,* 1–3.

Resnick, H. S., Kilpatrick, D. G., & Dansky, B. S., Saunders, B. E., & Best, C. L.

(1993). Prevalence of civilian trauma and post-traumatic stress disorder in a representative national sample of women. *Journal of Consulting and Clinical Psychology, 61*, 984–991.

Roessler, T. A., & McKenzie, N. (1994). Effects of childhood trauma on psychological functioning in adults sexually abused as children. *Journal of Nervous and Mental Disorders, 182*, 145–150.

Rose, S. M., Peabody, C. G., & Stratigeas, B. (1991). Undetected abuse among intensive case management clients. *Hospital and Community Psychiatry, 42*, 499–503.

Ross, C. A., Anderson, G., & Clark, P. (1994). Childhood abuse and the positive symptoms of schizophrenia. *Hospital and Community Psychiatry, 45*, 489–491.

Rundell, J. R., Ursano, R. J., Holloway, H. C., & Silberman, E. K. (1989). Psychiatric responses to trauma. *Hospital and Community Psychiatry, 40*, 68–74.

Russell, D. E. H. (1986). *The secret trauma: Incest in the lives of girls and women.* New York: Basic Books.

Saunders, B. E., Villeponteaux, L. A., Lipovsky, J. A., Kilpatrick, D. G., & Veronen, L. J. (1992). Child sexual assault as a risk factor for mental disorders among women: A community survey. *Journal of Interpersonal Violence, 7*, 189–204.

Sautter, F. J., Brailey, K., Uddo, M. M., Hamilton, M. F., Beard, M. G., & Borges, A. H. (1999). PTSD and comorbid psychotic disorder: Comparison with veterans diagnosed with PTSD or psychotic disorder. *Journal of Traumatic Stress, 12*, 73–88.

Scheidt, S. D. (1994). Great expectations: Challenges for women as mental health administrators. *Journal of Mental Health Administration, 21*, 419–429.

Schinnar, A. P., Rothbard, A. B., Kanter, R., & Jung, Y. S. (1990). An empirical literature review of definitions of severe and persistent mental illness. *American Journal of Psychiatry, 147*, 1602–1608.

Searles, P., & Berger, R. J. (1987). Factors associated with a history of childhood sexual experience in a nonclinical female population. *Journal of the American Academy of Child Psychiatry, 23*, 215–218.

Seidel, R. W., Gusman, F. D., & Abueg, F. R. (1994). Theoretical and practical foundations of an inpatient post-traumatic stress disorder and alcoholism treatment program. *Psychotherapy, 31*, 67–78.

Solomon, S. D. (1997). Psychosocial treatment of posttraumatic stress disorder. *In Session: Psychotherapy in Practice, 3*, 27–41.

Solomon, P., Draine, J., & Delaney, M. A. (1995). The working alliance and consumer case management. *Journal of Mental Health Administration, 22*, 126–134.

Sorenson, S. B., Stein, J. A., Siegel, J. M., Golding, J. M., & Burnam, M. A. (1987). Prevalence of adult sexual assault: The Los Angeles Epidemiologic Catchment Area study. *American Journal of Epidemiology, 126*, 1154–1164.

Stewart, S. H. (1996). Alcohol abuse in individuals exposed to trauma: A critical review. *Psychological Bulletin, 120*, 83–112.

Stewart, S. H., Pihl, R. O., Conrod, P. J., & Dongier, M. (1998). Functional associations among trauma, PTSD and substance-related disorders. *Addictive Behaviors, 6*, 797–812.

Stowe, H., & Harris, M. (1997). A social skills approach to trauma recovery. In M. Harris & C. L. Landis (Eds.), *Sexual abuse in the lives of women diagnosed with serious mental illness* (pp. 91–108). Amsterdam: Harwood Academic Publishers.

Straube, E. R., & Öhman (1990). Functional role of the different autonomic nervous system activity patterns found in schizophrenia: A new model. In E. R. Straube

& K. Hahlweg (Eds.), *Schizophrenia: Concepts, vulnerability, and intervention* (pp. 135–157). Berlin: Springer-Verlag.

Strauss, J. S., & Carpenter, W. T. (1977). Prediction of outcome in schizophrenia: III. Five-year outcome and its predictors. *Archives of General Psychiatry, 34,* 159–163.

Swett, C., & Halpert, M. (1993). Reported history of physical and sexual abuse in relation to dissociation and other symptomatology in women psychiatric inpatients. *Journal of Interpersonal Violence, 8,* 545–555.

Switzer, G. E., Dew, M. A., Thompson, K., Goycoolea, J. M., Derricott, T., & Mullins, S. D. (1999). Posttraumatic stress disorder and service utilization among urban mental health center clients. *Journal of Traumatic Stress, 12,* 25–39.

Symonds, M. (1982). Victim responses to terror: Understanding and treatment. In F. Ochberg & D. Soskis (Eds.), *Victims of terrorism* (pp. 95–103). Boulder, CO: Westview Press.

Talbot, N. L., Houghtalen, R. P., Cyrulik, S., Betz, A., Barkun, M., Duberstein, P. R., & Wynne, L. C. (1998). Women's safety in recovery: Group therapy for patients with a history of childhood sexual abuse. *Psychiatric Services, 49,* 213–217.

Triffleman, E. G., Marmar, C. R., Delucchi, K. L., & Ronfeldt, H. (1995). Childhood trauma and posttraumatic stress disorder in substance abuse inpatients. *Journal of Nervous and Mental Disease, 183,* 172–176.

van der Kolk, B. A. (1987). The psychological consequences of overwhelming life experiences. In B. A. van der Kolk (Ed.), *Psychological trauma* (pp. 1–30). Washington, DC: American Psychiatric Press.

Wakefield, H., & Underwager, R. (1992). Recovered memories of alleged sexual abuse: Lawsuits against parents. *Behavioral Sciences and the Law, 10,* 483–507.

Waldfogel, S., & Mueser, K. T. (1988). Another case of chronic PTSD with auditory hallucinations. *American Journal of Psychiatry, 145,* 13–14.

Wyatt, G. E. (1985). The sexual abuse of Afro-American and White-American women in childhood. *Child Abuse and Neglect, 9,* 507–519.

Wyatt, G. E., Guthrie, D., & Notgrass, C. M. (1992). Differential effects of women's child sexual abuse and subsequent sexual revictimization. *Journal of Consulting and Clinical Psychology, 60,* 167–173.

Zahn, T. P. (1986). Psychophysiological approaches to psychopathology. In M. G. H. Coles, E. Donchin, & S. W. Porges (Eds.), *Psychophysiology: Systems, processes and applications.* New York: Guilford Press.

IV

CASE HISTORY ANALYSIS AND PRACTICAL CONSIDERATIONS

15

Case History Analysis of the Treatments for PTSD: Lessons Learned

JACOB D. LINDY, JOHN P. WILSON,
and MATTHEW J. FRIEDMAN

This book casts a broad net over the field of trauma therapy. In this chapter, we attempt a synthesis through the more narrow view of the case histories in this book. What can we glean from the clinical work of experts in the field that may inform us about the indications for and the limitations of the various approaches? How do core approaches work differently to affect posttraumatic stress disorder (PTSD) and its allostatic forms? How can core approaches work in a complementary or sequential way?

In the concluding section of this chapter we look at the same case histories to examine common underlying features among the core approaches: Are there similar ways in which patients feel improved? Are there common ways in which clinicians work?

We return to the tetrahedral model of PTSD presented in Chapter 2, reviewing it in the light of specific clinical cases. In doing so we place the core approaches in relationship with each other: What is unique about each method? How do the interventions of the different modes work? How does entry into the complex world of PTSD through one portal lead the patient and clinician to discover other aspects of the disorder? How do the different approaches work together, either adjunctively or sequentially?

The 27 case histories reported in this book, *in toto*, do not form a representative or random sample on which we can test hypotheses, nor does our data easily lend itself to a definitive meta-analysis. But they do provide rich illustrations which teach us how practitioners of the differing core approaches think about their patients and what it is in their approach that works. Further, because we asked therapists to fill in certain uniform details about the traumas of their patients, the details of interventions that mattered most, and the presenting symptoms, we seek here to uncover patterns among treatment choices which may warrant further research.

Often, proponents of the various approaches at this point in our history seek to expand the usefulness of their approach to a wider scope and wider range of patients with PTSD. But emphasizing only the widening scope of each modality gives little help to the clinician trying at a given moment in time to determine the best fit between his or her patient and the various approaches.

CASES REPORTED

The book contains 27 case histories (which are summarized in Appendix 15.1 at the end of this chapter), as follows: psychopharmacological treatment, cases 23 and 24; psychoanalytic/psychodynamic therapy, cases 14–20; cognitive-behavioral therapy, cases 21 and 22; constructivist therapy, cases 4 and 5; dual diagnosis, case 25; culturally specific treatment, cases 1–3; family and couple therapy, cases 9–13; and groups therapy, cases 6–8.

MATCH BETWEEN TREATMENT APPROACH AND ACCESS TO PTSD CORE PHENOMENOLOGY

In Chapter 2 (Figures 2.2 and 2.3), we presented a tetrahedral model of core PTSD phenomenology and its relation to ego states and object relations. This provides five portals through which differing treatment approaches can meaningfully engage the core issues for the client with PTSD: P-1 engages the client around object relations, attachment, intimacy, and interpersonal relations; P-2 engages the client in response to symptoms of hyperarousal and physiological reactivity; P-3 engages the client's avoidance, detachment, and numbing; P-4 engages the client's altered ego states, self-structure, and identity configuration; and P-5 engages the client in areas of intrusion and reexperiencing.

The clinical presentations which therapists first engage their clients with PTSD, that is, the portal through which treatment begins, varies to some degree with the core approach. For those clients who entered treatment in hopes of altering disturbed patterns in interpersonal relations (P-1), especially intimacy and attachment (cases 4, 5, 6, 9, 10, 11, 13 and 20), therapists used group, family and individual psychodynamic and constructivist approaches. For example, Sam (case 6), a Vietnam war veteran fearing his tendency to sabotage relationships, homicidal revenge fantasies, and experience of any affect as being out of control, would damage his relation with his child, chose the group setting to obtain help. While his pathology contained multiple traumas and pathology amenable to different core approaches, his presenting difficulty matched best with the group approach.

When clients presented with symptoms of hyperarousal and physiological reactivity (P-2), as in cases 1, 2, 14, and 24, the therapist was apt to prescribe medication when using the psychobiological approach alone or in conjunction with either psychodynamic psychotherapy or culturally specific treatment. For example, DG (case 24), coincident with the pain and physical debilitation in adulthood, developed traumatic nightmares and startle/hypervigilant reactions of earlier childhood abuse. While earlier antidepressants had not helped, his psychiatrist prescribed beta-blockers to assist the allostatic load on the adrenergic system. Medication helped hyperarousal in other settings as well. For example, Phong (case 2), a 64-year-old Vietnamese man, sought help for nightmares, headaches, insomnia, and isolation. Phong was a war veteran and former officer, he had been held prisoner for 12 years in Vietnam by the communists. His wife and children were killed in the same war. His therapist, part of a culturally specific setting, was well suited to offer Phong immediate attention to his physiological hyperactivity with medication and cultural support through P-2.

In case histories (cases 7, 12, 18, and 25) where engagement with the client was primarily through P-3 (symptoms of avoidance, detachment, and numbing), the therapists employed group, family, individual psychodynamic, and dual diagnosis modes. For example, an American veteran of the Vietnam War (case 12) whose worst trauma in Vietnam occurred at Christmas time, withdrew into his room or "bunker" rather than be with his family during the holiday. The family felt shut out at just the most important time to be making contact. At his family's urging he was able to engage family therapy as a core approach well suited for presenting problems of P-3. There, his therapist engaged the family's dilemma with most meaningful results.

The clients who presented with altered ego states and self-structure were treated in a culturally specific setting, and by individual therapists offering constructivist, psychodynamic, and dissociative identity disorder approaches (cases 3, 4, 19, and 26). For example, Ms. A (case 4), a woman traumatized in childhood by parental neglect, abuse by a neighbor, and sexual abuse by a priest presented with a threatened sexual identity and difficulty in relationships, especially trust. Her sense of herself was as vulnerable and unsafe, and in response she was hypercritical of others to compensate for low self-esteem.

The constructivist approach engaged her presenting problems and her complex PTSD as well. For Mihai (case 19), whose symptoms of guilt, shame and nightmares grew worse as right-wing views gained renewed strength after the recent revolutions in Romania, his central issue revolved around the integrity of his identity. Memories returned of his imprisonment as a 20-year-old for his political views, when he was tortured, forced to torture others, and brainwashed during the Stalin era. His therapist was able to use a psychodynamic approach to engage him around the central issue of retaining one's self under overwhelming pressure to yield.

When the portal through which the patient presented was the reexperiencing and intrusion dimension of the disorder (P-5: cases 15, 16, 17, 21, 22, and 23) the approach was cognitive-behavioral engagement, one of the psychodynamic therapies, and medication. Those who, after some trust building, were able to narrate their trauma in a reasonably coherent script were well suited for the cognitive-behavioral approach. For example, Alice (case 21) complained of recurrent intrusive images of her being assaulted and raped with its possible consequences (fear of HIV), nightmares, avoidance of public places and transportation, and all contact with strangers. She was irritable, hypervigilant, and depressed. Her cognitive-behavioral therapist was well equipped to engage her reexperiencing symptoms through an imaging plan and dosed behavioral techniques, well suited for P-5.

On the other hand, those patients whose initial presentation was of reenactments which could not be described by the patient and which could only be clinically inferred tended toward the psychoanalytic approach. For example, Tina (case 17) presented with trauma-related somatic re-enactments (seizure-like movements repeating her 8-year-old son's movements before his death). She was unable at that time to verbalize a coherent story of the trauma history. Her psychodynamic therapist provided great relief when he was able to translate her seizure-like behavior into meaningful expressions of her grief and trauma. The psychoanalytic approach was well suited for the patient unable to verbalize her reexperiencing phenomenon (P-5).

Rarely were the portals unidimensional. Once one aspect of the disorder was engaged, often others would be as well. For example, a client having engaged around hyperarousal or numbing might move on to address interpersonal relations. Or, having first engaged problems in intimacy, the treatment would go on to uncover the impact of reexperiencing on those relationships and on the self-structure. Where the core treatment engaged reexperiencing, it invariably also addressed hyperarousal and avoidance as well. For example, in the case just mentioned of Tina, after work on the somatic reenactments of her son's death, she revealed a lifelong pattern of masochistic relationships. Exploring this interpersonal dimension of her life in turn led to memories of detachment and numbing, and finally to a new set of childhood traumas involving incest from her father and retaliatory enemas from her mother. With the recovery of these memories came new symptoms of dissociation and fragmented self-states. An allostatic adaptation to the childhood sequence emerged where she retained sanity only through a fantasy of her angel-like goodness shielding her from her pain.

With regard to the portals of entry, the core approaches form clusters. Regarding P-1 (interpersonal symptoms) the psychodynamic therapies—individual, group, and family dynamic therapies—engage easily. This same grouping of therapies can engage detachment and avoidance. Physiological hyperarousal (P-2) is the province of psychobiology. Often hyperarousal is also connected to reexperiencing symptoms (P-5). When these symptoms are related to a specific trauma memory, the cognitive-behavioral approach fits, and when the memories are indistinct, individual psychodynamic treatment is the choice. Finally, where it is damaged self-structure (P-4) which is the presenting condition, constructivist and analytic approaches engage best.

Culturally specific settings attend to highly traumatized patients with multiple traumas, so physiological hyperarousal (P-2) and damaged self-structure (P-4) are prominent portals of entry.

RECOVERY ENVIRONMENT,
OUTREACH, AND REFERRAL

Implicit in the case histories is the importance of specific sensitivity to a given trauma by the clinician and by the service setting itself. Survivors of natural disaster, for example, may find themselves in service settings which are not attuned to trauma. For example, the initial psychiatric diagnosis of Clyde, a 22-year-old man with depression, failed to uncover the presence of PTSD case 25 (dual diagnosis). In fact, he was treated unsuccessfully with electroconvulsive therapy (ECT). Later, in a PTSD-sensitive environment, history was obtained that his friends and their family were incinerated in a bushfire when he was age 8. In fact, he was experiencing intrusive images of a bushfire endangering his current city and his family home, and the diagnosis of PTSD had been missed.

The above case also illustrates a point of outreach. It is important to remember that the delivery of professional mental health care to the traumatized survivor is a relatively new phenomenon. Not long ago, PTSD patients were described as a "reluctant population" (Lindy, Grace, & Green, 1981) and outreach was considered indispensable to the success of any therapeutic effort. Among the cases presented by expert therapists in this book, we find that community outreach is practiced in each of the public, private, and academic settings in which the therapist contributors work. Indeed, without it, many of the clients whose treatments are described in this book might not have had access to a PTSD-sensitive environment. This is particularly true in the cross-cultural settings for traumatized Asian American immigrants and those refugees seeking political asylum.

SOURCE OF REFERRAL

The search for help often comes first from someone living with the PTSD patient rather than from the patient him- or herself. Given a reluctance to recognize or face the origins of the problems, some of our clients or patients find themselves able to accept the idea of treatment only when accompanied by others whom they trust. We were interested to see which core approaches matched with these referral patterns. Clients entering group, family, and couples therapy were often assigned to this approach in response to the pain and difficulties which other family members were having in relating to them. For example, Sam (case 6), a combat veteran with PTSD, presented with intrusive and numbing symptoms, family problems, and alcohol and self-medication problems. In Vietnam he had been ambushed, saw his buddy killed in front of him, engaged in body counts, and witnessed many deaths of civilians. With a history of aversive responses to other treatments, his main focus was on his family problems as he was attempting to rejoin his wife and daughter.

In contrast to the above, individual psychodynamic therapies and cognitive-behavioral therapies were more likely to be on the basis of referral from another professional. Constructivist therapies were self-referrals. Medication occurred in all categories of referral, as medication was frequently a complementary treatment approach.

REFERRALS OF INDIRECT PTSD

Sometimes it is in the indirect survivor, the family member or friend of the traumatized person, who has developed symptoms and seeks help for him- or herself. We were interested in which approach seemed to adapt best to these circumstances.

In two cases, the identified patient was not the traumatized survivor but his indirectly traumatized child. In both of these instances it was the family therapy setting which was attentive to the multigenerational impact of trauma. For example, a 4-year-old child (case 10) presented in her nursery school with oppositional behavior, tantrums, separation anxiety, and nightmares. The parents learned that the child was searching for her father's missing eye which he lost in Vietnam, although this had never been discussed in the family. The family therapist provided an ideal setting in which the father could explain to his daughter the emotional pain of the loss of his eye in an explosion during the war, and also explain that he was getting the help he needed for that pain. The daughter felt reassured that her perceptions about her father were correct (he had been having an anniversary reaction to the loss) and that he could still be a whole giving father even without his eye.

CHARACTERISTICS OF THE TRAUMA EXPERIENCE

In the following subsections, we examine characteristics of the traumatic events themselves and their match with core approaches. In doing so we peruse the case studies for patterns in the characteristics of the trauma, its acuteness or chronicity, its repetitiveness, its location, the presence of concomitant loss, and the roles and identifications of the survivor within the trauma context.

Trauma Population

Among our case histories, war veterans who experienced their trauma in a small-unit context tended to match with the group approach. Incest survivors who experienced their trauma in the home tended to match with individual constructivist or psychodynamic approaches. Victims of a well-defined episode of civilian violence or rape matched with the cognitive behavioral approach. Survivors of natural disasters are reported in dual diagnosis, cognitive-behavioral therapy, and among the psychodynamic cases. Of course there is much overlap as well. In fact, many expert clinicians chose cases to demonstrate the widening scope of the validity of their approach. A patient with early childhood trauma was successfully treated with medication, and another through group work, whereas war veterans without early childhood trauma were among those treated successfully by analytic therapists. Nonetheless, the overall tendencies are worth noting.

Acuteness versus Chronicity of Trauma Response

Experts in most core approaches chose to illustrate their points with cases where trauma occurred between 10 and 25 years ago. In contrast, experts in the cognitive-behavioral approach chose cases within the past year or so.

Single versus Repetitive and Brief versus Prolonged Trauma

The cases selected by authors of chapters representing the various core approaches divide sharply on the issue of chronicity.

In 21 cases, trauma was multiple and prolonged; in 3 cases, trauma was single and relatively brief. In either category, the traumas were severe. For example, Ven (case 1, a culturally specific treatment setting), a Cambodian refugee of the Pol Pot (Khmer Rouge) terror, is widowed and experienced her son's decapitation and the death by starvation of two children through the Khmer Rouge political terror. Of the single events, one was an assault/rape, the second a shooting in the abdomen. The 21 multiple and prolonged traumas were treated by the full spectrum of core approaches save for cognitive-behavioral therapy; those in the single-event category were treated only with the cognitive-behavioral approach.

Isolated Individual Trauma versus Community Trauma

In the majority of cases, trauma occurred to the client in a community context such as political persecution, war, or natural disaster. Those who experienced trauma in a community context tended to be treated in a community context, that is, culturally specific settings or by group and family approaches, settings in which similarly impacted survivors can express thoughts and feelings.

On the other hand, a little more than one-third received their traumas in isolated settings, without a community of similarly traumatized survivors. In many of the cases in this isolated category, the perpetrator of trauma was an emotionally significant person in the survivor's life, as in child abuse or incest. Among those cases where the trauma occurred in isolation, treatments were more likely in an individual context by constructivists, analytic therapists, or cognitive-behavioral therapists.

In isolated traumas, the perpetrator was most often a person whom the victim knew and toward whom he or she had intensely ambivalent feelings. These clients were treated by therapists using the constructivist and psychodynamic approaches, both of which engage the nuances of interpersonal relations and damaged self-states. The constructivist therapies in particular focused on empowering the client to form healthier, stronger boundaries (i.e., the intrapsychic site of the trauma in these particular cases; see the *Modes of Therapeutic Action* section below for case illustrations).

Loss and Delayed Grief

Significant loss (death of family members or close friends) is often part of the trauma experience, especially for children. Indeed, two-thirds of the case histories reported in this book record loss as part of the picture. In nine cases, the loss was striking—such as being forced to watch a husband being decapitated, or seeing one's best friend killed, or a child witnessing her mother's murder by a boyfriend.

Of those patients with striking losses, delayed grief became a focus of work in the analytic therapies. Of those where the striking loss was addressed in nonspecific supportive terms, the patients were seen in culturally specific settings.

Of note are two cases where the death was primarily the result of the patient's own action, that is, the patient was in the role of perpetrator. These were seen in dynamic treatments—one individual (see case 18 below) and one group.

Trauma Role

Symptoms of the clients in all of the approaches related back to their experiences of being overwhelmed in the trauma situation. Where the specifics of these trauma memories are recalled in depth, it is most often in the role of victim. But some occupied primarily other roles such as rescuer, supporter, or perpetrator.

While most patients' symptoms make sense as a result of their own experience in the trauma situation, some through unconscious identification with another in the trauma situation make sense only in light of the second person's trauma experience. For example, a 2-year-old boy simply played with the curls in his hair, attempting to visualize his mother's pretty hair when in fact he was responding to images of her bloodied hair after she was shot in the head in front of him. In case 18, Abraham's symptoms of loss also took a bodily form. This Vietnam veteran, father of a 13-year-old boy, carried himself hunched over with a somber visage as though he carried the living dead. In dynamic psychotherapy, his therapist finally learned that this striking posture contained Abraham's delusion that another 13-year-old boy, the one whom he had shot in a free-fire zone but held in his arms while dying, was still alive on his shoulder, influencing his current life.

The Trauma Experience Remembered
Clearly versus Indistinctly

In constructivist and psychodynamic approaches, therapists do not require patients to have conscious knowledge of the details of trauma experiences before the work itself can begin. The therapist assumes that the client may be unaware of a certain trauma either through unconscious repression or through disavowal, where details of the trauma may be hidden via strong affects such as shame or guilt. In children, levels of cognitive and emotional development will affect the child's ability to use words. In some of these therapies, the capacity to tell the story of the trauma is a treatment goal in and of itself. In contrast, cognitive-behavioral treatment protocols, imaging or exposure, require narration of the trauma as a starting point.

DEMOGRAPHIC FACTORS
IN THE HISTORY ANALYSIS

Race

A disturbing pattern regarding race emerges. Most case illustrations where race is mentioned involve whites, except where a culturally specific treatment program has been established. Therapists are mostly also white. While these numbers by no means capture the state of affairs in our field, they do indicate a pattern which we, as clinicians, need to be more sensitive to and find new solutions for. We know that there is great need to find and demonstrate suitable approaches to nonwhite trauma clients in the general population, and we need nonwhite therapists to join in carrying them out.

Sex

There are several noteworthy patterns regarding sex in the match between therapists and clients in the differing core approaches. Constructivist therapists, mostly women, treated women assaulted mostly by adult men, whereas group therapists, mostly men, treated male war veterans who were exposed to trauma at the hands of mostly enemy men as young adults and adolescents. The affinity generally seems to be toward a therapist and therapeutic setting of the same sex as the client. Two of three cases reported in which the clinician ran into difficulty as the treatment itself began to feel unsafe were situations where the male therapists were treating women whose perpetrators had been men.

Marital Status

Half of the clients are married, and distribution between married, and unmarried clients among the approaches appears even. It is worth noting that two of three clients in the culturally specific settings are widowed as part of the trauma experience itself, having lost their spouses in the political terror which caused their own PTSD. It is curious that completed analytically treated patients are more often married, perhaps suggesting that spousal support may be an ingredient in sustaining this treatment.

Age

In terms of the age of traumatization, specialists in child trauma of course provided the right fit for children, although some children with indirect PTSD appeared within the family treatment context. Among those who are now adults but whose trauma occurred in early childhood, both constructivist and psychodynamic approaches seemed to fit well.

MODES OF THERAPEUTIC ACTION

In the following subsections we use the case histories to identify unique modes of action of the core approaches and to see if we can find reasonable hypotheses for the tendencies discussed above which tend to match different trauma circumstances with different core approaches.

From the vantage point of the therapist, experts in the different approaches hypothesize differently about the aspect of the disorder that is being engaged and how the therapist's understanding and interventions lead to change in that engaged segment of the whole.

Cognitive-Behavioral Approaches

Cognitive-behavioral therapists attend to the intrusive effects of reexperiencing and provide practical means of extinguishing these phenomena. They provide a way for clients to frame and reframe the narrative of their traumatic experiences. The clinician proceeds on the basis that desensitization to traumatic stimuli attenuate those stimuli, restoring a pretraumatic equilibrium, both psychologically and physiologically. They reduce target symptoms of PTSD by habituating reexperiencing phenomena both within the safety of the therapeutic space and in environments which evoke pathological reactions. This improves the survivor's available energy to invest in healthy relationships and in self-development. The task both during the therapy sessions and in assignments at home is to overcome avoidance of traumatic memory by challenges that are specific, modulated, and of sufficient duration to achieve attenuation. For example, Alice (case 21) experienced unbidden thoughts and images as well as nightmares of her experience of being assaulted in an alleyway, robbed, and raped vaginally and anally. She was preoccupied with fears of HIV infection and could not enter public places or contact strangers. After mastering deep breathing exercises, she developed with her counselor a series of *in vivo* exercises from least difficult to most difficult. Her counselor encouraged her to tell the story of her rape, record it, and listen to the recording. Anxiety measured highest as she became aware of rage that she could contract HIV from the event. The counselor encouraged her to focus on fear rather than anger to get over this hurdle in imaginal listening. The treatment led to a vast reduction in PTSD symptoms in nine visits.

Group Therapy

The group therapist finds that the alienation of the trauma survivor is most directly engaged by members of a similarly traumatized yet recovering peer group. Group members offer the client a uniquely effective means of engagement. The group offers acceptance, empathy, support, and useful suggestions regarding adaptation. The therapist and cotherapist as well as other group members educate the client regarding the nature of PTSD. The group provides immediate feedback on ways in which pathology affects others. For example, Sam (case 6), a Vietnam war veteran, entered group therapy fearing that his lethality and self-loathing would destroy his effort to rejoin his wife and child. He found that the group members' understanding ("Family know how to push your button") and empathy (having been through similar experiences) enabled them to accept his feelings and fears. They were also practically helpful, getting him back to Alcoholics Anonymous (AA) and coming up with alternative strategies for dealing with hypervigilance.

Also, some dynamic groups address irrational expectations of the therapists as in transference and countertransference. Here again, group members can normalize and underline idiosyncracies regarding expectations of its members in this regard.

Constructivist Self-Developmental Theory

The constructivist therapist is careful to assess the patient's sense of self and bases the effect of the treatment on ways in which the therapeutic relationship bears on this sense of self. Since violation of boundaries is central in the traumas of childhood in complex PTSD (e.g., abuse, incest), it is only reasonable that the boundary between the client and the therapist becomes loaded, the site around which change may occur. This takes place when the patient can accept and verbalize wishes and when the therapist can appropriately—yet flexibly—negotiate new solutions. This enables new schemas to take hold. For example, Ms. C. (case 5), overwhelmed by a paranoid mother as a child and a traumatizing husband as an adult, felt that the 45-minute session did not meet her needs. Together with her therapist, she renegotiated this boundary of the therapy frame and altered it to 90 minutes per session, demonstrating her power to influence a boundary in a way which better met her needs.

Psychodynamic Approaches

For the analytic therapist, understanding, mastery, and meaning are core objectives which match the patient's needs regarding impaired relationships and a damaged sense of self. These are as much the focus of the therapeutic work as are manifest symptoms. It is the nature of the repetition compulsion that the important aspects of the trauma, conscious and unconscious, will tend to repeat themselves in the therapeutic space. Much of the memories so obtained will be new to the patient's awareness. As this occurs, it is the relationship, through the managing of the frame with interpretation, which is the site of therapeutic action. This is true in maintaining healthy aspects of the relationship in the therapeutic alliance as well as in the interpretation of its irrational components (as in transference, countertransference, and enactments). The here and now of the therapeutic setting, after the patient experiences it as safe enough, gains all the intensity of the trauma itself and includes the defensive operations which the patient has unconsciously used to cope with the trauma's effects. Reflection, interpretation, and empathy are crucial to the success of this method. Education and medication are often complementary. The task of monitoring countertransference is immense; the consequences of not monitoring it may derail a treatment, and finding the right balance is always important. For example, with Mihai (case 19, discussed earlier) empathically appreciating his need to yield while being brainwashed by Stalinist torturers could only be understood and communicated after the therapist was able to recognize by self-analysis that same tendency to yield existed in himself. In the case of Annette (case 16), the therapist was unaware of a countertransference in which he was the therapeutically overzealous mother. Annette's presenting symptom was her excessive preoccupation with the bowel habits of her 3-year-old child. She had repressed her own memory of being traumatized as a child by her mother's terrifying enemas (motivated by her mother's fear that Annette would develop the fatal illness of her sibling). All this came to light when her therapist commented that they would have to "go deeper" and responded to her anxiety by getting the patient a glass of water. Hearing the faucet, Annette dissociated, writhing on the floor as if being administered an enema. Later, understanding and translating (reconstructing) the traumatic enemas of childhood was possible when the therapist discovered that, through his therapeutic zeal, he had become, in the transference, the traumatizing mother. Discovering and working through her own trauma memories helped Annette with the current fears regarding her children and permitted the reworking of a number of key relationships.

Treatment of Families and Couples

For the family/couples therapist, especially useful is the capacity for the therapist to create a climate where family members can elucidate the ways in which PTSD interferes with intimacy. The couples therapist works to find creative ways to restore intimacy through genuine empathy and reciprocity once both parties understand the suffering of the other. The family therapist diagnoses problems in marital and family dysfunction such as enmeshment, boundary problems, or interference with intimacy, educates family members about the disorder of PTSD, and assists them (including the client) to reframe their impasse in terms of a dialectic dilemma in empathic terms, capable of creative solutions rather than a deadlock. For example, a Vietnam combat veteran (case 12), whose worst trauma in Vietnam occurred at Christmas time, withdrew into his room or "bunker" rather than be with his family during the holiday. The family felt shut out at just the most important time to be making contact. In family therapy, the therapist helped the family reframe this dialectic dilemma into a need to do something together which honored servicemen at that time of year. They successfully evolved a plan to serve a soup kitchen as a family.

Psychopharmacological Approaches to Cross-Cultural Treatment

Sometimes, the totality of losses, traumas, and dislocations in traumatized persons who have been political refugees is hard to imagine. The combined

approach which uses support by medication, socialization, and cultural reso-
nance, while keeping a safe distance from activating more trauma than the
patient can endure to remember, is most effective. For example, Christina
(case 3), a 25-year-old widowed graduate student, was struggling with suicidal thoughts, not eating or sleeping, and unable to find anything in life which
stirred hope. She had experienced multiple traumas in an African civil war.
Her husband was decapitated; she was raped, their home burned, and her
parents presumed killed, although their bodies had not been found. Her therapist was able to engage her damaged sense of self and hopelessness (P-4) by
participating in her advocacy for political asylum within a culturally specific
setting.

Uncovering, Suppressing, and Coping with Trauma Memory

The modes of therapy for PTSD fall along a spectrum as regards the stated
value of suppressing versus uncovering trauma memory. Several therapeutic
approaches focus on suppressive techniques. Medication, for example, suppresses hyperalert neurohormonal systems, reducing the frequency and impact of intrusive memory. Supportive groups are designed, via group acceptance, education, support, and centrality of daily living, suppress trauma
memory; culturally specific trauma settings, as in case 3 of Christina (just
discussed), employ medication and support within a culturally consonant setting which suppresses trauma memory. We see the same in work with the severely mentally ill. Therapists using the cognitive-behavioral approach emphasize the uncovering of the traumatic memory so that with cognitive and
behavioral exercises it can become attenuated. Psychodynamic approaches
strive for a balance between trauma narration, when the patient is ready,
and suppression of traumatic memory when such memory, disrupts ego
function. Constructivists work gradually and in the present so that new
schemas can replace old ones; psychoanalytic therapists let daily occurrences
be the clues that old traumas still organize new events, so that insight, empathic self-understanding, and internalization of function can restore altered
intrapsychic systems; and family therapists attend to the trauma itself only
insofar as dialectic dilemmas may be confronted and reframed in the here
and now rather than avoided. The balance between expressive and suppressive techniques in a given case is often a delicate one, and the sensitive therapist utilizing any approach may at times chose aspects of either. For example, selective serotonin reuptake inhibitors (SSRIs) may allow trauma memory to emerge with clarity. Analytic therapists may reinforce defenses in order to dose the emerging of trauma memory. Cognitive-behavioral
therapists may substitute a more tolerable supportive/suppressive affect such
as fear for the disruptive potential of rage (see case 21, Alice) so that a procedure can continue rather than be disrupted. Indeed the timing of sup-

pressive versus uncovering or expressive aspects of treatment is an art in many of the approaches described.

The Voice of Change

Within a given approach, change occurs when the clients feel that they now possesses knowledge or mastery which they did not earlier possess. What is the new source, voice, or perspective which traumatized clients are able to internalize as authentic and therefore enables them to change, and what is it about PTSD that makes this perspective so authentic?

1. *Group therapy.* Because the subjective experience of trauma is beyond understanding in the usual sense, peers who have undergone the same or similar trauma may be heard by the survivor as a truly authentic voice whereas others may not. In the group treatment cases, it is the observations by other group members which seem to have the greatest valence.

2. *Family therapy.* The isolation and alienation which often accompany PTSD drives away those who care most about the client. In contrast to experts, it may be one's own family member (e.g., a child) who may break through barriers in ways others cannot—say, to clarify the need for treatment or to empathize with the suffering from PTSD.

3. *Cognitive-behavioral therapy.* Here the client's own trauma descriptions, literally his or her own voice on tape, stirs affect and new memory. Also, newly experienced physiological mastery carries strong authentic weight.

4. *Analytic and constructivist therapies.* The internalized voice of analytic therapists gains authenticity as they pass the patients' unconscious tests of them and as they use transference, countertransference, and reenactment constructively to forward mastery and healing. The process for constructivist therapies is similar.

5. *Psychopharmacological therapy.* For patients collaborating with their physicians in finding the right psychopharmacological intervention, the patients feel empowered when their expertise in describing their situation is matched by the clinicians' expertise in finding the right medication and dosage.

Ultimately, in all the approaches it is each client's acceptance of his or her own voice which mitigates change. We emphasize here that the site of recovery from the psychological effects of trauma is not our office, our words, or the words of others in our settings, nor our prescriptions, behaviors, or technologies. Rather, the site of recovery is within the biopsychosocial space of the survivor. By locating recovery in the survivor rather than in our technique, we can see that various core approaches may offer assistance at specific points in time in the course of the disorder and its recovery. Even in the same survivor, approaches may assist recovery at certain times by supportive/suppressive means and at other times by expressive means. Alternatively our approaches may harm recovery when we apply the wrong method at the wrong time. In the end, we strive like our clients not only to remove symptoms but to restore those healthy psychological functions and adaptive biological systems which have been damaged subsequent to the trauma.

IMPORTANCE OF THE RELATIONSHIP WITH THE THERAPIST

While all modes depend upon the generally benign and hopeful presence of an expert/authority, there are some approaches where this is the exclusive realm of the relationship: (1) in culturally specific trauma settings, the doctor/leader occupies a wise-man role familiar to the villagers of Southeast Asia; (2) in cognitive-behavioral therapy, in the supportive–suppressive groups and in the use of medication, there are efforts to sustain the positive benign authority and to interfere with tendencies to the contrary as resistances to the treatment.

Several modalities utilize the relationship with the therapist to convey more than the positive general alliance; indeed, they use specific irrational components projected on to the therapist as an avenue for further work on the trauma itself. Psychoanalytic constructivist and dynamic family/group therapies follow these precepts. The understanding and use of such transference phenomena differ somewhat among the approaches. Constructivists offer a new object relationship around which core issues can be more healthfully negotiated. Through a growing regard for self, the clients recognize and express their needs and the therapists within the constraints of their role negotiate a response which goes a significant distance toward meeting those needs. In group and family settings, trusted individuals can point out the irrational nature of transference reactions which the client is having; they can point out the nature and effects of trauma reliving on the client and on those close to him or her. The psychoanalytic perspective offers the widest use of transference phenomena, as in this approach the relationship is key to healing.

COMMONALITIES AMONG THE APPROACHES

While the foregoing discussion has noted distinguishing features in the core approaches, we are left with the conclusion that they have many features in common. All of the core approaches seek to have the patient claim "authority over traumatic memories" (Herman, 1992). All approaches seek to reduce symptoms, to improve function, to improve relationships, to achieve better understanding of oneself, and to promote a more positive appraisal of self and the world.

While technical efforts to achieve these ends with the core approaches involve differences, they share the many nonspecific aspects of the treatment relationship which include listening, empathy, structure, and dosage. The relationship must be caring, respectful, and uncompromisingly ethical. In the end, all approaches embrace the notion of self-empowerment and mastery.

Similarities in Process: Safety, Disclosure, and Reconnection

To a remarkable extent all the approaches concern themselves whether overtly or covertly with the three phases of treatment, variously called (1) safety, building the alliance, trust, and relaxation training; (2) disclosure, trauma narrative, trauma script, and imaginal exposure; and (3) reconnection, self-continuity and meaning, integration, and synthesis.

A Few Purists

Among the experts writing chapters in this book, there are few who are not open to the valid addition of techniques which have historically been associated with other core approaches. Those who rely primarily on pharmacotherapy attend to the dynamics of the working alliance; psychodynamic therapists utilize cognitive reframing and medication; behaviorists use cognitive techniques; group clinicians make transference interpretations; clinicians treating patients with dual (or triple) diagnosis may prescribe medication and utilize cognitive-behavioral and psychodynamic therapies in the same patient. Indeed, the climate of the field has been such as to encourage the sharing of knowledge among experts for the common good of the trauma survivor.

Common Difficulties

In the cases described in this book, therapists using cognitive-behavioral, psychopharmacological, constructivist, and psychoanalytic approaches all identified difficult moments in their cases. In each instance the patient at least temporarily experienced loss of safety and control within the treatment. For example, one client felt unsafe and refused to return after her cognitive-behavioral therapist prolonged an *in vivo* exposure by staying with the client in a dark closet longer than the patient feared was tolerable. In one case a psychoanalytic therapist, urging the patient to go deeper, precipitated a troubling reenactment. In one constructivist case the patient momentarily felt unsafe when the therapist refused to answer a personal question regarding her sexual orientation. The psychopharmacologist identified the contradictory impact of psychological and neurophysiological aspects of the same case such that the same medications were safe during the day but unsafe at night.

One group therapist conveyed concern that the termination process for one group member might risk reexposure to an unsafe world without the support of the group. In all the above cases, the client had moved at least temporarily from a more safe to a less safe state. The means of addressing these temporary periods of loss of safety vary with the different approaches.

SUMMARY

From the case histories in this book we infer certain patterns of practice among expert trauma clinicians that provide clues to the relative indications for and limitations of the core approaches to PTSD. The cognitive-behavioral approach is especially useful if the portal of entry is a reexperiencing of a defined traumatic memory, such as rape or violence, which is capable of being put into words. It is also especially useful when the trauma is a single event and relatively recent, and when the client's role is that of victim. The approach is salient in such cases because the client directly confronts those fears which cause the symptoms and, by attenuating them, gains mastery over them.

The constructivist approach engages interpersonal and self-state aspects of the client's current and past life. This approach addresses itself to patients with complex PTSD who are victims of childhood abuse, often sexual. Their memories are often indistinct at first, and the perpetrator is someone about whom the client has strongly ambivalent feelings. The trauma has occurred in an isolated setting with profound effects on current life and relationships. The treatment directly engages schemas of self-esteem, and the therapist provides a healthy model in both regulation of self-esteem and management of boundaries, so that intimate relations may develop with hope and trust rather than suspicion.

The psychodynamic spectrum of approaches (individual, family, and group) respond well to clients who present with avoidance/detachment, interpersonal problems, and damaged self-states. Traumas include war, torture, incest, and natural disaster. Traumas are usually multiple, include significant losses, and have occurred some years in the past. Dynamic treatments are particularly suited when the patient is experiencing guilt regarding his or her role as the perceived perpetrator or when symptoms of reexperiencing represent the suffering of others in the trauma situation.

The psychopharmacological approach is well suited for patients who present with symptoms of physiological hyperarousal and the reexperiencing symptoms of PTSD. It may work well in conjunction with all other approaches. It is particularly recommended in culturally specific settings, the severely mentally ill, and dual (or triple) diagnosis.

The group approach highlights opportunities to work on interpersonal aspects of trauma, detachment, alienation, avoidance, and loss. In this book, patients discussed were largely war veterans, although any community of trauma survivors is well suited for this modality. Groups rebuild acceptance in self and trust in others where trauma has disrupted it.

The family approach like others in the dynamic cluster appeals to patients with interpersonal and avoidance/detachment presentation. Family members rather than the person with PTSD may mobilize the treatment. It is a setting well designed to reestablish communication where trauma has wrought breaks in intimate relations. Further, the setting is well suited for family members who themselves suffer PTSD indirectly from their affected relative.

Of course, the patterns we describe here come from the limited database of the case histories in this book and the experience of the editors. In our view, these clinical patterns are of practical use for the reader of this book and deserve the attention of researchers in the future to test them rigorously.

Thoughtful clinicians who wish to avail their patients of the best possible fit between the presenting situation (both overt symptoms and the interpersonal and intrapsychic difficulties) and the core treatments available need to take a careful history, elaborate the presenting symptoms, and inquire sensitively about the nature of the trauma as the client is now able to describe it. Such efforts will put clinicians in a position to make good use of the final two chapters of this book.

REFERENCES

Herman, J. L. (1992). *Trauma and recovery*. New York: Basic Books.
Lindy, J. D., Grace, M. C., & Green, B. L. (1981). Survivors: Outreach to a reluctant population. *American Journal of Orthopsychiatry, 51*(3), 468–478.

APPENDIX 15.1

Name	Age	Demographics	Symptoms	Trauma and loss	No. of years Posttrauma	Medications	Treatment forms	Status
Cross-Cultural:								
Case 1 Ven (Ch. 11)	49	Female Widowed Cambodian refugee	Trouble sleeping Trembling Pain Bilateral numbness Chronic	One son decapitated Two children starved Husband killed and legs cut off	23	Doxepin Clonidine Fluoxetine	Socialization groups	Improved Vulnerable
Case 2 Phong (Ch. 11)	64	Male Single Vietnam refugee Colonel	Headaches Trouble sleeping Nightmares Alone Chronic	Political prisoner, 12 years Wife and children killed	? 7	Fluoxetine Trazodone Clonidine	Socialization groups	Partial improvement
Case 3 Christina (Ch. 11)	25	Female Widowed Zaire refugee Student	Poor sleep Poor appetite No enjoyment in life Suicidal ideas Subacute	Husband decapitated Parents presumed killed Raped Home burned	?	Imipramine Clonidine Propranolol	Individual support Psychotherapy Religious community support Political asylum	Improved
Complex PTSD								
Case 4 Ms. A (Ch. 9)	45	Female Married Professional	Dissociated Not in tune Relation difficulty Threatened identity Chronic	Parental neglect Child abuse by neighbor Child abuse by priest, ages 4–6	> 30		Individual long-term psychotherapy	Improved

Case	Age	Status	Presenting problems	Trauma history			Treatment	Outcome
Case 5 Ms. C (Ch. 9)	40s	Female Divorced	Depressed, alone Unsatisfied in relations Unsatisfied in work Chronic	Mother's paranoid illness Abusive relationship with husband, 20 years	> 5	None	Individual long-term psychotherapy	Improved
Case 6 Sam (Ch. 8)	50	Male Remarried, twice Veteran	Unable to parent Sabotaged relationships Feared loss of control Anger, numbness, alcohol	Abused by mother's boyfriend Abandoned by father Abusive foster home Vietnam firefights Wounded with shrapnel Chronic	> 25	?	Group treatment Dynamic	Improved
Case 7 John (Ch. 8)	50	Male Married Veteran	Isolated Self-destructive alcohol use Unable to get anything out of life	Atrocities Horrific death of best friend	?	?	Family therapy	Family improved John is questionable
Group, cognitive-behavioral								
Case 8 Mark	48	Male Divorced Veteran	Disagreement with supervisor Discomfort around others	Explosion which injured friends Heavy combat Nightmares	25	?	Group cognitive- behavioral	Improved

Family/couples

Case 9: Family where father avoids 13-year-old girl having killed child that same age in Vietnam (Ch. 13)

Case 10: 4-year-old child is searching for father's missing eye from Vietnam (Ch. 13)

Case 11: Mother of combat veteran depressed and guilty for hospitalizing homicidal son (Ch. 13)

Case 12: Combat veteran and wife "living separate lives" because PTSD not understood (Ch. 13)

Case 13: Couple unable to connect; depressed at anniversary of friend's death (Ch. 13)

(continued)

405

APPENDIX 15.1 *cont.*

Name	Age	Demographics	Symptoms	Trauma and loss	No. of years Posttrauma	Medications	Treatment forms	Status
PTSD and SMI								
No cases								
Psychoanalytic								
Case 14 Frank (Ch. 5)	50	Male Married Veteran	Fatigue Unable to rest	Reconnaissance Search-and-destroy missions		On medications	Analytic	Improved
Case 15 Rob (Ch. 5)	50	Male Married Veteran	Impulsive Suspicious Nightmares	Scout		On medications	Analytic	Improved
Case 16 Annette (Ch. 5)	35	Female Married Work at home	Impaired parenting Anxiety	Traumatic enemas as a child		None	Analytic	Improved
Case 17 Tina (Ch. 5)	Mid-40s	Female married Counselor	Somatic reenactment Masochistic relationships Suicidal	Death of child Incest as child		Fluoxetine	Analytic	Mild improvement
Case 18 Abraham (Ch. 5)	37	Male Married Veteran	Numbness Alienation Blocked emotions with son	Search and destroy missions Killed Vietnamese boy and grandfather		Imipramine	Analytic	Improved

Case 19 Mihai (Ch. 5)	69	Male	Married	Political prisoner	Brainwashing Imprisonment Torture	Guilt Shame Nightmares			Analytic	Improved
Case 20 Kelly (Ch. 9)	48	Female	Married	Counselor	Childhood physical abuse Childhood sexual abuse	Cut off from feelings		None	Analytic	Some improvement
Cognitive-behavioral										
Case 21 Alice (Ch. 7)	58	Female	Divorced/ African/ American	Real estate agent	Robbed Raped vaginally and anally	Intrusive thoughts Nightmares Trouble sleeping Intense physical/emotional reactions	1		Cognitive-behavioral	Improved
Case 22 Rebecca (Ch. 7)	34	Female	Single	Restaurant manager	Shot Stalked	Recurrent thoughts Nightmares Intense physical/emotional responses Unable to work/drive by restaurant	6 months		Cognitive-behavioral	No change
Psychopharmacology										
Case 23 KM (Ch. 4)	42	Female		Executive	Childhood sexual abuse	Dissociative episodes	> 30	Clonidine Guanfacine	Pharmacological	Improved

(continued)

APPENDIX 15.1 *cont.*

Name	Age	Demographics	Symptoms	Trauma and loss	No. of years Posttrauma	Medications	Treatment forms	Status
Case 24 DG (Ch. 4)	55	Male Disabled	Nightmares Startle reactions	Childhood sexual abuse Childhood physical abuse Problems with intimacy	> 30	Beta-blocker	Pharmacological	Partial improvement
Case 25 Clyde (Ch. 10)	Early 20s	Male Student	Depression Intrusive images	Bushfire	14	Monoamine oxidase inhibitor	Cognitive-behavioral Analytic	Improved

16

Practical Considerations in the Treatment of PTSD: Guidelines for Practitioners

JOHN P. WILSON, MATTHEW J. FRIEDMAN,
and JACOB D. LINDY

An organismic holistic approach to the treatment of posttraumatic stress disorder (PTSD) underscores its complexity as a psychological syndrome. There is a range and diversity of traumatic stressors which are embedded in and define the nature of a particular traumatic event. The consequence of trauma is a specific intrapsychic organization of ego states and allostatic adaptation which controls symptom manifestation. As such, the practical choice of how to intervene to assist victims of trauma confronts the practitioner with decision points as to alternative interventions and psychotherapeutic approaches.

Acute interventions following a disaster, for example, may require a crisis intervention, short-term cognitive behavior therapy or a form of stress debriefing to normalize the expectable stress response sequelae (Raphael & Wilson, 2000; Horowitz, 1986). At the other end of the spectrum, complex PTSD may require intensive, prolonged psychotherapy and adjunctive pharmacotherapy to facilitate the rebuilding of shattered lives and narcissistically damaged ego states and persons (Watkins & Watkins, 1997; see our Chapter 2, this volume, for a discussion). Moreover, the trauma population being helped may require specialized treatment for PTSD depending on the characteristics which define the client (e.g., children, families, refugees, disaster victims, or persons with preexisting severe mental illness who have suffered trauma leading to PTSD). Thus, the treatment goals for PTSD have varying objectives depending on the treatment approach for PTSD, the trauma population being served, and the nature and complexity of the posttraumatic phenomenology. One practical advantage of the organismic model of PTSD and dissociative phenomena presented in Part I of this volume is that it allows the practitioner flexibility in discerning the unique configuration of PTSD in a client and the five portals of entry (see Figures 2.2 and 2.3 in Chapter 2) by which to consider how to reach the configuration of PTSD phenomenology as a dynamic, organismic process.

As a general overview, Table 16.1 lists the 11 core treatment approaches discussed in Parts I and II and their treatment goals. For each of the treatment approaches for PTSD, the five major dimensions of PTSD derived from the allostatic tetrahedral model of PTSD are presented: (1) psychobiological (DSM-IV D criteria); (2) traumatic memory (DSM-IV B criteria); (3) avoidance, numbing, denial, and detachment (DSM-IV C criteria); (4) self-structure, ego states, and identity; and (5) PTSD and interpersonal relations.

For each of the five major dimensions of PTSD derived from the allostatic tetrahedral model is a scale which indicates the degree of relevance of each of the treatment approaches to the five dimensions of PTSD phenomenology. As Table 16.1 indicates, the scale has four rating points: (0) not applicable, (+) somewhat relevant, (++) moderately relevant, and (+++) highly relevant. By contrasting and comparing the scale points it is possible to discern areas of similarity and dissimilarity between the 11 core treatment approaches. By examining the specific treatment goals for the core approaches, both conceptual and pragmatic differences can be evaluated by the practitioner for a PTSD client. For example, acute interventions in response to critical incident events and disasters address the psychobiological components of PTSD (i.e., reduction of hyperarousal and confronting avoidance, denial, and numbing symptoms) but typically do not attempt to "treat," "intervene," or "deal" with the trauma's impact to the self-structure, ego states, or postevent interpersonal relationships (Wilson & Raphael, 2000). On the other hand, the core treatment approaches for complex PTSD and the treatment of families and couples are all highly relevant to how trauma has impacted interpersonal relations and avoidance, denial, and numbing aspects of PTSD.

Table 16.1 can be useful to the practitioner as a guide for decision making. More than one treatment approach may be indicated, depending on the configuration of the PTSD phenomenology. For example, psychopharmacological approaches may be useful to many of the treatment goals. In this regard, pharmacological approaches may be a primary modality or as one useful, and sometimes necessary, to bolster the effectiveness of a very different treatment modality, such as those discussed by Kinzie in Chapter 11, this volume, for the treatment of trauma clients from non-Western cultures.

TABLE 16.1. Treatment Approaches for PTSD and Their Goals

Core treatment approaches for PTSD	Dimensions of PTSD derived from the Tetrahedral model					Treatment goals
	I. Psychobiological	II. Traumatic memory	III. Avoidance, numbing, denial, and coping	IV. Self-structure, ego states, and identity	V. Interpersonal relations	
Psychopharmacotherapy	+++	++	+++	0	0	Facilitate normalization toward homeostasis
Psychodynamic	+	+++	+++	+++	++	Restore toward normal intrapsychic functioning
Acute interventions	++	+	++	0	0	Reestablish a normal stress response pattern
Cognitive-behavioral	++	+++	+++	++	+	Gain authority over traumatic memories
Group psychotherapy	0	+++	+++	+	+++	Facilitate normalization of PTSD responses and enhance capacity for healthy relationships
Complex PTSD	0	+++	+++	+++	++	Restore a positive self-schema of effective coping
Dual diagnosis	+++	+++	+++	++	++	Determine treatment that fosters recovery from Axis I and Axis II disorders
Cross-cultural	++	+	+++	+	++	Foster recovery within an embedded cultural framework
Children	++	+++	+++	+	+++	Foster trauma recovery to overcome interruption of normal development
Families and couples	0	++	+++	+	+++	Restore healthy attachments, relationships, and capacity for intimacy
Severe mental illness and PTSD	0	+	++	0	+++	Facilitate social reintegration and support for activities of daily living

Note. +, somewhat relevant; ++, moderately relevant; +++, highly relevant; 0, not applicable.

In the following sections, we summarize the key features of the treatment approaches as a synopsis guideline for use by practitioners. Our goal is to present the essential features of each of the 11 treatment approaches for PTSD and highlight how they may be used by the clinical practitioner who faces choice points regarding strategies and methods for treating PTSD. As such, this chapter is not intended to be directive nor comprehensive. Rather, it is to provide a framework for clinical understanding, case assessment, and empowerment of the client's recovery.

TREATMENT APPROACHES FOR PTSD AND SPECIAL TRAUMA POPULATIONS

Psychopharmacotherapy for PTSD

Pharmacotherapy is often targeted at psychobiological allostatic load in PTSD (see Friedman, Chapter 4, this volume, for a discussion). The treatment goal of various medications for PTSD is the restoration of homeostasis or normalization toward it. We should note that by definition allostasis is a changed but stable systemic and integrated stress response process within organismic functioning. The restoration of or normalization toward homeostasis reflects better and more functional levels of posttraumatic adaptation—one in which maladaptive allostatic subtypes (i.e., "repeated hits," "lack of adaptation," "prolonged stress," "inadequate response," and "combined-fusion" patterns—see Chapter 1 for a discussion) are modulated or attenuated, thus producing changed psychobiological and behavioral outcomes in which PTSD related behaviors are far less disruptive. As Table 16.1 illustrates, psychopharmacotherapy of PTSD is highly relevant to three of the five core dimensions of PTSD (i.e., psychobiological symptoms; traumatic memory; and avoidance, numbing, and denial) but has little direct relevance to restoration of self-structure, ego states, and identity or to improvement of interpersonal and object relations. Nevertheless, practitioners should consider medications for PTSD as a rational and useful adjunct to psychotherapeutic efforts within a framework of holistic organismic functioning of PTSD.

Psychodynamic Approaches to PTSD

The treatment goals of psychodynamic approaches to PTSD are to restore normal intrapsychic functioning. Such approaches place emphasis on unconscious and ego-defensive dynamics in the specific configuration of ego states in PTSD. Allostatic psychodynamic approaches to PTSD recognize that ego defenses (e.g., repression, denial, disavowal, suppression, or projection) are organized around affects which have been dysregulated by traumatic experiences. In that regard, ego-control mechanisms have been overwhelmed, rendered insufficient in function, or rigidified as intrapsychic processes. Through the analysis of trauma specific transference (TST) processes (Wilson & Lindy, 1994) the therapist gains insight into how traumatized ego states are crystallized around defenses designed to ward off distressing intrusive thoughts, feelings, and images of the traumatic event. Dysregulated painful emotions caused by trauma are intrapsychically linked to cognitive processes of information processing and defensive efforts to "control" and "dose" the degree of pain attached to the memory of the trauma.

By tradition, psychodynamic approaches to the treatment of PTSD (Lindy, 1993) place emphasis on levels of conscious awareness (LCA) of dysregulated psychobiological processes. Allostasis as a form of organismic stress response does not discriminate between mind–body phenomena. Allostasis is also dysregulation of cognitive processes and therefore includes altered states of conscious awareness about traumatic material. Altered states of conscious awareness span the spectrum from dissociated mental states to hyperalert/ hypervigilant cognitive functioning and include degrees of unconscious mental and behavioral activities. Arthur S. Blank, Jr. (1985), for example, listed clinically derived criteria for the "unconscious flashback" in PTSD. Similarly, Niederland (1964) described case histories which illustrate unconscious guilt and punishment themes in PTSD for Holocaust survivors. Wilson and Lindy (1994) presented case histories of PTSD patients who manifest unconscious forms of self-recrimination and self-blame, as well as unconscious suicidal ideation and unconscious shame, anger, and humiliation among victims of torture and war trauma. Considered from the perspective of allostatic dysregulations, there can be unconscious forms of behavior evident for any affect which is attached to painful traumatic memories. Hence, in TST reactions (which unfold and present in many diverse ways in psychotherapy) the critical task of the practitioner is to decode the meaning of the unconscious transference projection at that moment (i.e., *in situ*) in terms of its significance for the patient. Successful analysis of TST projections yields interpretations that identify defenses against traumatic injuries to the self. In this regard it is meaningful to speak of restoring normal intrapsychic functioning as the central goal of treatment from a psychodynamic perspective.

Acute Interventions for PTSD

Acute interventions for PTSD are those which typically occur in the immediate wake of trauma. Such interventions following a traumatic event include crisis interventions, stress debriefings, and short-term counseling (Raphael & Wilson, 2000) as well as brief cognitive-behavioral therapy (CBT) (Bryant, Harvey, Dang, Sackville, & Basten, 1998; Bryant, Sackville, Dang, Moulds, & Guthrie, 1999; Foa, Hearst-Ikeda, & Perry, 1995). Where exposure to death, dying, and human suffering is part of the traumatic event, the issue of traumatic bereavement is important and an acute intervention may be necessary to facilitate the bereavement process. Moreover, as noted by Raphael and Dobson in Chapter 6, this volume, acute interventions may need to recognize that acute stress disorder (ASD), or symptoms thereof, may be precursors to "full-blown" PTSD at a later time. Thus, acute interventions for stress reactions, ASD or PTSD, must be adapted to address a broad spectrum of critical incident events (e.g., natural disasters, school shootings, motor vehicle accidents, bank robberies, or hostage situations) which challenge the practitioner as to how to best provide assistance. In that regard, the overall treatment goal of acute intervention procedures is to reestablish the normal stress response. Indeed, as noted by Raphael and Dobson in Chapter 6, this volume, there are at least seven primary purposes of acute posttrauma interventions: (1) providing assistance, aid, and counseling to restore homeostasis and reduce allostatic dysregulations, especially those associated with acute stress response symptoms of hyperarousal, intrusive recollections, avoidance, numbing, dissociation, denial, psychic overload, daze, disorientation, and loss of capacity for normal coping; (2) providing education as to the nature of ASD, PTSD, and expectable psychological reactions following a traumatic or highly stressful life event; (3) targeting a specific set of intervention techniques (e.g., critical incident stress debriefing or CBT) to facilitate a return to normal functioning; (4) targeting interventions to assist with the processing of the event as soon as possible in order to (5) prevent longer-term adverse effects on coping and adaptation; (6) targeting interventions to treat identifiable disorders, problems, or crises that are disruptive to healthy coping; and (7) targeting interventions to facilitate the resolution of ASD, PTSD, or other indicators of stress response syndromes with phasic stages (e.g., denial, avoidance, intrusion, working through, and cognitive restructuring).

As Table 16.1 illustrates, acute interventions are primarily directed to the psychobiological and avoidance symptoms of ASD and PTSD. Because they are acute interventions, they are *not* targeted specifically at ego-state functions or interpersonal relationships. In the broadest sense, the various types of acute interventions described by Raphael and Dobson in Chapter 6 (e.g., psychological first aid, crisis intervention, military models of debriefing, grief work, critical incident stress debriefings, or CBT) are oriented toward reestablishing the normal stress response sequence and promoting positive coping.

The concept of acute interventions focuses on early responses to trauma victims. Clinical lore and disaster research (e.g., Smith & North, 1993) provide evidence that rapid intervention following a disaster is helpful in stabilizing and normalizing the expectable stress response to overwhelming life events. However, there is a dearth of scientific studies on the short- and long-term effectiveness of early interventions. For example, Rose and Bisson (1998) reviewed six studies which employed randomized controlled trials and found only two with positive (i.e., salutary) outcomes. Moreover, two studies found negative effects of intervention. Richard A. Byrant and his colleagues

(1998, 1999) examined the treatment of ASD in several studies which compared CBT to supportive counseling for civilian trauma survivors and found that CBT was more effective than supportive counseling at follow-up intervals (i.e., 6 months or longer). Similar findings were obtained by Foa et al. (1995) for victims of sexual assault who were treated with CBT. In a study of the prevention of postrape psychopathology, Resnick, Acierno, Holmes, Kilpatrick, and Jager (1999), evaluated women who had been raped within 72 hours of the sexual assault and found that the level of distress at the time of their medical–forensic examination predicted PTSD symptomatology 6 weeks later. Further, a structured educational intervention prior to the forensic examination appeared to reduce the stress experienced during the medical procedure.

A recent comprehensive review of the literature on psychological debriefings (Raphael & Wilson, 2000) has noted that acute interventions take many forms (e.g., short-term cognitive behavioral treatments, critical incident stress debriefings, supportive counseling, community-based crisis intervention, disaster relief, or trauma action teams for civilian disasters). Further, there are not enough comparative scientific data by which to evaluate the efficacy of such procedures for the treatment of ASD or PTSD. Nevertheless, acute interventions are and will be necessary in many disaster situations (e.g., the bombing of the Oklahoma City federal building, body retrieval in natural and technological disasters), and so compassionate clinical care should "do no harm" while controlled scientific studies generate data to assess effective and noneffective interventions.

Cognitive-Behavioral Treatment for PTSD

Cognitive behavioral treatments for PTSD include a range of methods and techniques to assist patients in processing and overcoming the debilitating aspects of PTSD. At the heart of the different methods are the treatment goals of gaining authority over traumatic memories through exposure and by correcting or reframing disturbed memories, beliefs, interpretations, and emotions.

As Table 16.1 indicates, CBTs target all five of the core PTSD dimensions and have the most relevance to three areas: (1) traumatic memories; (2) avoidance, numbing, and denial; and (3) stressor impacts to the self-structure, ego states, and personal identity. Further, evidence reviewed in Chapter 7 of this volume by Zoellner, Fitzgibbons, and Foa suggests that CBT affects the psychobiological (e.g., hyperarousal) aspects of PTSD as well as the interpersonal domain of objects relations (e.g., reducing fear of others, detachment, or estrangement tendencies).

The practitioner considering the use of CBT for PTSD treatment has various therapeutic tools available in terms of targeting treatment and making assessments as to how to use one of the five portals of entry into PTSD phenomenology reflected in the tetrahedral models presented by us in Chapter 2, this volume. The strength and elegance of CBT is that it is based on scientific principles of learning and conditioned responses to threat, fear, and other anxiety-inducing states. These techniques include (1) exposure treatments, (2) anxiety management, (3) cognitive therapy and reprocessing, (4) systematic desensitization, (5) assertiveness training, (6) biofeedback, and (7) combined techniques.

Complex PTSD: Treatment Considerations

"Complex PTSD" is a term that has been employed in the past two decades to indicate that the phenomenology of PTSD extends beyond the diagnostic criteria set forth in DSM-IV. For the practitioner, it is important to note that the logic of that diagnostic manual of the American Psychiatric Association (1994) was to create algorithms for differential diagnosis of mental disorders. The diagnostic algorithms are, in essence, the minimal set of criteria by which to define a disorder and, in turn, distinguish it from others. In terms of PTSD, researchers and clinicians have come to the realization that PTSD is *not* a unidimensional construct (see our Chapters 1 and 2, this volume, for a discussion). The concept of complex PTSD supersedes the categories of DSM-IV (i.e., behaviors, symptoms, emotional states, cognitive schemas) and defines symptoms observed among trauma survivors that extend beyond its official diagnostic criteria.

Among other authors, Judith Herman (1992) initially has proposed six dimensions of symptoms to explicate the concept of complex PTSD. These dimensions reflect the following alterations in different levels of psychological functioning and are entirely consistent with our tetrahedral allostatic model of PTSD: (1) alteration in affect regulation, (2) alteration in consciousness, (3) alteration in self-perception, (4) alteration in perception of the perpetrator or cause of traumatic injury, (5) alteration in relations with others (e.g., isolation, impulsivity), and (6) alteration in systems of meaning.

Practitioners who treat complex PTSD face a formidable task since they must decide how to support the client while dealing with multifaceted psychological symptoms at each of the five core dimensions we have listed in Table 16.1. As the table illustrates, treatment approaches to complex PTSD are highly relevant to ameliorating traumatic memories, avoidance behaviors, and damage to the self-structure, ego states, and identity. Similarly, treatment approaches to complex PTSD inevitably must address how the disorder impacts interpersonal and object relations. However, unlike the approach of the more cognitive-behavioral therapeutic techniques, the treatment of complex PTSD is not directly concerned with the psychobiological components of PTSD.

In Chapter 9, this volume, Laurie Ann Pearlman describes how the treatment of complex PTSD can be approached by constructivist self-developmental theory (CSDT). CSDT enables the practitioner to assess cognitive schemas of the client that have been altered by experiences of interpersonal abuse, violence, and other types of trauma. Cognitive schemas pertain to the client's basic needs for security, self-esteem, and self-efficacy. In this regard, the primary treatment goal of CSDT is to restore positive self-schemas of effective coping, an objective that is most closely aligned with the goals of psychodynamic treatment approaches.

In CSDT approaches to complex PTSD, Pearlman suggests that clinical work involves six interrelated processes: (1) identifying areas of schema disruption; (2) exploring the sources of disruption; (3) exploring the meanings of the disrupted schema; (4) exploring the defensive nature of disrupted schema; (5) therapeutically challenging the disrupted schema in nurturing ways, and (6) facilitating positive life experiences which will restore a self-schema of positive coping. Consistent with the allostatic model of dysregulated organismic functioning presented in Part I of this volume, treatment of complex PTSD is directed toward ameliorating the six areas of psychological disruption identified by Herman (1992), listed above. CSDT and other approaches to the treatment of complex PTSD attempts to (1) restore organismic integrity, unity, and coherence within the self; (2) restore the client's firm belief in his or her efficacy to cope successfully with the environment; and (3) restore his or her positive worldview and belief that life is meaningful.

Issues in the Dual Diagnosis of PTSD

The issue of comorbidity in the treatment of PTSD has grown in importance as the number of scientific studies yield data by which to inform practitioners about the linkage between PTSD and other disorders. In terms of treatment goals, Table 16.1 indicates that for PTSD and dual diagnosis, the object is to facilitate recovery from Axis I and Axis II disorders. While such a treatment goal seems obvious and straightforward, the clinical nuances of case management are much more complex.

For practitioners, there are several conceptual paradigms that should be considered when they are formulating a treatment plan. First, PTSD may be the only diagnosis that requires one or more of the treatments that we have discussed throughout this book. Second, the client may have had an Axis I or Axis II psychiatric disorder prior to the development of PTSD. Third, the client may develop PTSD and another Axis I disorder as a result of trauma (e.g., major depression or substance abuse as a form of self-medication). Where substance abuse is a form of self-medication for PTSD, the client may be at significant risk for addiction, a factor that complicates the treatment plan. Fourth, as a result of trauma, the individual may have a transformation of his or her basic personality structure and manifest characteristics that may be difficult to distinguish from the features of a personality disorder (e.g., suspicion, mistrust, guardedness, isolation, irritability, and anger). Alterations in basic personality processes induced by trauma have been referred to as PTPDs (i.e., posttraumatic personality disorder), underscoring the point that the individual experiences a life-altering traumatic event that, in essence, reshaped his or her personality traits into relatively stable patterns of behavior and coping that were not present before the trauma.

In a recent review of the literature on the epidemiology of PTSD, Breslau (1998) concluded as follows:

> Most community residents with PTSD have at least one other psychiatric disorder in their lifetime. Recent analyses that have addressed etiologic questions regarding the observed lifetime co-morbidities in PTSD have suggested several pathways: (1) PTSD increases the risk of first onset major depression and drug use disorder; (2) exposure to traumatic events per se, in the absence of PTSD, does not increase the risk of these disorders; (3) pre-existing major depression and anxiety disorder increase the vulnerability to PTSD following trauma; and (4) major depression increases the probability of exposure to trauma. (p. 26)

Epidemiological data (Breslau, 1998) show that among those with PTSD, 36.6% had lifetime major depression; 58.1% had a lifetime anxiety disorder other than PTSD; 31.2% had lifetime alcohol abuse disorder; and 21.5% had lifetime drug abuse disorder. Similar findings are summarized in Chapter 10, by McFarlane, pointing to the reality that individuals with PTSD are at risk for depression, alcohol and drug abuse, and other anxiety disorders (e.g., panic disorders; generalized anxiety disorder).

In conclusion, the treatment of comorbidity in PTSD requires combined treatment methods. As noted by Friedman (2000), "clinicians most commonly add pharmacotherapy to individual and group therapy—drug treatment not only ameliorates psychobiological abnormalities associated with PTSD, but may provide sufficient symptom reduction for clients to participate in [trauma-focused treatment]" (p. 34).

Cross-Cultural Treatments for PTSD

In Chapter 11, Kinzie presents a clinical guideline for optimal cross-cultural treatment of PTSD. As Table 16.1 illustrates, we have formulated the treatment goal as that of fostering recovery within an embedded cultural framework. This treatment objective expresses the view that an understanding of cultural differences is important when a clinician is treating a client from a non-Western culture. Culture represents the internalization of values, customs, mores, and culturally rooted beliefs as well as "rules" pertaining to social interaction and self-presentation. As discussed by Friedman in Chapter 4, this volume, recent research publications (e.g., Marsella, Friedman, Gerrity & Scurfield, 1996; Kinzie, 1988, 1993; Wilson, 1989) have underscored the wide-range of cultural differences that influence how the patient processes traumatic memories and his or her capacity and willingness to form a trusting therapeutic alliance. So how do practitioners address the critical questions of cultural diversity in the treatment of PTSD?

Kinzie (see Chapter 11, this volume) and his associates at the University of Oregon Health Sciences Center have had nearly two decades of experience in working with culturally diverse populations with PTSD (e.g., Vietnamese, Cambodians, Laotians, Thais, and Congolese). Based on the need to provide the best possible service to these populations, Kinzie and his colleagues have evolved a multicultural treatment program that grew out of the need to address the spectrum of psychiatric disorders in which their patients had suffered because of severe trauma. As Table 16.1 indicates, of the five core dimensions of PTSD, cross-cultural treatment approaches primarily target the psychobiological aspects and the avoidance, denial, and numbing components of posttraumatic adaptation. However, the targeting of these symptom clusters is done with medications and psychoeducational techniques which recognize the importance of fostering recovery within an *embedded cultural framework*. Stated differently, in order to be effective, the therapist must know how to "step into the culture" of the client while at the same time suspending his or her own culturally shaped beliefs and values. Clearly, this is a skill that requires training, experience, and a capacity for sustained empathic atunement (Wilson & Lindy, 1994).

As a capsule summary, we have condensed the elements of the cross-cultural treatment of PTSD proposed Kinzie in Chapter 11 as follows:

- The treatment of comorbidity is paramount. Many cross-cultural clients present with a dual diagnosis and complex PTSD.
- Interpretations of bilingual staff members are important to treatment goals and understanding cultural differences.
- Easy access to the program without bureaucratic hassle is important to achieve acceptance and regular utilization of the service by cross-cultural clients.
- Acceptance of the program by the refugee, ethnic, or minority client is important to credibility with the target population.
- The program should have links to other social and medical services that are readily accessible.
- Medical (i.e., physical) and psychological needs should be carefully evaluated. Special sensitivity may be required for populations who have been physically injured or tortured by perpetrators. Since physicians assist in the torture process in some countries, posttraumatic physical examinations may be very difficult. The mere presence of a physician may trigger traumatic memories (Agger & Jensen, 1993; Juhler, 1993).
- Patients should be given opportunities to provide feedback to the program staff regarding the quality and standards of care.

- The staff needs to understand multicultural diversity and to have a broad base of competence when working with refugee or minority populations.

The development of a treatment program for culturally diverse clients with PTSD who may also have a dual diagnosis is not an easy task. It should not come as a surprise that the treatment process itself requires innovation, flexibility, and a knowledge of how to best promote recovery within an embedded cultural framework. In Chapter 11, this volume, Kinzie highlights some of the primary concerns, which include the following: (1) establishment of safety; (2) continuity of care; (3) obtaining a complete trauma history; (4) sensitivity as to the issue of when to "open up" the trauma story or when to let it remain "sealed over"; and (5) maintenance of a secure environment at the place of treatment, thereby minimizing "triggering cues" for posttraumatic stress associated with persons in position of power and authority.

Treatment of PTSD in Children

The treatment of posttraumatic states in children and adolescents focuses on trauma's impact to psychological development. The primary treatment goal is to promote trauma recovery to overcome the interruption of normal development. As Table 16.1 indicates, this treatment goal is, overall, most relevant to the PTSD clusters of traumatic memory; avoidance, numbing, and denial; and interpersonal and object relations. Because of age-related factors associated with epigenetic development, the treatment of the psychobiological components of PTSD is somewhat relevant and medications may be warranted (although there is little pharmacological research with children to guide us at this time; Friedman, 2000).

Among the crucial issues in the treatment of PTSD in children is understanding the specific stage and developmental tasks which are normative in the processes of healthy maturation. Moreover, ego development is a continuous process and through it the self-structure emerges with a sense of personal identity (Wilson, 1989; Erikson, 1968). The treatment of children and adolescents with a history of trauma must be sensitive to how it has affected self-worth, self-esteem, the organization of ego states (including defenses against distressing traumatic memory), and the configuration of identity. Trauma which occurs during the formative years can cause a fracturing of the self (e.g., dissociative identity disorder) or give rise to abnormal character and personality processes that may be at least as injurious as physical damage to the body. From the point of allostasis, both physical and psychic injuries cause psychobiological alterations in organismic functioning and disrupt normal development.

Kathleen Nader presents in Chapter 12, this volume, a detailed and comprehensive overview of treatment methods for children and adolescents with a history of trauma. Since a review of each of the alternative treatment methods (e.g., play therapy) is beyond the scope of this discussion, it is important to note that they revolve around four major themes: (1) repeated review of the event, (2) reprocessing or redefinition of memories, (3) restoration of a sense of competence and relative sense of safety, and (4) increase in sense of control. These four themes are consistent with the treatment goals for the other core therapies for PTSD listed in Table 16.1. This is not surprising since Nader reviews the alternative treatments for which there are scientific outcome data. For example, repeated review of the event is consistent with cognitive-behavioral exposure and cognitive restructuring techniques as well as approaches to dual diagnosis. The reprocessing or redefinition of memories has elements of both CBT and psychodynamic approaches. Similarly, the restoration of a sense of competence and a relative sense of safety is congruent with the objective of complex PTSD treatment. Finally, increasing a sense of self-control may be achieved by individual, family, group, or play therapies. Nevertheless, no matter which treatment options are adopted for working with children and adolescents with a history of trauma, there are recurring trends that define useful PTSD treatment:

- The child needs to feel safe, supported, and in a protected environment.
- The child must be permitted to progress in processing trauma at his or her pace. Regressions, relapses, and false gains do occur and should not be construed as failure. PTSD symptoms wax and wane over time.
- The developmental age or phase of ego development will differentially influence the impact of a given trauma. Traumatization may result in acceleration, fixation, or regression in normal development (Wilson, 1989; Erikson, 1950, 1968).
- The link between trauma and subsequent personality development is not well known. Theoretically and clinically, it is understood that trauma can alter personality characteristics in ways that give rise to developmental and personality disorders. In some exceptionally gifted individuals, trauma may give rise to psychosocial acceleration in ego processes (Wilson, 1989) or produce fractures in the self that may be expressed in art, creative endeavors, and compensatory achievement-oriented activities.
- Early trauma and victimization may make the person especially vulnerable to later interpersonal crises (Wilson, Harel, & Kahana, 1988, 1989). The issue of stress vulnerability and resiliency has become a focal point for psychoeducational interventions (Flannery, 1990) that seek to enhance resilient coping.

The long-term consequences of traumatization in childhood and adolescence are not fully understood at this time. The existing research literature suggests that there is a broad range of potential adverse outcomes. As Nader points out in Chapter 12, this volume, children improve with time and PTSD symptoms lessen. Damage to the internal organization of ego states may result in what some have termed narcissistic injury, a bruising or fracturing of the soul, or a loss of self-sameness and continuity to an individuals existence in time, space, and culture.

Treatment Approaches for Families and Couples

It is an unfortunate truism that traumatic events occur in the lives of families and couples. Individual families or couples may be involved in a life-threatening event (a motor vehicle accident, natural disaster, criminal assault, terminal illness, etc.) in which a member of the couple or family becomes afflicted with PTSD. The clinical question for the practitioner is how to best formulate a treatment plan that will assist the psychically injured client, couple or one or more members of a family.

In Table 16.1 we have stated the treatment goal for families and couples as that of restoring healthy attachments, relationships, and the capacity for intimacy. Moreover, as noted in the table and by Laurie Harkness and Nola Zador in Chapter 13, this volume, treatment typically concerns the core triad PTSD symptoms and their effects on interpersonal functioning. As these authors state: "First, the reexperiencing cluster (i.e., the disturbance in memory) *affects the survivors' ability to be present in the present.* Second, the numbing and avoidance symptoms interfere with the individual's capacity to identify, modulate, and express feelings. Third, the hyperarousal symptoms impact on the survivor's sense of safety and capacity to trust" (p. 336; emphasis added). Once present, the PTSD symptoms in a couple or family can have systemic effects, impacting the family structure, affect expression, decision making, communication patterns, and patterns of behavior and control.

In Chapter 13, Harkness and Zador suggest that once PTSD is present in a couple or family, the impact on interpersonal relations may be seen in two areas: (1) anger management and problems with aggression; and (2) tendencies toward isolation, withdrawal, and emotional detachment. Clearly, aggression and detachment reflect allostatic dysregulations of arousal and affect. On the one hand, anger and aggression are "attack" modes of dealing with conflict, distress, or other aspects of PTSD. Hyperarousal and dysregulated angry affect is behavior directed toward others in an attempt to effect emotional discharge or achieve some subjective sense of control in a situation. On the other hand, detachment is behavior that leads to tendencies to move away from others, often in an attempt to create security through actions that minimize contact or interactions with others. Avoidance in interpersonal transactions also reflects allostatic dysregulation of affect, but unlike the attack mode of anger toward others, detachment is more likely to be associated with anxiety, fears, and thoughts of hopelessness, helplessness, and depressive psychiatric symptoms (Harkness, 1993).

In terms of treatment options, Wilson and Kurtz (1997) reviewed the various approaches from the literature on couple and marital therapies. They note that the goals of family assessment within the clinical context differ somewhat from the goals of scientific inquiry (since the objective is treatment orientation rather than research based on controlled trials). The functions of assessing PTSD in a clinical setting with families are as follows: (1) screening and initial evaluation; (2) definition of the client's problem, which may include diagnosis, labeling, or qualification of its severity; (3) planning or establishing treatment goals; and (4) monitoring treatment progress and evaluation of treatment outcome" (p. 350). In a similar vein, Harkness and Zador suggest (see Chapter 13, this volume) that while there are many models for working with PTSD in families and couples, there are several key components for successful PTSD treatment in these populations:

- Psychoeducational information about trauma, PTSD, and its effects on individuals, couples, and families
- Disclosure of the trauma story and its manifestation at the individual, dyadic, or group level
- Identification of the different ways that PTSD has impacted relationships
- Establishing boundaries and processes that facilitate safety in the context of a trusting therapeutic relationship and among dyads or family members
- Identification and screening for potential problem areas such as substance abuse, domestic violence, the presence of weapons, and homicidal and suicidal potentialities
- Assessment and identification of themes that emerge in couples/families around roles in the trauma associated with feelings of shame, guilt, responsibility, anger, blame, and areas of personal and social vulnerability
- Disclosure and working through of unintegrated traumatic material in ways that preserve couple/family unity and healthy relationships
- Assessment of the impact of trauma and its probable long-term consequences to the couple/family

As regards the final point, in some cases, as depicted in the Paramount film *Ordinary People* (1980), a family trauma may cause a split between parents and children or, in turn, lead to estrangement between partners when denial or blame override the healing forces present in the situation. Moreover, as Danieli's (1994) work has shown, traumatized families may exhibit transgenerational effects which have trajectories and consequences between and among generations. As Harkness and Zador note in Chapter 13, some couples/families struggle with dialectical dilemmas in which "families become polarized and live parallel lives, both the family and the survivor feel alone, misunderstood, and unsupported. This polarization is a consequence of the inability to understand, integrate, appreciate, and move on beyond the dialectical dilemma" (p. 349).

It is evident that the treatment of PTSD in couples/families is a multifaceted phenomenon. Since families/couples are bonded social units, the impact of trauma is primarily to the overall stability and cohesiveness of the unit itself. What makes assessment and treatment difficult is that the traumatic event can set in motion changes in the social structure of the family. Roles, interpersonal patterns of coping with trauma, communication and decision-making processes can, and typically do, change when PTSD afflicts the heart of relational patterns. Thus, it is reasonable to speak of the treatment goal as that of restoring healthy attachments, relationships and capacity for intimacy.

Group Psychotherapy for PTSD

In group psychotherapy, there is an implicit assumption that by "being together" survivors of trauma can find opportunities to share and exchange aspects of their traumatic and life experiences with kindred souls. In the context of a group, much like that of a family, social bonds can be forged which provide avenues of friendship, trust, and opportunities for genuine self-disclosure of personal concerns. As such, group psychotherapy is a social-psychological process which is subject to the dynamics of small-group interaction. Each group is unique and defined by the personality characteristics of its members who bring their trauma histories to the group (Aronoff & Wilson, 1985). As a social process, the dynamics of the group are expectable in terms of the evolution of social structure, role differentiation, leadership, socioemotional, and task-oriented behaviors. What makes group psychotherapy unique in terms of the treatment of PTSD is that trauma survivors seek a social process in which to feel secure enough to disclose distressing and painful aspects of their trauma with others in a social milieu of trust, affiliation, commonality of experience, and a tacit knowledge that the other members understand the emotional burden of PTSD and its consequences to their lives. In that regard, the commonality of PTSD's legacy produces a trauma-response pattern which includes a "language system" between the survivor members about the psychological nuances and subtleties of their experiences. Indeed, it is common clinical knowledge that survivors have a belief (or cognitive schema) that "if you weren't there, you wouldn't understand," and are therefore reticent about disclosing information concerning the stressful experiences they endured. In a group of survivors of the same traumatic event there is a tacit understanding of the commonly shared aspects of personal problems associated with that event which facilitates communication.

Nevertheless, the group setting is an arena in which reenactments and reliving phenomena occur. Where trauma involved another person and especially the loss of another survivor during the trauma, interpersonal dynamics may get acted out with other survivors in the group in an attempt to forge closure. In an overly simplified sense, it is possible to say that group psychotherapy creates a milieu in which multiple transference projections (Wilson & Lindy, 1994) can be expressed vis-à-vis interpersonal dynamics. Moreover, as the brilliant sociologist Philip Slater (1959) observed, small groups are "microcosms of reality." In terms of the treatment of PTSD, small therapeutic groups can be microcosms of reality that not only encapsulate the emotional "tone" of individual psychic trauma but afford a means by which to examine and observe the self in the process of active enactments and reenactments of life as it was "then" (i.e., during the trauma) and as expressed "now," in day-to-day living within the group. In an existential sense (Yalom, 1985), the microcosm of the group is a mirror of the client's life and how it has shaped personality, coping with trauma and the nature of relatedness to others. In Table 16.1 we identify the treatment goal of group psychotherapy as the normalization of PTSD response and the enhanced capacity for healthy relationships.

The practitioner considering using group psychotherapy for PTSD or referring a client to a trauma-focused group, should evaluate the potential benefits and liabilities of this treatment modality. Group treatment is not for every trauma survivor, and there are practical considerations to be evaluated before encouraging a PTSD client to attend group treatment.

First of all, it is useful to consider the potential advantages of group psychotherapy that might be beneficial to healing. What is germane to the process of PTSD focal group psychotherapy? What are the social mechanisms and processes that assist group members in the processing and integration of their individual trauma history? What is it about participation in the group, as a social process, that facilitates healing? What is it about the affiliative quality of a group that helps to restore the healthy capacity to cope and relate to others in a salutary manner?

In Chapter 8, this volume, Foy et al. list five basic factors common to group psychotherapy for PTSD:

> (1) homogeneous membership in the group by survivors of the same type of trauma (e.g., combat veterans or sexual assault survivors); (2) acknowledgment and validation of the traumatic exposure; (3) normalization of traumatic responses; (4) utilization of the presence of other individuals with a similar traumatic history to dispel the notion that the therapist cannot be helpful to the survivors because he or she has not shared the experience; and (5) the adoption of a nonjudgmental stance toward behavior required for survival at the time of the trauma. Incorporating these principles facilitates the development of a psychologically safe, respectful, therapeutic environment. (p. 4)

Foy et al. note that the specific therapeutic approaches stem from different theoretical orientations, such as cognitive-behavioral, psychodynamic, supportive, or other frameworks, as to the structure and process of small group interactions for the treatment of PTSD. Furthermore, they note that there are less than 20 scientific studies of group psychotherapy outcomes, most of which provide evidence that this treatment modality is helpful to PTSD clients. But what is it about the process of involvement in group treatment for PTSD that facilitates healing?

While the available scientific data are less adequate than one would ideally prefer, clinical experience, considered together with the robust scientific literature on small-group processes (e.g., Aronoff & Wilson, 1985; Bales, 1979), provides clues as to the mechanisms in PTSD focus groups as to their therapeutic efficacy. These points are summarized as follows:

- When properly organized, based on screening for the psychological "fitness" of members, groups provide a safe place to commune with fellow survivors.
- Homogeneous trauma-focused groups enable the members to speak with each other without fear of misunderstanding or being judged by others (i.e., nonsurvivors) who do not have a psychological context by which to interpret the specifics of a person's trauma story.
- The group provides a setting for attachment, bonding, and identification with others and their emotional difficulties associated with PTSD.
- The group process encourages self-disclosure of the trauma history and PTSD's disruptive legacy to healthy psychosocial functioning. Self-disclosure has been shown to be predictive of current positive mental health status (Kahana, Harel, & Kahana, 1988; Harel, Wilson, & Kahana, 1993; Wilson, Harel, & Kahana, 1988, 1989). Self-disclosure in the context of a safe therapeutic setting contravenes stigmatization, alienation, detachment, and isolation from others.
- Participation in the group reinforces each member's personal identity as a survivor who can relate to and perceive fellow survivors as sharing a historical-cultural framework of traumatic experience (war veterans, refugees, victims of disaster or personal violence, etc.).
- The group provides a social process of acceptance and validation of the traumatic experience which is typically not available in normal transactions in society.
- Participation in the group enhances the perception of personal and social resources to aid in coping.
- Involvement in the group increases the capacity to process unassimilated traumatic memories and the capacity to find meaning in the traumatic experience and life afterward.

- The group process creates a social-psychological structure of interaction in which connection, bonding, and caring can occur within a significant community of friends and fellow survivors.
- The involvement in homogeneous groups facilitates a sense of group identity and each member's sense of self as a survivor. The sense of group identity is important (war veterans, sex abuse survivors, survivors of a school terrorist attack, etc.) because it not only validates the commonality of the experience but anchors it both contextually and sociohistorically in the life of each participant.
- A therapeutic group and involvement with others provide models of recovery, problem solving, conflict resolution, and ways of mastering maladaptive behaviors associated with PTSD. In this regard, groups provide arenas for learning alternative behaviors in terms of healthy coping and adaptation after traumatization.
- Time-limited groups encourage the participant to become proactive and take responsibility for changing maladaptive behavior. The development and initiation of proactive self-care often leads to an increase in an internal locus of control, sense of efficacy, and altruistic behaviors (Harel et al., 1993; Wilson et al., 1989; Wilson, Harel, & Kahana, 1988).

In conclusion, it may be seen that group psychotherapy is a different modality of treatment from the other 11 presented in Table 16.1. As a group process, this treatment process facilitates the normalization of PTSD as a stress response syndrome and enhances the capacity of healthy bonding, attachments, and modes of interpersonal behavior.

Severe Mental Illness and PTSD Treatment

The severe mental illnesses (SMI) such as schizophrenia, major depression, delusional disorders, psychotic disorders, and bipolar disorders have been the traditional province of modern psychiatry. The complexity of severe mental illness gave rise to nosological systems of classification and scientific studies of their etiology and pathological sequelae. As noted by Kim T. Mueser and Stanley D. Rosenberg in Chapter 14, this volume, recent epidemiological and national comorbidity studies have discovered that lifetime exposure to a traumatic event is quite prevalent in U.S. society, with population estimates ranging between 39% and 56%. Thus, the question naturally arises as to the relationship between trauma exposure and the development of SMI. Further, if there is a correlation between trauma exposure and SMI, is there also a relationship between SMI and PTSD in the history of the patient's illness?

In terms of an operational definition of SMI, Mueser and Rosenberg (Chapter 14) define the condition as follows:

> Severe mental illness is a general term used to describe individuals with psychiatric disorders that have a profound impact on functioning in a wide range of domains, such as the ability to work, to care for oneself and live independently in the community, and to maintain rewarding interpersonal relationship. . . . Psychotic symptoms such as hallucinations or delusions are common but not universal in this population. Due to their difficulties working and living independently in the community, patients with SMI frequently receive disability income, such as Social Security Disability Income (SSDI) or Social Security Supplemental Income (SSSI)." (p. 356)

In the simplest formulations then, SMI is associated with impairment in functioning, a fact well known to practitioners who work with such patients. But what if the person with SMI also has a history of trauma and the symptoms of PTSD? As Mueser and Rosenberg note, "only three studies have examined PTSD in patients with SMI, but each study suggests notably higher rates of PTSD" (Chapter 14, p. 358). Moreover, the results of these studies revealed that PTSD was not only underdiagnosed in SMI patients but their clinical records lacked information as to the specificity of their trauma histories and lacked diagnostic codes for PTSD. Clearly, the underdiagnoses and infrequent documentation trauma histories, as well as lack of a DSM-IV diagnosis (of 309.81) for the PTSD, had treatment implications. Most notably was the tendency to focus on the SMI and not to explore the patient's trauma history and PTSD symptomatology. As noted earlier in this chapter, dual diagnosis is not uncommon in PTSD, especially major depression and substance abuse. However, in the case of SMI, it is as if the patient's clinical status is being viewed through the "lens" of SMI rather than focusing the lens more carefully to sharpen the resolution enough to "see" PTSD and its relation to SMI. Mueser and Rosenberg in Chapter 14 hypothesize as follows:

> PTSD is mainly responsible for the relationship between trauma and more severe clinical presentation in patients with SMI. PTSD is given a central mediating role in this model because the symptoms which define PTSD, as well as its common clinical correlations, can be theoretically linked to a worse prognosis of SMI. PTSD is hypothesized to both directly and indirectly increase symptom severity and risk of relapse in patients with SMI. PTSD can directly affect SMI through increased avoidance behavior, distress related to reexperiencing the trauma, and physiological overarousal. Common correlates of PTSD can also indirectly affect SMI, including retraumatization, a poor working alliance, and substance abuse. (pp. 360–361)

The treatment of patients with SMI and PTSD is at least as complex and difficult as that reviewed for dual diagnosis and complex PTSD. The combination of PTSD and SMI presents a challenge to practitioners because of the severity of the psychiatric disorder and the manner in which PTSD overlaps with some of the symptoms of SMI (e.g., hallucinations, intrusive thoughts, images and feelings; suspicion, doubt, mistrust, guardedness; reticence of self-disclosure; secretiveness; depressive vegetative symptoms; and hyperarousal states with emotional lability; see Chapter 2 for a discussion of the 65 PTSD symptoms in the core five dimensions derived from the allostatic tetrahedral model). Moreover, not only is there the possibility of SMI/PTSD symptom overlap, but as Mueser and Rosenberg note, PTSD mediates and to some extent "drives" SMI behavioral manifestations.

At present there are not enough scientifically controlled studies of SMI/PTSD treatment. Mueser and Rosenberg suggest some practical guidelines for practitioners and those working in institutional settings with PTSD embedded within SMI.

- Combined treatment approaches for SMI and PTSD are useful. As with other PTSD comorbidity approaches, SMI/PTSD requires a formulation as to how to address the multilayered complexity of the patient with a history of trauma, PTSD, and the development of SMI.
- The timing and phasing of PTSD therapy using cognitive-behavioral, pharmacological, or psychodynamic core PTSD treatments requires (1) careful assessment of the patient's mental status, (2) his or her capacity to tolerate a core PTSD treatment, and (3) the risk of SMI by exposure of the trauma material.
- Psychoeducation and support for the activities of daily living is crucial to contravene the debilitating symptoms of SMI.
- The routine case management of a patient should include a comprehensive trauma history, adequate psychological and psychometric assessment, and proper charting of the history and PTSD diagnosis in the file.
- Service provision requires carefully coordinated cooperation between mental health providers in order to match the needed services to the patient's needs so as to achieve optimal rehabilitation strategies.
- Given the complexity of SMI/PTSD, long-term care is likely, and it is expectable that relapse, episodic manifestations of PTSD, and chronicity of SMI will occur.
- Standardization yet flexible interventions for SMI/PTSD need to be developed, evaluated, and subjected to scientific study as part of comprehensive rehabilitation—treatment programs.

In conclusion, Table 16.1 indicates that the primary treatment goal for SMI and PTSD is social reintegration and support for the activities of daily living.

REFERENCES

Agger, I., & Jensen, S. (1993). The psychosexual trauma of torture. In J. P. Wilson & B. Raphael (Eds.), *International handbook of traumatic stress syndromes* (pp. 703–715). New York: Plenum Press.

American Psychiatric Association. (1994). *Diagnositc and statistical manual of mental disorders* (4th ed.). Washington, DC: Author.

Aronoff, J., & Wilson, J. P. (1985). *Personality in the social process*. Hillsdale, NJ: Erlbaum.

Bales, R. F. (1979). *Personality and interpersonal behavior*. New York: Holt, Rinehart & Winston.

Blank, A. S., Jr. (1985). The unconscious flashback to the war in Vietnam veterans: Clinical mystery, legal defense, and community problem. In S. M. Sonnenberg, A. S. Blank, Jr., & J. A. Talbott (Eds.), *The trauma of war: Stress and recovery in Vietnam veterans*. Washington, DC: American Psychiatric Press.

Breslau, N. (1998). Epidemiology of trauma and posttraumatic stress disorder. In R. Yehuda (Ed.). *Psychological trauma* (pp. 1–27). Washington, DC: American Psychiatric Press.

Bryant, R. A., Harvey, A. G., Dang, S. T., Sackville, T., & Basten, C. (1998). Treatment of acute stress disorder: A comparison of cognitive-behavioral therapy and supportive counseling. *Journal of Consulting and Clinical Psychology, 66*(5), 862–866.

Bryant, R. A., Sackville, T., Dang, S. T., Moulds, M., & Guthrie, R. (1999). Treating acute stress disorder: An evaluation of cognitive-behavior therapy and supportive counseling techniques. *American Journal of Psychiatry, 156*(11), 1780–1786.

Danieli, Y. (Ed.). (1994). *International handbook of multigenerational legacies of trauma*. New York: Plenum Press.

Erikson, E. (1950). *Childhood and society*. New York: Norton.

Erikson, E. (1968). *Identity, youth and crisis*. New York: Norton.

Flannery, R. B. (1990). *Becoming stress resistant*. New York: Continuum Press.

Foa, E., Hearst-Ikeda, D., & Perry, J. (1995). Evaluation of a brief cognitive-behavioral program for the prevention of chronic PTSD in recent assault victims. *Journal of Consulting and Clinical Psychology, 63*(6), 948–955.

Friedman, M. J. (2000). *Posttraumatic stress disorders*. Kansas City, MO: Compact Clinicals.

Harel, Z., Wilson, J. P., & Kahana, B. (1993). War and remembrance: The legacy of Pearl Harbor. In J. P. Wilson & B. Raphael (Eds.), *International handbook of traumatic stress syndromes* (pp. 263–275). New York: Plenum Press.

Harkness, L. L. (1993). Transgenerational transmission of war-related trauma. In J. P. Wilson & B. Raphael (Eds.), *International handbook of traumatic stress syndromes* (pp. 635–643). New York: Plenum Press.

Herman, J. (1992). *Trauma and recovery*. New York: Basic Books.

Horowitz, M. (1986). *Stress response syndromes*. Northvale, NJ: Aronson.

Juhler, M. (1993). Medical diagnosis and treatment of torture survivors. *International handbook of traumatic stress syndromes*. New York: Plenum Press.

Kahana, B., Harel, Z., & Kahana, B. (1988). Predictors of psychological well-being among survivors of the Holocaust. In J. P. Wilson, Z. Harel, & B. Kahana (Eds.), *Human adaptation to extreme stress: From the Holocaust to Vietnam* (pp. 171–192). New York: Plenum Press.

Kinzie, J. D. (1988). The psychiatric effects of massive trauma on Cambodian refugees. In J. P. Wilson, Z. Harel, & B. Kahana (Eds.), *Human adaptation to extreme stress: From the Holocaust to Vietnam* (pp. 305–317). New York: Plenum Press.

Kinzie, J. D. (1993). Posttraumatic effects and their treatment among Southeast Asian refugees. In J. P. Wilson & B. Raphael (Eds.), *International handbook of traumatic stress syndromes*. New York: Plenum Press.

Lindy, J. D. (1993). Focal psychoanalytic psychotherapy of posttraumatic stress disorder. In J. P. Wilson & B. Raphael (Eds.), *International handbook of traumatic stress syndromes* (pp. 803–811). New York: Plenum Press.

Marsella, A. J., Friedman, M. J., Gerrity, E., & Scurfield, R. M. (Eds.). (1996). *Ethnocultural aspects of post-traumatic stress disorder: Issues, research and applications*. Washington, DC: American Psychological Association Press.

Niederland, W. G. (1964). Psychiatric disorders among persecution victims: A contribution to the understanding of concentration camp pathology and its aftermath. *Journal of Nervous and Mental Disease, 139,* 458–474.

Ordinary people [film]. (1980). Hollywood, CA: Paramount Studios.

Raphael, B., & Wilson, J. P. (2000). *Psychological debriefings: Theory, practice, evidence.* Cambridge, UK: Cambridge University Press.

Resnick, H. A., Acierno, R., Holmes, M., Kilpatrick, D., & Jager, N. (1999). Prevention of post-rape psychopathology: Preliminary findings of a controlled acute rape treatment study. *Journal of Anxiety Disorders, 13*(4), 359–370.

Rose, S., & Bisson, J. (1998). Brief early psychological interventions following trauma: A systematic review of the literature. *Journal of Traumatic Stress, 11*(4), 697–710.

Slater, P. (1959). *Microcosm.* New York: Wiley.

Smith, E. M., & North, C. S. (1993). Posttraumatic stress disorder in natural disasters and technological accidents. In J. P. Wilson & B. Raphael (Eds.), *International handbook of traumatic stress syndromes* (pp. 405–419). New York: Plenum Press.

Watkins, J. G., & Watkins, H. H. (1997). *Ego states.* New York: Norton.

Wilson, J. P. (Ed.). (1989). *Trauma, transformation and healing.* New York: Brunner/Mazel.

Wilson, J. P., Harel, Z., & Kahana, B. (Eds.). (1988). *Human adaptation to extreme stress: From the Holocaust to Vietnam.* New York: Plenum Press.

Wilson, J. P., Harel, Z., & Kahana, B. (1989). The day of infamy: The legacy of Pearl Harbor. In J. P. Wilson (Ed.), *Trauma, transformation and healing* (pp. 129–159). New York: Brunner/Mazel.

Wilson, J. P., & Kurtz, R. (1997). Assessing PTSD in couples and families. In J. P. Wilson & T. M. Keane (Eds.), *Assessing psychological trauma and PTSD* (pp. 349–373). New York: Guilford Press.

Wilson, J. P., & Lindy, J. D. (1994). *Countertransference in the treatment of PTSD.* New York: Guilford Press.

Wilson, J. P., & Raphael, B. (2000). *Psychological debriefings.* Cambridge, UK: Cambridge Press.

Yalom, I. D. (1985). *The theory and practice of group psychotherapy* (3rd ed.). New York: Basic Books.

17

Respecting the Trauma Membrane: Above All, Do No Harm

JACOB D. LINDY and JOHN P. WILSON

In witnessing the mental health response to trauma and its aftermath for the past 30 years or so, we have seen a pendulum shift: from a time when mental health clinicians and scientists—and their diagnostic nomenclature—turned a blind eye toward trauma to a time when aggressive mental health responses are offered sometimes without request, at nearly all phases of this difficult and often chronic condition (Raphael & Wilson, 2000). It is as though the mental health community, once an avoidant anti-war (type I, Wilson & Lindy, 1994) countertransference community, has moved to a therapeutically over-ambitious (type II) countertransference position.

While some 30 years ago those of us out in the field said to our colleagues, "Please come out from your ivory towers into the disaster community where trauma is going unrecognized and untreated," now we are saying to our colleagues, "Slow down, consider the person, the trauma and its context, and above all do no harm." Clearly, the advancement of knowledge has led to a deeper understanding of post-traumatic stress disorder (PTSD) and with it a new awareness of the needs for interventions and ethical precautions.

Encouraged by the beliefs that talking helps and that the expression of emotion is a universal good, emergency workers in the field of disaster now sometimes urge the recently traumatized patient to "Tell me exactly what happened" and to experience now warded-off affect states: "Tell me exactly how it felt." In fact, the trauma survivor may be using quite appropriate emergency defenses such as denial and disbelief, defenses quite possibly linked with emergency release of neurohormones (see Raphael & Wilson, 2000, for a discussion of types of debriefing and their use).

In time-limited psychotherapy shortly after the trauma, a clinician feeling the pressures from third-party payers may demand that the client integrate previously undigested psychic duress too soon, as though it were within the patient's potential to accomplish within the time frame designated by the managed care provisions and limited insurance coverage. Time pressures and the urge to "uncover" trauma's injury to the client poses risks in the treatment process.

Later, during court proceedings, the survivor is likely to be questioned in great detail about the trauma events by people, even forensic mental health professionals with whom they have no relationship and some of whom proceed without concern for the impact of the rekindling of overwhelming affect. But who can guarantee that no harm occurs in the courtroom and legal system of justice?

Along with these aggressive approaches has gone a decrease in appreciation for the value of ego defenses, those unconscious activities by which the psychically injured protect themselves until they have the resources to face and work through pain. Today, as we respond from the pendulum's swing, it is timely to reconsider the role of defenses in traumatic states, their adaptive functioning, and the therapist's role in valuing them. We would do well to heed the old medical maxim, "Above all do no harm."

DO NO HARM IN DIAGNOSING

Just as we did a disservice some 30 years ago (i.e., pre-DSM-III until about 1985) by not giving survivors of trauma a legitimate diagnostic label if symptoms lasted more than 3 months, we take the public health risk today of denying services to a wide variety of people with posttraumatic conditions because their symptom picture falls outside criteria of PTSD. Trauma may cause PTSD, but it can lead to symptoms, personal struggles, and conflicts which defy psychiatric labels per se but may require psychotherapy. Indeed the condition which did not exist 30 years ago is now "written in stone" in a variety of contexts and scientific arenas (Friedman, 2000).

In this regard, rigid application of DSM-IV excludes at least four important posttrauma populations who need our study and care:

1. *Posttraumatic states may be incorporated into character structure in such a way that PTSD is no longer the presenting issue.* For example, a former flight controller, now a tax adviser, came to treatment at the request of his wife, who had noted a decline in his interpersonal interests save for a group of clients all of

whom were in the process of settling estates. The interest was obsessive and grim. One by one he paid attention only to the needs of these suffering families but without personal satisfaction or relief. His interpersonal world had become encapsulated in a posttrauma circumstance. The patient had been a flight controller when he was involved in guiding an aircraft to a crash landing in which some passenger died or were injured. He was convinced he had not done his job properly and was responsible for the deaths and the suffering of the passengers who were injured in the airplane crash, as well as of the families of the victims. He did not present with the intrusive, physiological, or classical numbing signs of PTSD. Rather, his world was realigned in a grim and tragic way as he unconsciously atoned for his trauma-related decisions.

A number of survivors of the Buffalo Creek dam collapse in 1972 who were followed 20 years later showed restricted lives, preoccupied with the loss through catastrophe of close family members, and ritualistically preserving life as it was before the massive flood which hit this rural coal-mining valley in West Virginia. These survivors failed to meet criteria for PTSD, but their lives and character were significantly affected by it (Honig, Grace, Lindy, Newman, & Titchener, 1993).

2. *Posttraumatic states may be heavily influenced by concomitant grief and by culture sufficient to alter the presenting clinical picture.* For example, following the genocide in which 800,000 out of a population of 6 million were slaughtered in a 4-month period in Rwanda in 1994, the local populace came to call suffering survivors by the Kenyarwandan name, *ihahamuka*, a state of being without life.[1] Yet, when one of the country's two psychiatrists studied these people, few met the criteria of PTSD (Hagengimana, 1999). Rather, having lost parents, spouses, and children, these persons (often women) were overcome with frozen grief[2] which masked PTSD and other syndromes. Further, a cultural overlay which included witchcraft and somatization of emotional concerns made the presenting pictures look more like organic illness and irrational fear than like classic PTSD.

3. Because *certain victimized persons are still in the traumatizing situation*, as for example battered wives, and politically harassed individuals escaping but not yet free of totalitarian regimes, the symptom picture may differ from classic PTSD (see Herman, 1993; van der Kolk, 1994). Suspicion, indecisiveness, and anxiety with regard to ambivalently held objects may carry the day. In PTSD, dreams may take a variety of forms, some of which may cover traumatic ones, and reenactments may be real experiences rather than irrationally distorted ones.

4. *Some trauma is set off in our technological age simply by widespread information,* such as TV reports about people's exposure to chromosome-changing toxic agents and radioactivity. These conditions have a distinctly somatic and paranoid picture. Intrusions are of fantasied happenings like explosions or de-

formed offspring. Discontinuity is one of dread regarding the next generation. Increasingly these syndromes deserve our attention and are reasonably
considered as related to PTSD (Green, Lindy, & Grace, 1999).

DO NO HARM IN TREATMENT PLANNING

Today, in contrast to some 30 years ago, there are many treatment options offered for PTSD (Matsakis, 1997; Friedman, 2000; Wilson, 1994). One of the
purposes of this book is to assist the clinician in determining which method
may be best for his or her patient. In Chapter 15 we reviewed the many cases
presented in this book and examined how the choice of the most appropriate
treatment method is a function of many variables including type duration
and repetition of trauma, type of pathology, chronicity, concomitant diagnosis, etc. Our point here is simply that there are multiple portals of entry with
the core treatment approaches which can be utilized in the treatment of posttraumatic states, including posttraumatic stress disorders and allied conditions (Breslau, 1998).

1. Where posttraumatic character change is the presenting problem one
should consider strongly the psychodynamic approach. Posttraumatic character change is a persistent realignment of object relations and pathogenic
fantasies which have developed posttrauma. These changes constrict and define the person, and will likely be activated in the transference. In this way
they may be open to interpretation and working through. Indeed, posttrauma character change is one of the specific indications for psychodynamic
treatment of PTSD.

2. Among PTSD patients who present through the portal of specific
symptom clusters (see our Chapter 2, this volume), rather than with character change, there is a group worth noting who are particularly helped in analytic psychotherapy (Lindy, 1993). In these cases of PTSD, the patient's dominant symptoms, when considered from within the trauma context, belong
not to the patient's own threat to life experience but rather to the experience
of another, often a victim in the trauma with a worse or fatal outcome. For
example, a survivor of a supper club fire developed urinary urgency, the
physical sensation belonging to her friend who had excused herself to go to
the lavatory moments before fire killed the friend. The patient did extremely
well in a time-limited dynamic psychotherapy. A Vietnam veteran with psy-
chogenic chest pain, who was haunted by memories of a little girl with a
crushed chest who had been run over by his truck, also did well in focal psychoanalytic treatment (Lindy, 1993; Wilson & Lindy, 1994).

This issue of role displacement in the trauma configuration is also true
of traumatic dreams, fantasies, and somatic symptoms. From a dynamic perspective, the unconscious need to take on the suffering of another in the trau-

ma scene may represent a particular ego organization which may benefit from analytic psychotherapy (Lindy, 1993; Krystal, 1988, 1993).

DO NO HARM IN INTERVENING: TRAUMA AND DEFENSE IN THE CLINICAL SITUATION

As therapists, we do not so much begin to treat our trauma survivor patients on the basis of our own initiative, but rather we begin when they invite us to enter the space covered by the trauma membrane. As we noted in Chapter 2, there are five portals of entry into PTSD ego spaces and the understanding of the client's psychological reality as shaped by trauma. The trauma membrane, initially a barrier designed by friends and kin to protect the traumatically impaired survivor, becomes in time an internally based structure, a semipermeable membrane which covers the space left in the repression barrier by the trauma experiences (Lindy, 1985). Being invited under this membrane (i.e., as a therapist) comes as we pass tests regarding our knowledge concerning the trauma circumstance, and also pass tests of trustworthiness. Survivors continue a similar process of testing us and then inviting us throughout the therapy into their phenomenal reality. In fact, clients want us to understand their "inner reality" of traumatization but use ego defenses to protect their perceived and experienced sense of vulnerability. When we accept that invitation, at any given moment, as therapists we are aware of three elements influencing our tactical decisions as to where and how to guide the therapy: (1) we remember the relevant traumatic details which the survivor has already shared; (2) we are concerned with the dilemmas in his or her current life or transference life which he or she conveys within a general affect state; and (3) we observe the trauma-protecting defenses which guard against taking on too much in the next step. As therapists, we are tempted to ignore the third element, the trauma-protecting defenses. Instead, we attend only to these questions: What is the next layer of detail in the trauma? What is the dynamic meaning of the current object of interest to the patient? What is next in the trauma story? But by proceeding to what is next, what is deeper, we may inadvertently attack the defense, plunging the survivor back into the trauma itself, while ignoring the affect state and ego defense of the present. Such is the dialectic risk in treating PTSD. For the analytic psychotherapist such action risks harm, the harm of precipitating more trauma than one can deal with at the moment, the harm of damaging the working alliance, the harm of damaging the newly reforming defenses and their ability to replace the trauma membrane. The awareness of such potential harm signals, in different ways, the value of supervision and consultation in such critical junctures in psychotherapy.

Trauma by definition overwhelms the protective capacity of defenses, it disrupts the stimulus barrier (Freud, 1955/1920); it tears a hole in the survivors' belief in their capacity to cope with whatever befalls them. Posttraumatically, the survivor dreads a repeat of that state of being overwhelmed and works hard to protect him- or herself from such a repetition. What begins to form in the place of the tear in the repression barrier is at first a thin layer or trauma membrane designed to keep noxious (i.e., trauma-reminding stimuli) away and to let in only those sources of stimuli which will soothe the wound. Gradually, the lining of this membrane becomes slightly thicker as defenses specifically responding to the trauma or later defenses characteristic of the premorbid personality advance like layers of new epithelium in a healing but still "open" wound. These theoretical metaphors underline cautionary principles which should guide the therapist. From a technical point of view, the therapist is concerned lest his or her intervention pierce the newly forming protective barrier.

CASE ILLUSTRATIONS

Margaret is a 35-year-old woman whose father attacked her when angry and violated sexual boundaries with her. She works as a school counselor and brings into her sessions repeated stories of children being abused physically and sexually by parents. In the stories she is the strident and haughty yet ineffective counselor who splits off her own terrified feelings.

In another instance, Michael, referred for work inhibition and an absence of positive relationships, was the victim of his older foster brother's repeated choking him as a small child to the point of passing out and the victim of the brother's performing anal intercourse on him at the same time. Now, paradoxically, he mocks and teases his male therapist threatening to grab his notes, or steal an object from his desk. These threats, at times playful and at other times menacing, make the therapist anxious, then furious. He feels that the patient's childish attacks are an insult to the therapy.

In circumstances such as these the therapist is often frustrated, prone to a countertransference response, and as a result is in a position to cause harm. Returning to the case of Margaret, who defended against trauma with haughtiness, the therapist may think to himself: you speak of others rather than yourself; you pose as powerful accuser covering your own experience as the timidly abused; your tales of the failures of others to confront trauma are endless; isn't it time that you addressed the helplessness and abuse you experienced as a child? Yet if he were to act on such thoughts, the interventions might risk harm by penetrating defenses without appreciating their value both now and in the past, how they came to be, and what functions they serve.

Or, as in the case of Michael, where the patient has turned passive into active, the therapist in his anger at having his own boundaries penetrated may angrily snap back, "You [his patient] are willfully breaking the treat-

ment's boundaries; stop it, you are behaving like a bad and vengeful child."
In such a circumstance, Michael's defense of turning passive to active would
have catapulted the therapist into a harmful countertransference, speaking
like the attacking foster brother.

In these circumstances what kinds of interventions would "do no
harm"? With countertransference in tow, Margaret's therapist could show interest in the stories of the abused children: "What was it like for the victims,
and how does it feel relating their stories while being powerless to influence
the situation despite your best efforts?" This could lead to: "It is so difficult
here exploring these traumatic situations about which you have such very
deep feelings." Such interventions respect the cause of defensive haughtiness
while facilitating the patient's choice to allow the therapist to engage the next
deeper level.

With Michael, the therapist, with countertransference in tow, might
point out that it is no fun feeling helpless as one is being mercilessly teased or
threatened to the point of having one's privacy invaded; and that that situation must be one which is uncomfortably familiar to him. Again, the intervention respects the origin of the defensive turning active into passive without attacking it.

We know that in the natural history of efforts to manage trauma, survivors substitute various combinations of defenses to fill the hole in the ego's
protective barrier. Shortly before and in the midst of trauma there may be
gross denial and disbelief: "This can't be happening to me; I'm in a dream
and tomorrow when I awaken, the horror will be gone." In its most extreme
case, when the trauma is too severe and too often and the ego too immature,
there may be dissociation to the point of ego fragmentation, with the fragments over time having the potential to become separate centers of initiative.
One fragment trying to preserve an essential tie to the perpetrating figure
might turn on the self saying, "It was I who brought on these monstrous happenings"; another might say, "I'll kill you for damaging that child"; another
might persecute in return for the assault; another might cower in terror; yet
another might identify with the perpetrator, becoming a murderer or a harlot
of unsurpassed magnificence. These defensive fragments in the most extreme
case, as in dissociative disorder, represent one form of pathological adaptation to being overwhelmed by trauma. Disavowing the trauma represents a
continuance of the initial denial and disbelief: "I know that these terrible
things happened to me, but if I act and think as if nothing has changed I can
go about my life and function, although with considerably less energy and affective commitment." What was initially a trauma membrane has now become a line of disavowal.

For many survivors, gradual accretions of other defenses supplement
the disavowal. Among these are efforts to isolate, to displace somatize, to
turn passive into active and less pathological forms of dissociation. Narcissistic aspects of the trauma also call into play narcissistic defenses, haughti-

ness, or reactively omnipotent or grandiose fantasies. Early on, even apparent sublimations can have such drivenness that they do not easily fall in the area of conflict-free egofunctioning, while later on, more neutralized sublimations may indicate that the working through of the trauma has been more complete.

While trauma always sits in the room with the patient and clinician in terms of the potential for reenactment, in a more palpable way it is the patient's fragile newly forming defenses against that trauma which are most crucial to him or her at the time and the most relevant subject of the therapist's interest. These defenses may have been precisely those emergency defenses which were present at the time of the trauma. For example, Tina (see Chapters 5 and 15, case 17) on experiencing part of her trauma in the office with the therapist, literally got up and pinned her back against the opposite wall. She later explained that when she was pinned down in the actual sexual trauma as a child, this out-of-body dissociation was the way she protected herself. Or emerging defenses at the time of being overwhelmed by the original trauma may be the resumption of older ones. For example, one patient having lost her family and belongings in a natural disaster, sat for hours counting and arranging small trinkets recovered from the house, trying to rearrange her broken world. Such patients do not need mental health workers to plunge past these defenses, dismissing them as irrelevant, or to delve further as if the defenses were interfering with the real work of recovering the content of traumatic memory. Rather, these situations call for empathy with the tremendous effort to maintain cohesion in the face of traumatic overload. Taking charge, testing the therapist to see if one can tease or threaten beyond the limits, rearranging things carefully while knowing that elsewhere they are in such disorder, all these are fragile and pathological defenses at the site of the trauma membrane. They sit in the room and demand being dealt with.

So long as defenses are in the service of reinforcing disavowal, the therapist does not have permission to make links to the trauma situation. So long as the therapist is guided by a strategy of digging out the trauma content, he or she is at risk of plunging past these fragile defenses and exacerbating not a dosed trauma segment but an overwhelming traumatic reenactment and a potential fracture of the therapeutic alliance—in short, of causing harm.

On the other hand, if we are guided by an appreciation of how the patient is trying to manage the pressure of the trauma memory in the present with these defenses we are more likely to be empathic with his real present struggle that the trauma will break through and find him unprepared. By gaining trust, respect for dosage, we prepare the ground for the patient's own decision to open up trauma content.

Much of the literature on the therapy of traumatic state appropriately focuses on the necessity of building a safe environment and trust (Wilson & Lindy, 1994). This is not an activity limited to the initial phase of the therapy, and it is easily violated at any stage of therapy. At any point in the treatment our interventions demonstrate our trustworthiness. When as a result of intervention the patient feels he has more ability and energy to work, capacity for empathy for himself and others, and more understanding of the traumatic situation, then our interventions continue to engender trust. When clinical intervention break defenses (often in an acting out of a countertransference) and precipitate an overwhelming of the psychic balance, we have damaged that safe space. Our fingers are metaphorically on the window to the trauma, opening it only so far as the patient is ready to tolerate. And we measure this readiness, as does he in the relative strength and flexibility of those defenses. This is the central message of "do no harm."

Later during the consolidating phase of treatment we will watch as the survivor regains aspects of himself lost since the trauma: his sense of humor; his creative impulse; his capacity for affection; his energy for work; and his compassion for others in a similar plight. But if we are watching carefully we will also see that defenses gain in maturation and usefulness. Some of these will be traits that made up the client's pretraumatic character. Others will be new posttraumatic changes in personality process. For healthier defenses as they gain force and familiarity now take on stronger traits in the client's everyday life. What were fragile and ineffective traits trying to block traumatic content, such as isolation, become constructive competence in work tasks. Projections might become a capacity for empathy; paranoid traits might become insistence on moral principles and an appropriate demand for protection and loyalty.

TRAUMA AND DEFENSE IN THE NATURAL SETTING: LESSONS TO BE LEARNED

While we researchers in the PTSD field have done much to quantify and factor-analyze the prevalence of symptom clusters of clinical and nonclinical populations following exposure to trauma, we have done little to study in single cases how traumatic experiences become detoxified in nontreatment settings. As investigators we must better understand trauma-binding defenses in nonclinical populations which successfully encapsulate trauma sufficiently to permit return of function and gradual working through via reactivation at expectable points in natural life activities: anniversaries, developmental phases of children, parents and self, etc.

If we are most likely to do harm to our trauma patients when we do not understand or respect the role of defense in the healing of the condition, then we must learn more about the natural history of defense in relation to trauma containment or encapsulation. This was one of the reasons we embarked on follow-up interviews of children who were in the Buffalo Creek dam break and flood in 1972. Could we learn something of how defenses worked in survivors who did not develop PTSD (Honig et al., 1993)?

Louise, a 28-year-old divorced woman now living far from her childhood home, had experienced the disaster at Buffalo Creek as an 8-year-old child. In the course of a routine research interview about her current life, health, and symptoms, her experience in the flood and childhood health and symptoms, she answered questions almost cheerfully. Her affect was primarily in the present, which was challenged but happy. She was especially happy being interviewed in that it reminded her of home. It also reminded her of the interviews some 20 years earlier by attorneys and psychiatrists, which had been part of her awakening to an outside world. In fact one of the effects of the flood was to allow her to live with relatives outside the hollow, and begin her trek to a broader life experience. In her first narration of the flood experience, she explained that her uncle carried her up the mountain to safety. But when the interviewer asked her to draw her experiences in the flood and to comment on the drawings as she was proceeding, an odd event occurred. She inadvertently unmasked a previously buried trauma detail, the sight of a truncated baby.

Louise remembered being carried up the mountain by her uncle since her leg was in a cast from a broken ankle. At some point in the climb he passed Louise to her grandmother. Now it became clear what had happened in that moment. Her uncle had seen a mud-caked baby and turned Louise over to her grandmother so that he could determine whether the baby were alive and what should be done with it next. Previously Louise had only remembered Grandma's shoulder and her blanket and their reassuring and protective function. Only now was she remembering the detail which had caused her uncle to transfer her suddenly to Grandma. It was the horrific sight of the baby with the truncated body which that blanket hid from her. Internally she had constructed an encapsulating symbol, Grandma's blanket, which served to isolate the traumatic image and protect her from the psychological consequences of the sight. In fact, she had seen the baby and been puzzled, then terrified, by what she saw. Some of the horror returned now in the interview.

During the flood, Louise had been exposed to the destruction of her home and community, the near death of her mother and family, and a grotesque image of a dead mud-caked baby, but clearly there were efforts by her uncle and grandmother to protect her. She was unaware that the older siblings absorbed her mother's crisis and took on guilt in regard to it. Grandma unconsciously extended the impact of her shielding symbol, Grandma's blanket, so that there was retrograde suppression of the visual stimulus. In no recounting of the flood had Louise ever remembered this traumatic detail. In retrospect she noted that Grandma's blanket, which she did remember vividly, had later in her childhood become associated with a vague sense of unease. At the time of the original interview Louise was functioning slightly below school level but gave no evidence of PTSD. At a follow-up interview again no PTSD was observed on standardized tests. Defenses had served Louise well.

Cases such as these will teach us much of the mechanisms of sequestering and working through of trauma. Informed with such data, our own work will likely be respectful of the value of defenses which sequester effectively, and cautious lest we disturb them with our good intentions.

DO NO HARM TERMINATING

PTSD, especially complex PTSD, may be a lifelong condition with integration limited and treatment necessary on an intermittent rather than constant basis. In these circumstances, we may harm patients by asserting that brief treatments will cure (Raphael & Wilson, 2000).

The building of a therapeutic alliance is central to the development of trust, the establishment of a safe space, and the working though of trauma. We should do no harm by placing trauma patients in clinical settings where there are frequent turnovers of therapists. Stability through consistency is an important theme in posttraumatic therapies.

The closeness which develops in the successful treatment of patients with PTSD, like the attachment of fellow survivors, is one that is lasting and also gratifying. Therapists feeling that their treatment should continue indefinitely may be experiencing a positive attachment countertransference resistance to termination. We risk doing harm when we as therapists fall into the seductive trap that we are the only ones who can be of help to a particular survivor/patient.

In order to maintain a level perspective regarding the pressures on termination, the therapist should be using specific criteria in determining when attention to the trauma has been sufficient; a useful end point might be the resumption of engagement in phase-appropriate task, rather than the complete elimination of symptoms.

When attending to the patient's everyday life has been part of the treatment throughout, relative stability in that area is easier to assess than when the present-life activities has been split off as though not central to the treatment effort.

THE HARM WE DID; THE HARM WE'RE DOING

Looking back historically, analytic therapists may have caused harm some 30 years ago when they prematurely attributed symptoms in adolescents and adults to events in early childhood rather than recognizing the pain of current trauma (Simon, 1992). Unwittingly they said to their trauma patients, "Neither I nor my theory can bear the intensity of your current pain." Analytic therapists may have caused harm some 30 years ago by treating reports of childhood sexual abuse as though they were fantasies rather than real. Unwittingly they said, "Neither I nor my theory can endure the idea that these horrendous events may have really happened." However, with 100 years of clinical wisdom, we now know that denials of the past are not limited to medical practitioners or patients.

In today's atmosphere therapists risk doing different kinds of harm. Because the trauma is now seen as all too real, therapists risk hraming patients when they deprive them of an unconscious life which surrounds trauma with necessary irrational defenses and compensatory fantasies. Finally, in certain cases, we can cause harm by focusing exclusively on the trauma before us, which blinds us from seeing more buried and as yet unacknowledged traumas that may have laid the groundwork for this one (Wilson & Lindy, 1994).

SUMMARY

In the past three decades the pendulum has swung in the management of the survivor with posttrauma pathology from a period of professional isolation to a period of professional zeal. While we cannot help patients whose illnesses we do not recognize, study, or treat, once we do engage our therapeutic energies we would do well to follow the old medical maxim, "Do no harm." In doing no harm, the therapist working with PTSD needs sensitivity, sustained empathic efforts, and patience. The therapist's clinical sensitivity must be attuned to the necessary role of defenses in the patient to protect the injured spaces of the ego which require guarding until psychological safety is achieved. As the case histories presented above illustrate, the PTSD client will find unique ways to test the therapist's trust, groundedness, and capacity to create a safe environment. Trauma-specific transference reactions are expectable and will tax countertransference processes in the therapist (Wilson & Lindy, 1994). Psychodynamic approaches to posttraumatic therapy recognize multiple ways that the challenge of "doing no harm" is evident throughout the process of providing proper care, from diagnosis to treatment to termination.

NOTES

1. Robert J. Lifton (1967) observed a similar phenomenon among Japanese survivors of the atomic bomb at Hiroshima were labled by the post-bomb society as *hibakusha* or atomic-disease-affected persons whose psychic reality was a state of being somewhere between life and death.

2. Again, Robert J. Lifton (1967) found frozen grief to be a common postbomb reaction among those who survived the atomic bomb at Hiroshima. Frozen or impacted grief was strongly associated with death and survivor guilt among victims.

REFERENCES

Breslau, N. (1998). Epidemiology of trauma and posttraumatic stress disorder. In R. Yohuda (Ed.), *Psychological trauma* (pp. 1–27). Washington, DC: American Psychiatric Press.

Freud, S. (1955). *Beyond the pleasure principle* (pp. 29–33). Standard Edition, Vol. 18. London: Hogarth Press. (Original work published 1920)

Friedman, M. J. (2000). *Post-traumatic stress disorders*. Kansas City, MO: Compact Clinicals.

Green, B. L., Lindy, J. D., & Grace, M. C. (1994). Psychological effects of toxic contamination: Informed of radioactive contamination syndrome. In R. Ursano, B. McCaughey, & C. Fullerton (Eds.), *Individual and community responses to trauma and disaster: The structure of human chaos* (pp. 154–176). Cambridge, UK: Cambridge University Press.

Hagengimana, A. (2000). *Ihahamuka: A PTSD-like syndrome among survivors of the Rwandan genocide.* Manuscript in preparation.

Herman, J. (1992). *Trauma and recovery.* New York: Basic Books.

Herman, J. L. (1993). Sequelae of prolonged and repeated trauma: Evidence for a complex posttraumatic syndrome (DESNOS). In J. R. T. Davidson & E. D. Foa (Eds.), *Post traumatic stress disorder: DSM-IV and beyond* (pp. 213–228). Washington, DC: American Psychiatric Press.

Honig, R. G., Grace, M. C., Lindy, J. D., Newman, C. L., & Titchener, J. L. (1993). Portraits of survival: A twenty-year follow-up of the Buffalo Creek flood. *Psychoanalytic Study of the Child, 48,* 327–355.

Krystal, H. (1988). *Integration of self-healing.* Hillsdale, NJ: Analytic Press.

Lifton, R. J. (1967). *Death in life: Survivors of Hiroshima.* New York: Random House.

Lindy, J. (1988). *Vietnam: A casebook.* New York: Brunner/Mazel.

Lindy, J. (1993). Focal psychoanalytic psychotherapy of post-traumatic stress disorder. In J. P. Wilson & B. Raphael (Eds.), *International handbook of traumatic stress syndromes* (pp. 803–811). New York: Plenum Press.

Lindy, J. D. (1985) The trauma membrane and other concepts derived from psychotherapeutic work with survivors of natural disaster. *Psychiatric Annals, 15*(3), 153–160.

Lindy, J. D., Green, B. L., & Grace, M. C. (1992). Somatic reenactment in the treatment of posttraumatic stress disorder. In W. DeLoos & W. Op den Velde (Eds.), *Psychotherapy and psychosomatics of psychotrauma* (pp. 180–186). Basel: Karger.

Lindy, J. D., & Wilson, J. P. (1994). Empathic strain and therapist defense: Type I and type II CTR's. In J. P. Wilson & J. D. Lindy (Eds.), *Countertransference in the treatment of PTSD* (pp. 31–61). New York: Guilford Press.

Matsakis, A. (1997). *Trust after trauma.* Oakland, CA: New Harbinger Publications, Inc.

Raphael, B., & Wilson, J. P. (2000). *Psychological debriefing: Theory, practice, evidence.* Cambridge, UK: Cambridge University Press.

Simon, B., & Bullock, C. (1992). Incest, see under Oedipus Complex: The history of an error in psychoanalysis. *Journal of the American Psychoanalytic Association, 40,* 995–988.

Wilson, J. P. (1995). Traumatic events and PTSD prevention. In B. Raphael & A. D. Barrows (Eds.), *The handbook of preventative psychiatry* (pp. 281–296). Amsterdam: Elsevier.

Wilson, J. P., & Lindy, J. D. (1999). *Countertransference in the treatment of PTSD.* New York: Guilford Press.

Author Index

Subject Index